THE
HIGH BLOOD
PRESSURE
SOLUTION

HIGH BLOOD
PRESSURE
SOLUTION

NATURAL
PREVENTION
and *CURE* with
the *K FACTOR*

Richard D. Moore, M.D., Ph.D.

Healing Arts Press
Rochester, Vermont

Healing Arts Press
One Park Street
Rochester, Vermont 05767
www.InnerTraditions.com

Healing Arts Press is a division of Inner Traditions International

Note to the reader: This book is intended as an informational guide. The remedies, approaches, and techniques described herein are meant to supplement, and not to be a substitute for, professional medical care or treatment. They should not be used to treat a serious ailment without prior consultation with a qualified healthcare professional.

LIBRARY OF CONGRESS CATALOGING-IN-PUBLICATION DATA
Moore, Richard, M.D., Ph.D.
    The high blood pressure solution : natural prevention and cure with the K factor / Richard Moore.
        p. cm.
    Includes bibliographical references and index.
    ISBN 0-89281-446-2
    1. Hypertension—Diet therapy. 2. High-potassium diet. 3. Salt-free diet. 4. Potassium in the body. I. Title.
RC685.H8M569 1993
616.1'320654—dc20
                                                          92-46210
                                                          CIP

Printed and bound in the United States

10 9 8

Text design by Randi Jinkins

Contents

Acknowledgments vii

How to Use This Book ix

INTRODUCTION
The Revolution in High Blood Pressure 1

PART ONE

THE PROBLEM 15

CHAPTER 1
What Is High Blood Pressure? 19

CHAPTER 2
Drugs–The Usual Treatment 26

PART TWO

THE ANSWER: MOVING FROM THE MYTH OF
CONTROL TO A BALANCE WITH NATURE 43

CHAPTER 3
Hypertension: More than Just High Blood Pressure! 49

CHAPTER 4
The Action at the Cell Membrane 56

CHAPTER 5
High Blood Pressure Is Not Inevitable: Cultural Evidence 88

CHAPTER 6
Working with the Wisdom of the Body:
An Adequate K Factor Lowers Blood Pressure and Prolongs Life 100

CHAPTER 7
Variations on a Theme: The Importance of Fitness 119

CHAPTER 8
Other Factors that Influence Blood Pressure 127

PART THREE

THE PROGRAM 141

CHAPTER 9
Step One: See Your Doctor 147

CHAPTER 10
Step Two: Eat Right 153

CHAPTER 11
Step Three: Exercise 184

CHAPTER 12
Step Four: Help Your Body Find Its Proper Weight 210

PART FOUR
THE WORKBOOK 225

CHAPTER 13
The Workbook 226

PART FIVE
ADDITIONAL CONSIDERATIONS 249

CHAPTER 14
Why the Emphasis on Drugs? 250

CHAPTER 15
Additional Evidence: Low Dietary K Factor–
A Main Cause of Primary Hypertension 260

PART SIX
SALT, BLOOD PRESSURE REGULATION,
AND DRUG ACTION 277

CHAPTER 16
How Important Is Salt? 278

CHAPTER 17
How the Kidneys, Hormones, and Nervous System
Work Together to Control Blood Pressure 283

CHAPTER 18
Antihypertensive Drugs 299

PART SEVEN
FOR THE PHYSICIAN 311

CHAPTER 19
Information for the Physician 312

References 331
Index 367

Acknowledgments

No one can do anything worthwhile alone. Much of the research that led me to write this book could not have been done without the collaboration of several students, two excellent technicians, and four bright, dedicated young Ph.D.s I particularly appreciate the high quality of work done by Dr. Mark Fidelman and Dr. John Munford: their work on insulin (although we never even dreamed it at the time) has turned out to be directly relevant to hypertension.

Special appreciation goes to Barb, whose support enabled much of the research on insulin to come into this world, and to "good-time" Charlie, whose participation extended far beyond anything he might have imagined.

Dr. George Webb, my co-author of a previous version of this book, *The K Factor: Reversing and Preventing High Blood Pressure without Drugs,* was unable to assist with the writing of this present version due to prior commitments. But in spite of his busy schedule, George was very helpful in double checking some important points.

This book is dedicated to those pioneers who were way ahead of me in realizing that dietary potassium is part of the key to healthy blood pressure. Noteworthy is Dr. Walter Kempner, who in the late 1940s showed that a fruit-rice diet (which has a high K Factor) can reliably lower blood pressure back to the normal range. But especially significant is the work of Dr. Lewis Dahl—an acknowledged leader in hypertension research in his own day—who recognized long before I did that the ratio of dietary potassium to sodium is a key to hypertension.

Thanks also go to author Douglas Terman and to Dr. Lorin Mullins, who was my mentor at the physics department of Purdue University. Over the years, Lorin has offered constructive criticism and helped shape my scientific outlook. It is also important to me to acknowledge Dr. George Garceau (deceased), former Chief of Orthopedic Surgery at Indiana University School of Medicine, who not only showed me what a physician truly can be, but taught me that what is called "radical" may be conservative and what is called "conservative" may actually be radical.

I also want to express my appreciation for the generous time several physicians and scientists spent in reviewing parts of both this version and the previous version of this book. Because of the wide range of material covered, their constructive criticism in their respective areas of expertise was essential in order to ensure that the information presented is as sound and reliable as possible. They include:

Mark Cohen, Ph.D., Professor of Anthropology, SUNY, Plattsburgh, New York;

John Crabbé, M.D., University of Catholic Louvain, School of Medicine, Bruxelles (Chapters 4 and 7);

David Fisch, M.D., Southwest Cardiovascular Consultants, Houston, Texas (Chapters 18 and 19);

Robert Kochan, Ph.D., Biodynamics Laboratory, University of Wisconsin (Chapter 11);

Jarek Kolonowski, M.D., University of Catholic Louvain, School of Medicine, Bruxelles (Chapters 4 and 7);

Wayne A. Gavryck, M.D., Internal Medicine, Turners Falls, Massachusetts (Chapter 19);

Raj K. Gupta, Ph.D., Department of Physiology and Biophysics, Albert Einstein College of Medicine, Bronx, New York;

David W. Maughan, Ph.D., Department of Physiology and Biophysics, University of Vermont, College of Medicine (Chapter 16);

Lorin J. Mullins, Ph.D., Professor Emeritus, Department of Biophysics, University of Maryland School of Medicine (several chapters);

Ethan Sims, M.D., University of Vermont, College of Medicine (Chapters 4, 7, 9, and 12);

Ray Sjodin, Ph.D., Department of Biophysics, University of Maryland (Chapter 4);

Richard Steinhardt, Ph.D., Department of Zoology, University of California, Berkeley (Chapters 4 and 7);

Rachael Yeater, Ph.D., Human Performance Laboratory, West Virginia University (Chapter 11); and

Allan Walker, M.D., Internal Medicine, Plattsburgh, New York (Chapter 19).

I am especially grateful to Leslie Colket and Cannon Labrie of Inner Traditions for invaluable help in editing the manuscript. During the final stages of writing when I was becoming fatigued, Cannon's help was decisive. And as always, Publisher Ehud Sperling stimulates my thinking and helps extend its scope.

How to Use This Book

The message of this book is simple. Make sure your diet has a proper balance between potassium and sodium (as measured by the K Factor), get adequate exercise, keep reasonably trim, and avoid excess alcohol and not only will you not get hypertension, but if you already have it you can probably reverse it. In the months and years to come, you will also be hearing a similar message from the National High Blood Pressure Education Program.

This book explains how to accomplish these objectives.

But it does more, it will help you understand the evidence for our confidence that this is the proper approach to hypertension *and* it will help you to understand how these lifestyle changes affect your body. This knowledge should provide you with the motivation necessary for you to take the simple steps described here.

In that spirit, the book is written so any interested reader, regardless of familiarity and/or education in this area, can follow the story. At the same time, it has the detail and documentation one would expect to find in a book for professionals. Thus, it respects the intelligence of the reader and should reassure you that everything here is already in the scientific and medical literature and is very well substantiated. In the true scientific spirit, I don't want anyone to take what I say for granted.

This is also an unusual book in that it is written not just for the layperson but also for physicians.

There are two reasons for this. Although all the evidence presented here is already published, it is published only in bits and pieces and is often buried in highly detailed reports. Because of this, even most people in the medical profession are unaware of how the parts fit together into the whole picture.

Another reason is so that it can be used to help you and your doctor work *together.* Your physician will find it especially useful because it will provide you with the background necessary for her/him to adequately discuss your problems with you.

Thus, the book is written for both you *and* your doctor.

Because of this, *The High Blood Pressure Solution* has been organized to be read several ways. The Introduction is a brief summary of the whole book, so be sure to read all of it.

Parts One and Two are introductory; they tell you what the problem is, and what the answer is. The program proposed in Part Three will be more effective if you become familiar with this information. You must read Chapters 1 and 3 in their entirety. In Chapter 1, be sure to note that the experts now recognize that what we previously called "normal" blood pressure is not a healthy or "optimal" blood pressure! Chapter 3 will open your eyes to the fact that hypertension involves much more than just elevated blood pressure.

After that, you can read Chapters 4 through 8 straight through, skip part or all of any given chapter and read its summary, or read only the summaries at the end of each chapter. If you read Chapter 4 on the cell, I suggest you scan it first and look at the illustrations to get the general picture. This chapter documents that the problems in hypertension not only involve, but *begin* in, the cell. Many readers will find the cultural evidence in Chapter 5 fascinating. Chapter 6, especially the first few pages, presents the evidence for the effectiveness of increasing the dietary K Factor. You will see that increasing the K Factor by amounts too small to affect blood pressure has been shown—both in experimental animals and in humans—to decrease strokes. Chapter 7 about fitness will show you how all these factors are connected and help convince you of the importance of moderate exercise and watching your weight. Chapter 8 will answer your questions about alcohol, stress, and other factors. In any case, it is essential to read the summary of Part Two.

In Part Three you will find the program, a series of step-by-step instructions about how to work with your doctor to prevent or to cure your hypertension—not just treat the symptom of elevated blood pressure. You can read this material before, during, or after you become acquainted with the material in Parts One and Two. If you are going to embark on the program, it is essential that you read the introduction to Part Three, as well as Chapter 9 in its entirety, first. Be certain to read pages 173 to 176 in Chapter 10 before starting to increase your dietary K Factor.

Part Four includes a workbook to help you keep track of your progress in the program. Also included are recommendations for food shopping and a useful table that lists the amounts of sodium and potassium as well as the K Factor for most foods.

In Part Five, I discuss why it has taken so long to realize that changes in nutrition, weight, exercise, and alcohol consumption are the key to hypertension. Additional evidence is also provided for those who want to go into more detail.

Part Six provides information about salt, about the role of the kidneys and hormones in the development of elevated blood pressure, and about what drugs do and how they do it. While reading these chapters will deepen your understanding of the program and how it works, they are not "required reading."

Part Seven is written to assist your physician in working with you.

You can begin your journey to normal blood pressure and good health *today*. **See your doctor before taking any of the steps outlined in this book.**

The Revolution in High Blood Pressure

... among the most important contributors to the ... prevalence of high blood pressure are: a high sodium chloride intake many times beyond human physiologic needs, overweight, physical inactivity, excessive alcohol consumption, and an inadequate intake of potassium.

from the 1993 Working Group Report
for Prevention of Hypertension
supported by the National Heart,
Lung, and Blood Institute[1]

We are in the midst of a major shift in our approach to high blood pressure. This revolution is based upon new insights into the fundamental causes of this widespread condition. We know that the problem involves more than just elevated blood pressure. We also know that in the vast majority of cases, hypertension is preventable. This new perspective gives us the guidelines for solving a major health problem and in the process significantly cutting health care costs.

In 1986, Dr. George Webb and I wrote *The K Factor: Reversing and Preventing High Blood Pressure Without Drugs,* a previous version of this book.[2] We concluded that there are three key factors for naturally preventing or treating hypertension:

• Diet, especially the K Factor (increasing potassium and lowering sodium)
• Weight control
• Exercise

Even then, the scientific evidence supporting our conclusions was overpowering, being based upon over three hundred published studies. As you can see, our recommendations in 1986 were identical (except for concern with excessive alcohol consumption) with those of the 1993 report of the Working Group for Prevention of Hypertension supported by the National Heart, Lung, and Blood Institute, quoted above.

In the *K Factor,* we also concluded:

> There is now overpowering evidence that high blood pressure, one of the major health problems in the United States today, is usually an unnecessary disease that can easily be avoided . . .

In the 1993 Working Group Report, the medical authorities also take a *new* position that hypertension is preventable. This report states:

> . . . this is an appropriate time for the National High Blood Pressure Education Program (NHBPEP) in conjunction with other interested parties to initiate a national campaign whose specific goal is the primary prevention of high blood pressure.[3]

In a related report, these authorities recognize that hypertension can often be treated without drugs.

The realization that hypertension is preventable is just part of a new perspective that amounts to a revolution in our understanding of this condition.

THE NEW PERSPECTIVE

The new revolutionary view of hypertension is based upon four related insights into the true nature of high blood pressure:

1. There is a lot more to hypertension than just elevated blood pressure. The high blood pressure is a sure sign that there is an imbalance throughout the whole body. This imbalance often involves increased blood cholesterol, decreased effectiveness of insulin, and a tendency to have high blood sugar levels. In the last analysis, these abnormalities are the result of imbalances within the living cell.

Because these problems involve much more than elevated blood pressure, we should stop calling this condition high blood pressure and instead call it by its other name—hypertension. Calling it high blood pressure* tends to focus our attention on correcting only part of the problem—the blood pressure—without addressing the other abnormalities.

---

*Throughout this book, I still intermittently use the phrase "high blood pressure" because most people are not yet used to the term "hypertension."

For example, although lowering blood pressure with drugs definitely reduces strokes and stroke-related death, the evidence that this significantly decreases overall mortality is debatable (see Chapter 2). On the other hand, even a small increase in dietary potassium (and thus the K Factor—K is the symbol for potassium) has been found to significantly decrease stroke-related deaths even when it doesn't lower blood pressure (see Chapter 6). Moreover—and surprising to many—the extra potassium has been shown to lower blood cholesterol levels.

2. A blood pressure in the previously defined "normal" range is *not* healthy. We now realize that a blood pressure of 120/80—which is still called normal—is not optimal because it is too high for maximum protection against strokes and heart attacks. As a result, development of complications from hypertension can begin even when blood pressure is in the so-called normal range.

This fact is reflected in the 1993 Report on primary prevention of hypertension by the Working Group of the National High Blood Pressure Education Program (NHBPEP), which points out that:

> . . . vascular complications can occur *prior* to the onset of established hypertension because the blood pressure-cardiovascular disease risk relationship is continuous and progressive, even within the normotensive [normal] blood pressure range [emphasis mine].[4]

Thus, typical Americans who feel comfortable because their blood pressure is "normal" (say 120/80) are living with a false sense of security. The 1993 Report quoted above should help shake all of us out of our complacency.

Some of you may have bought this book for a relative or a friend who has hypertension, but feel it is not for you because you have "normal" blood pressure. But if your blood pressure is above 110/70, *this book is for you too.*

3. Whereas we used to think that if you had inherited the wrong genes you would inevitably get high blood pressure, we now realize that 95% of the cases occur because of readily correctable mistakes in the processing and preparation of food. Lack of moderate exercise, being overweight, and drinking too much alcohol also contribute.

4. Because hypertension is not inevitable but is due to mistakes in what we eat and what we do, it can be prevented, reversed, and in some cases even cured by eliminating these same mistakes. This is a disease condition that can be practically wiped out!

Waiting until the blood pressure is elevated and then using drugs to lower it is like locking the barn after the horse is out: it is obviously better to prevent the problem in the first place. However, when the blood pressure has become elevated, an adequate increase of the dietary K Factor can usually lower it—especially if combined with proper exercise and weight control.

Thus the revolution in our understanding of hypertension is a tremendously significant development. Implementation of the prevention strategy proposed by the Working Group of the National High Blood Pressure Education Program (NHBPEP) offers the possibility of not only eliminating up to 80% of the strokes in the United States but also significantly reducing heart attacks, kidney disease, blindness, and other consequences of hypertension.

In addition to the health benefits, this prevention campaign could eventually save most of the several billion dollars per year currently spent in the treatment of hypertension *and its consequences.* This could significantly reduce the exploding medical care costs in the United States, which at the end of 1992 amounted to about 13% of the gross domestic product (GDP), or approximately $800 billion— about 70% of the entire federal budget![5] In 1940, medical care cost us $4 billion, which was just 4% of our GDP. Moreover, it is estimated that if the present trend continues, costs will rise above the trillion-dollar per year level by 1995 and the two trillion-dollar per year level by the year 2000![6] This level of cost for medical care would amount to $30,000 annually for a family of four. Clearly this second trillion will not be available.

The treatment of hypertension contributes significantly to these medical costs. The cost of treating hypertension in the United States is several billion dollars a year.[7]

THE PROGRAM

The key nutritional changes pointed out in 1986 in The K Factor and in this book are virtually the same as those recommended by the 1993 Report on primary prevention of hypertension by the Working Group of the National High Blood Pressure Education Program (NHBPEP). According to this group, to reduce the prevalence of high blood pressure, the most important things to avoid are these:

> a high sodium chloride intake many times beyond human physiologic needs, overweight, physical inactivity, excessive alcohol consumption, and an inadequate intake of potassium.[8]

Avoiding both a high sodium intake and an inadequate intake of potassium is identical to keeping the dietary ratio of potassium to sodium—the K Factor—from being too low. Simple lifestyle changes can be effective in preventing and in treating hypertension: keeping the dietary K Factor up, losing excess weight, getting appropriate exercise, and avoiding excess alcohol consumption. The same changes are now recommended for initial treatment of most cases of hypertension by the Fifth Joint National Committee on Detection, Evaluation, and Treatment of High Blood Pressure (see Chapter 2).[9]

The key to prevention, and as claimed in this book to successful treatment, is not expensive and high-tech. Moreover, the required changes are not only few but uncomplicated. You don't have to go on a diet—in fact you can eat almost any type of food you want. Remember, the problem isn't so much what you eat but mistakes in how the food is processed and prepared. But to avoid these easily correctable mistakes, you do have to become informed about the nutritional principles outlined in this book.

THESE PRINCIPLES APPLY EVEN IF YOU ALREADY HAVE HYPERTENSION

For many, probably most, of those who already have hypertension, the new insights about lifestyle offer the possibility—right now—of working with their physicians to successfully treat their hypertension without drugs. This is especially true if their elevated blood pressure is detected early. In such cases, by removing the causes—an inadequate dietary K Factor, excess weight, inadequate exercise, or too much alcohol—the promise now exists of actually curing hypertension and thus preventing its dire consequences such as strokes and cardiovascular disease. Even if you do take drugs, the recommended lifestyle changes should give you further protection.

It is to be emphasized, however, that once they have occurred, no one can cure some of the complications of hypertension—strokes, blindness, and kidney disease, for example. But if the cause—improper lifestyle—of hypertension is corrected in time, one can not only restore blood pressure to normal but, more importantly, prevent the dire consequences of this common condition.

So make no mistake, if you have elevated blood pressure and do *nothing* about it—either ignore appropriate lifestyle changes, or use antihypertensive drugs— you are taking a huge and unnecessary chance of not just a sudden death but of becoming seriously incapacitated.

For those who find they do need to take antihypertensive drugs, the recommended lifestyle changes may be at least as important in reducing suffering and death. Although drug treatment does succeed in reducing some complications of hypertension, this success is by no means complete. As the Working Group of the National High Blood Pressure Education Program points out:

> Even those who derive optimal benefit from their antihypertensive treatment are likely to have a higher risk of morbidity [damage such as strokes and heart attacks] and mortality than their untreated "normotensive" counterparts with a similar level of blood pressure.[10]

In other words, even when drug treatment successfully lowers the blood pressure, this produces only a partial reduction in damage to health and in death. For example, it is well established that lowering blood pressure by drugs results in about a 40% reduction in strokes and in stroke-related death—a significant benefit. The flip side of this is that successfully lowering the blood pressure with drugs fails to prevent about 60% of strokes and stroke-related death.

But even increasing the dietary K Factor by eating just one banana a day may reduce strokes just as much. So there is reason to think that larger increases may produce even better results than drugs do.

THE SCIENTIFIC EVIDENCE FOR THE NEW APPROACH

How do we know this lifestyle approach is the answer? The authors of the two NIH-supported reports came to this view by a careful and extensive examination of hypertension in different human populations, studies of animals with hypertension, studies of humans designed to identify which dietary changes lower blood pressure, and studies of the effects of exercise, of weight loss, and of changing alcohol consumption. This evidence is summarized in Chapters 5, 6, 7, and 8.

The approach developed in this book also includes this same evidence, but its foundations go further—and deeper—all the way down to the workings of each living cell in your body.

What is this new foundation? In my view, the strongest evidence rests not on the empirical studies mentioned above, but upon a new biophysical understanding of how the living cell works as an indivisible—holistic if you wish—system which is inseparably connected to the whole body.

This new holistic scientific view of the living cell hinges upon the discovery that the membrane that surrounds each cell is not only an information processing system, but an energy distribution system. The energy is transported in the form of electricity, but rather than being carried by electrons, this electricity is carried by positively charged sodium atoms—the same sodium atoms in table salt.

If this electrical system runs down, changes occur that make it more likely that you will develop an imbalance in your blood cholesterol, an elevation in your blood sugar, an abnormal response to insulin—and elevated blood pressure. All of these abnormalities are likely to be found in people with hypertension and in people with adult-type diabetes. (If you find this hard to believe, read Chapters 4 and 7.)

This electrical system is charged up by the movement of sodium out of the cell in exchange for potassium coming in. In the living cell, potassium and sodium work in a reciprocal manner: when one goes up, the other must go down. So it's necessary to maintain a high ratio between potassium and sodium to prevent these bad consequences. Hence the *ratio* of potassium to sodium reflects the true state of affairs.

Thus, in people with high blood pressure, too little potassium in the diet is as bad and has essentially the same effect as too much sodium. Too much sodium and too little potassium can be deadly. Thus, the key to preventing hypertension is a proper balance between sodium and potassium. The K Factor is a measure of this balance.

The prediction that the dietary K Factor is a key to hypertension was made *before* we looked at clinical studies, population studies, and preliminary treatment trials that were already filed away in the library. Imagine our surprise that some years earlier, a few very astute physicians had already discovered this by increasing the ratio of potassium to sodium in the diet of animals with hypertension! Since then, a large number of studies have also verified that a proper dietary K Factor can both prevent hypertension and can lower blood pressure in those who already have it (see Chapters 5 and 6).

If we look at the K Factor of unprocessed food, we see where the problem lies. In our own bodies, the ratio of total potassium to sodium is high, with a value a little over 4.0 (that means four times as much potassium as sodium). The K Factor is also naturally high, about the same value, in animals and much higher in plants. So it is not surprising that the human race became adapted to eating food with a high K Factor. In fact, throughout the world, groups whose dietary K Factor is greater than 4.0 simply don't have the common form of hypertension.

Most of the food we eat has a high K Factor in its natural form. Indeed, if it weren't for mistakes in commercial food processing, use of table salt (sodium chloride), and boiling food to cook it (which washes out the potassium), it would actually be difficult to have a dietary K Factor of less than 4 *regardless of what you eat!* But by the time the commercial food processors are through with our food and we cook it at home, the K Factor is reduced almost *tenfold.*

So it's not so much *what* we eat, but the way it's prepared in the factory, in the restaurant, and in the home that causes problems. We have gotten into habits of food preparation that flip-flop the natural balance of potassium to sodium—actually reversing it. That's where the imbalance begins that leads to hypertension.

By their effect upon regulation of exchange of potassium with sodium within the body, lack of exercise and obesity compound the nutritional imbalance. As you will see later, a reason both weight reduction and exercise help return blood pressure to normal may well be that they assist the body's mechanisms that normally maintain a proper balance between potassium and sodium in each cell.

Although the 1993 Report of the Working Group of the National High Blood Pressure Education Program (NHBPEP) acknowledges the importance of the potassium to sodium ratio, or the K Factor, the Fifth Report of the Joint National Committee on Detection, Evaluation, and Treatment of High Blood Pressure[11] does not. This failure to explicitly endorse the importance of the potassium-to-sodium ratio is disappointing but not surprising in view of several flawed studies that I discuss in Chapter 6.

WHY HAVE THESE AUTHORITATIVE COMMITTEES MOVED SO SLOWLY?

There are striking examples of facts that have been ignored because the cultural climate was not ready to incorporate them into a consistent theme.

Ilya Prigogine and Isabelle Stengers[12]

I think there have been many reasons why the authorities have moved so slowly—chief among them the fact that "the cultural climate was not ready to incorporate them into a consistent theme."

The essence of fundamental science, such as the biophysical approach, is to find a consistent theme and test its validity by confirming its predictions. Indeed, the conclusions outlined in this book, using these new insights from basic science, were predicted over six years ago. Now, these same conclusions about lifestyle modifications are also affirmed in the 1993 Report of the Working Group of the National High Blood Pressure Education Program (NHBPEP).

New biophysical insights stand in contrast to the tendency of our culture to view nature as a mechanism—as a machine. Among other things, this has biased our thinking to automatically assume that high blood pressure is purely a mechanical problem. In this image, the problem is simply that too much pressure will make too much work for the heart and too much stress on the arteries in our heart, brain, and kidneys. It's rather like a mechanical water system: if the pressure gets too high either the pump will fail or the pipes will burst. Therefore the answer is simply to decrease the blood pressure and all the consequences of hypertension, such as strokes, increased chance of heart attack, kidney disease, and blindness should go away.

As it turns out, part of the problem *is* mechanical, which accounts for the clear ability of blood-pressure-lowering drugs to reduce strokes. Their effectiveness in decreasing heart attacks is less obvious, however, and even in reducing strokes, the success is only partial. Clearly, something more than mechanical effects are involved.

In the process of viewing nature as a machine, we have developed a fragmented way of looking at the world. We tend to see nature as composed of unrelated parts. So in considering problems like hypertension, there is a tendency to look at one thing at a time without realizing that in the body, indeed in all of nature, everything affects everything else.

Another reason is that physicians naturally, and understandably, are cautious in changing their views. Let's face it, making decisions about life-and-death matters is scary. It's an awesome responsibility to take a position that will affect the life of another, let alone the lives of hundreds of thousands. Remember too that physicians take the Hippocratic oath, and in spite of today's cynicism, I believe the vast majority take it quite seriously. "First of all, do no harm," becomes a standard for every action. This caution leads to a fear of doing something with which the physician is not familiar. This fear becomes all the greater if the procedure is different from accepted practice. So it is not easy to make changes that are contrary to the accepted practice. Legal considerations make this even worse, since malpractice suits are usually decided on the basis, not of scientific evidence, but of whether or not the physician was following the accepted, recommended practice.

So when I put on my M.D. hat, I can understand the caution and initial reluctance of the Joint National Committee to accept a major change in perspective. Its understandable that M.D.s* are especially reluctant to change approaches that are even partially successful and by the same token tend to consider something new as "radical."

But when I put on my Ph.D. hat and think as a scientist who has participated in the basic research upon which the message in this book stands, I see that this caution is misplaced. Indeed, the old "interventionist" approach that emphasizes drugs seems radical, and the new approach, founded upon basic science, seems truly conservative.

An approach based upon a modern scientific understanding of the living cell which leads us to realize that nature already had the answer—and that answer lies in a proper lifestyle that allows the cell to find its proper balance—seems to me the more conservative. In any case, eating more fruits and vegetables, exercising, losing weight, and avoiding alcohol can hardly be called a radical approach— especially when it is based not only upon experience and clinical studies, but upon solid scientific understanding of how the body works.

The Influence of Our Fragmented View of Reality upon the Development of Our New Perspective

But I think there are deeper reasons for our failure to recognize the true situation for so long. I address these more in Chapter 17, but here I will briefly give you an idea.

In our culture, we have deified technology in the sense that we automatically look to technology to save us from all problems. This has biased our scientific activities toward technological control instead of toward understanding and learning how to be in harmony and in balance with nature.

Like everyone else, I too have been influenced by this. During my internship 1n 1958, I prescribed drugs to people with hypertension. It seemed obvious that drugs were the answer to disease. Even after returning to graduate school in biophysics

---

*The Joint National Committee is composed not only of M.D.s, but R.N.s, O.D.s and people with backgrounds in statistics and public health.

and to full-time research, if I had been asked how to treat high blood pressure, I would have recommended drugs, probably diuretics.

The history of the revolution in our approach to hypertension illustrates how difficult it can be to change this kind of thinking. Even after my own research had clearly suggested that the ratio of potassium to sodium is the key to high blood pressure, I couldn't let go of my old habits of thought. It took three or four years and many conversations with other scientists for me to accept the evidence that most cases of hypertension are caused by what we do to ourselves and thus are preventable.

But I wasn't by any means the first to come to this new perspective, the origins of which can be traced at least as far back as 1928 when a Canadian physician, Dr. W. L. T. Addison, reported that increasing dietary potassium lowered blood pressure in his patients. Through the years, several American physicians, including Dr. Walter Kempner and Dr. Lewis Dahl, repeated the Canadian success in treating high blood pressure but were frustrated in their attempts to gain their colleagues' attention. In 1972, Dr. Dahl commented on this resistance:

> For reasons that are difficult to fathom, there appeared a great deal of antipathy to Kempner's reports as well as irrational disbelief in the effectiveness of the diet ... For those of you who are unfamiliar with the diet, let me define it as a low sodium, or a high potassium [emphasis mine], or a high carbohydrate, or a low protein, or a low fat, or a high fluid diet.[13]

Now the climate is shifting in the direction recommended in this book.

My involvement in this story began when my own research finally convinced me that a proper balance of potassium to sodium is required for healthy blood pressure. Having gone to medical school before getting my Ph.D. in biophysics, I naturally thought the people involved in research concerning high blood pressure would like to know more about this. So I attempted to talk with people in the organizations dedicated to research and treatment of high blood pressure. For the most part, they weren't interested.

It turned out that I wasn't the first to receive a cold shoulder from the medical experts. Dr. Lorin Mullins, then chairperson of the Department of Biophysics at the University of Maryland School of Medicine, had had similar experiences. Dr. Mullins, together with a couple of others, began urging me to write a book that would bring this knowledge to the public. After all, many foods such as potatoes and bananas are abundant in potassium, and increasing such food in the diet couldn't possibly hurt anyone—especially when it was quite clear that this could lower blood pressure.

I found help in a colleague, Dr. George Webb, of the University of Vermont, who had come to similar conclusions and had successfully treated his own hypertension by increasing the ratio of potassium to sodium in his diet. So George and I wrote *The K Factor: Reversing and Preventing High Blood Pressure without Drugs*.

A major publishing house expressed enthusiasm for the book and gave us a $50,000 advance. Early in 1986, this publisher announced in *Publishers Weekly* that *The K Factor* would be one of their top offerings for 1986 and stated their intention to spend $50,000 on advertising. Then the publisher sent me to five major cities to speak on radio and on TV. In the first weeks, over fourteen thousand copies were sold. When we next met to discuss further promotion, I was informed that they were not going to spend their advertising budget and that there would be no more speaking tours for me. The whole mood had changed.

Several months later, another book appeared from this same publisher that promoted drugs as the answer to high blood pressure. It looked hastily written and completely ignored a large study that had cast doubt on the effectiveness of antihypertensive drugs to reduce death (see Chapter 2). I confronted the person in charge and asked why they didn't put the other authors and myself on a talk show and let us argue it out. I pointed out they would obviously sell a lot of both books that way. That wouldn't be necessary, he replied.

The K Factor then faded into oblivion. Both George and I regularly received letters from individuals asking how they could get copies of the book. I lent my copy to someone and never got it back. I couldn't buy a replacement even from the publisher. For over three years I didn't even have a copy of my own book. Finally, a friend found an unsold copy for me in a bookstore in Alaska. *The K Factor* had virtually disappeared from the face of the earth.

Evidently, "the cultural climate was not ready to incorporate" the new view "into a consistent theme." But now the climate *has* begun to change.

BRINGING HEALTH CARE INTO THE TWENTY-FIRST CENTURY

As we near the end of the second millennium, we are living in a time when this fragmented view of reality is breaking down. The leading edge of science, particularly physics, biophysics, and the emerging science of complexity and chaos, has shown that nature is not so much made up of separate parts but is a seamless web in which everything has some effect, however small, on everything else.

This new scientific view of nature has taken us to the verge of a twenty-first-century health care approach. We now realize the human body is much more complex than a machine—much more complex than even the most advanced computer. A century ago, one of the pioneers of medical physiology, Walter Cannon, intuited that this complexity provides a problem-solving aspect to the human body and expressed this in the phrase "the wisdom of the body."

While we have been trying to figure out how to force ourselves into good health, Mother Nature and your body already have the answers.

In terms of treatment we must remember that, although they may assist the process, drugs don't heal—only the body can heal itself. Thus, the primary goal of therapy should always be to remove the cause of the disease and thus allow the wisdom of the body to restore its own balance.

If you treat your body properly, it will keep your blood pressure in the healthy range.

Working in Balance with Nature Instead of Trying to Control Nature: The Only Answer to Our Exploding Medical Costs

In addition to the fact that it is scientifically sound, there is a strong economic incentive to consider lifestyle alteration instead of drugs in the treatment of hypertension. In keeping with the hard financial realities of our "health care" crisis, the 1993 report of the Fifth Joint National Committee on Detection, Evaluation, and Treatment of High Blood Pressure (JNC 5 Report) points out that the cost of lifelong antihypertensive therapy (70% to 80% of which is due to drug costs) represents a significant component of the nation's financial commitment to health. Accordingly, the JNC 5 Report concludes that "for individual as well as societal reasons, minimizing cost must be an essential component of the health care provider's responsibility."[14]

I put the term "health care" in quotations precisely because we do not have a system with a health-oriented philosophy and focus. Rather, our system has been a "medical care system," which focuses upon disease and the use of medicines and technology as opposed to health and prevention. As long as we continue to focus on a disease instead of health, we are locking the barn after the horse has already gone.

No amount of insurance reform or government support will solve the present escalating health care crisis. As long as we continue down the path of trying to control disease—rather than prevent it by promoting health—our so-called "health care" system is doomed not only to fail in its own terms of promoting health, but to contribute to the financial bankruptcy of the country.

Working in Balance with Nature Instead of Trying to Control Nature: The Road to Health Instead of Disease

As far back as 500 B.C., Socrates affirmed this principle:

> Then, if we are not able to hunt the goose with one idea, with three
> we may take our prey; *Beauty, Symmetry [balance], Truth* are the
> three . . .[15]

Most ancient cultures recognized the importance of symmetry—of balance—in all things. In view of our new scientific perspective it is clear that the time has come for a return to the principle of balance. People need to find the balance within themselves and with nature and thus take charge of their own health. If nothing else, the looming financial collapse of the present medical care system will force this development.

Taking drugs instead of taking charge of our lives is part of a societal trend to surrender personal responsibility to powers outside of ourselves. And without taking charge of our lives, we can't find balance. On the other hand, prevention is based upon balance and reflects a mentality that is consistent with personal responsibility, independence, self-confidence, and empowerment.

In this context, the prevention of hypertension is more important even than it appears. Since the most healthy blood pressure is less than 110/70, the vast majority of Americans—who until now have been complacent about a blood pressure of 120/80—have blood pressure that is in the range associated with increased risk of stroke and of heart attack. Within this broader perspective, hypertension is a pandemic. But fortunately, now that we realize that the vast majority of cases of elevated blood pressure are due to lifestyle, this is a pandemic that can be prevented.

In keeping with the trend toward a cooperative approach, the recent decision of the Working Group of the National High Blood Pressure Education Program (NHBPEP) to launch a sustained national campaign to prevent hypertension is a heartening (pun intended) development. In my view, there is no longer any reasonable doubt that the lifestyle changes proposed by this group can, within a couple of decades, virtually wipe out the common type of hypertension.

The recent requirement by the FDA that labels on all processed foods clearly show calories, total fat, saturated fat, cholesterol, and sodium is a step in the right direction, but unfortunately it overlooks potassium. Many food processors, however, already list the amount of potassium. If we all work together—if we cooperate—there can be a future where hypertension is uncommon.

But to cooperate, to be responsible for our own health, we must be educated about the basics. An approach to health based upon fundamental scientific principles and upon the philosophy of working in balance with nature is the only way to bring health care into the twenty-first century—and the only way to truly contain exploding medical costs.

THE KEY TO THE SUCCESS OF THE REVOLUTION IS COOPERATION

Preventing high blood pressure will of necessity be a cooperative venture. Using the information in this book, physicians and patients can join together to solve this problem. After all, it is they, the physician and patient together, who are in the front lines where the decisions concerning each individual case must be made.

Those of you who have hypertension, or are concerned about getting it, will find that you are no longer alone in taking preventive steps. No longer do you need to feel that eating properly is a hopeless task. You are no longer alone in being concerned about how to reduce fat and table salt in your food. My colleague, Dr. George Webb (who has successfully treated his hypertension by the K Factor approach) tells me that chefs are using less sodium and they will use still less if you request that they do. When going to the salad bar, go for the fresh salads and look for fruits such as bananas; be wary of the canned salads. A baked potato without butter or sour cream is great. If you eat Chinese, ask the chef to not use soy sauce; get a vegetable dish; stir frying doesn't cause any loss of potassium.

So it is easier than ever before for you to take charge of your own nutrition. There is a support network emerging. Soon, eating food with a proper K Factor and not too much fat will become the norm.

But you don't have to wait for the prevention campaign sponsored by the National High Blood Pressure Education Program to take hold. With the information in this book, you can begin doing your part right now. By using the principles outlined in this book, you can choose food that is appropriate without imposing your nutritional restrictions on other people. And remember that even if you have "normal" blood pressure, it's probably too high. So why not make the proper lifestyle shift to decrease your risk of stroke or heart attack *right now.*

To start, after consulting with your doctor, just reduce the table salt you add to your food. As you will see, it is important to be off all table salt, both at the table and in your cooking, for one week before starting the schedule in Chapter 10. During this time, you can read the book through Part Three, stock your kitchen with appropriate foods and condiments, and *see your doctor to discuss this program before beginning.*

PART ONE

THE
PROBLEM

Hypertension is the major determinant of coronary heart disease, the chief cause of cerebrovascular disease [primarily strokes] and the commonest reason for initiating lifetime medication.

Nissmen and Stanley[1]

If you have high blood pressure, you have lots of company. On the basis of the 1988–91 National Health and Nutrition Examination Survey (HANES III), about 50 million adult Americans—almost one out of every four—suffer from high blood pressure, or hypertension.[2] This condition is the most common threat to health in the United States and continues to be the most serious health problem of American blacks.[3] As much as 25% of all deaths in black men and 50% of deaths in black women may be due to the consequences of hypertension.[4] Worldwide, perhaps as many as 500 million to one billion persons have hypertension.[5]

Hypertension is the major cause of strokes. High blood pressure kills tens of thousands of Americans every year through strokes and heart attacks. In addition, hypertension condemns additional thousands to a life of invalidism with paralysis, inability to speak or hear, heart failure, blindness, or kidney disease.

What makes hypertension doubly dangerous is that you can have it and still feel absolutely normal, or even feel great—until you are stricken with one of the grisly consequences of this "silent killer."

If the 50 million Americans afflicted by this condition could feel their blood pressure go up, the news media would be talking about the largest epidemic we have yet seen. Indeed, hypertension has reached epidemic proportions. And this epidemic is costing many billions of health care dollars a year to treat. That figure does not take into account the cost incurred when the consequences strike: the cost of premature deaths, of such incapacitating handicaps as deafness, or of being bedridden for life because of strokes or kidney disease, for example.

It is the thesis of this book that most of the dire human and economic conse-

16

quences of hypertension can be avoided. As you will see, the scientific evidence to support this claim has steadily accumulated over the past half century.

But if these factors have not been enough to force our society to reevaluate the prevention and treatment of hypertension, the looming health care crisis posed by ballooning medical costs will.

Twenty-five years ago, it looked as though drugs were the answer for hypertension; almost everyone thought that.

Within the medical establishment, however, there were a few lone voices of dissent. Dr. Walter Kempner, of Duke University Medical School, kept pointing out that his rice-fruit diet was a proven success for lowering elevated blood pressure.[6] Also, Dr. Lewis Dahl of the Brookhaven National Laboratory[7] and Dr. Lot Page of Tufts University School of Medicine[8] could point to evidence that too much sodium was part of the problem.

But in view of the potency of the new drugs—thiazide diuretics—in decreasing blood pressure, not many people wanted to be bothered with changing their eating habits. As a result, the production of drugs to treat hypertension grew into a multibillion-dollar-a-year industry. That's a lot of dollars! But attempting to prevent the terrible consequences of hypertension—the death, the paralysis—seemed worth it. So over the past quarter century, the use of drugs has become the accepted means of treating everyone with hypertension.

By now, a lot of doctors have grown skeptical of drugs. Besides the frequent unpleasant side effects, many patients on drugs complain they just don't feel good. But because of legal risks and lack of knowledge of a good alternative treatment, doctors continue to prescribe drugs for almost everyone with hypertension.

In 1982 came the first report that cast doubt upon the assumption that drugs are the answer to hypertension. This bombshell was an article in the *Journal of the American Medical Association*, citing evidence that aggressive use of drugs failed to help about half of all the people suffering from hypertension.[9] In some cases drug treatment actually increased their rate of death.

Then in 1985, just after Dr. George Webb and I finished the manuscript for the first version of this book, came the second shock. In the *British Medical Journal*, the Medical Research Council of Great Britian reported the results of the best and by far the largest study of drug treatment of hypertension ever conducted.[10] This study involved over 17,000 people with hypertension and followed the results of drug treatment over a period of five and a half years. The study confirmed that drug treatment can lower the elevated blood pressure in almost all patients. It also demonstrated that by so doing, drug treatment reduced fatal strokes by 34%. But the astonishing result was that although blood pressure was lowered into the "normal" range and stroke-related death was reduced, drug treatment of hypertension *did not reduce the overall rate of death.*

So far, no one has been able to successfully explain away this evidence, and the significance is beginning to sink in. A major rethinking of the whole problem is under way, with an increasing awareness of the importance of lifestyle choices, including nutrition, in both prevention and treatment. Indeed, this new awareness has led the National High Blood Pressure Education Program, which is sponsored by the National Heart, Lung, and Blood Institute, to call for a national campaign whose specific goal is the prevention of high blood pressure.[11]

In the last few years, the medical establishment has begun to back off from the blanket recommendation that everybody with hypertension be treated with drugs. For example, in late summer of 1985 the Vermont affiliate of the American Heart Association stated: "Changing one's lifestyle is the recommended method of controlling high blood pressure, but . . . may not be enough to control hypertension in everyone."[12] Then, in 1988, the Joint National Committee of Detection, Evaluation, and Treatment of High Blood Pressure recommended that patients with borderline hypertension (diastolic blood pressure between 90 and 94 mm Hg) "and who are otherwise at relatively low risk of developing cardiovascular disease should initially be treated with nonpharmacological [nondrug] approaches."[13]

More recently, in its 1993 Report, the Joint National Committee emphasized that the goal of treating people with hypertension is not just to lower the blood pressure but to prevent the death and damage to health associated with hypertension "by the least intrusive means possible," recommending that treatment of most people with hypertension begin with a three- to six-month period of modification in lifestyle.[14]

Before going into specifics about the nondrug approach described in this book, let's look at the types of hypertension that exist and the drugs commonly used to treat them. That's what Part I is about. It's important that you know these facts before deciding how to use the rest of the book.

CHAPTER 1

What Is High Blood Pressure?

WHAT IT ISN'T

High blood pressure, or *hypertension,* is not the same thing as heart disease, but it can make heart disease worse. By damaging its arteries and making the heart work too hard, hypertension can help trigger (or be a risk factor for) heart attacks.

Both heart disease and hypertension can kill you. Heart disease can cause you to spend the rest of your life with chest pain or shortness of breath. But not only does hypertension make heart disease more likely, it can cause you to "stroke out" so that—even if you survive—you spend the rest of your life partially paralyzed, unable to hear, or unable to speak.

There are some similarities in the causes of hypertension and coronary artery heart disease. For a long time, we have understood that coronary artery heart disease is due to mistakes in lifestyle, especially nutrition (particularly an overindulgence of dietary fat). In this book we present the evidence that most cases of hypertension are also due to mistakes in lifestyle—primarily nutrition, but also lack of exercise.

But there are also critical differences in their causes. An important cause of coronary artery heart disease is dietary fat and cholesterol. The most important contributor to hypertension, however, is a low ratio of potassium (K) to sodium (Na)—the K Factor—in the food people eat.

Also, high blood pressure is not the same thing as, nor is it due to, "hardening of the arteries"—a term that refers to the cumulative effects of age and poor nutrition, in addition to hypertension, upon the arteries.

Finally, hypertension is not a type of nervous tension.

WHAT IT IS

Whether or not your doctor decides you have hypertension depends on how high your blood pressure is. That's all there is to it.*

Blood pressure is the pressure the blood exerts against the walls of all your arteries (the large blood vessels that carry blood from your heart to your body's tissues). Your heart creates this blood pressure by pumping blood into the arteries. How can you tell if your blood pressure is too high? You can't—unless it's measured. In fact, about a third of the people with high blood pressure don't realize they have it.[1]

HOW IT'S MEASURED

Your doctor measures your blood pressure by inflating a cuff around your arm with enough pressure to squeeze the artery inside your arm shut. By releasing the pressure of the cuff and listening to the sounds of the pulsating blood as the artery reopens, your doctor can determine your blood pressure. (We'll describe how you can measure your own blood pressure in Part Four.)

WHAT THE NUMBERS MEAN

There are two different numbers that define your blood pressure, and each represents a pressure, the maximum and minimum during a complete pulse cycle. Every blood pressure reading is expressed by these two numbers.

As an example, a blood pressure reading of 120/80 ("120 over 80") is not a fraction, even though it looks like one. The first number is always greater than the second.

The first number is the *systolic blood pressure*—the maximum pressure reached in the arteries while the heart is contracting and thus pumping blood into them. Our example of systolic blood pressure is 120, considered "normal" for a young adult. It's actually 120 millimeters of mercury (mm Hg), which means the pressure is sufficient to push a column of mercury up a distance of 120 millimeters (mm), or about 5 inches. Hg is the chemical symbol for mercury, whose Latin (scientific) name is *hydragyrum,* or "water silver."

The second number is the *diastolic blood pressure*—the minimum pressure of the blood, which occurs while the heart is relaxing between beats. Our example of diastolic blood pressure is 80, which has been considered "normal" for a young adult.

---

*Because of new discoveries described in this book, in the future the blood levels of hormones such as insulin and renin may also be used to diagnose hypertension.

The graph in Figure 1 shows how the blood pressure in your arteries changes as the heart beats. The horizontal lines show the so-called "normal" values we used in our example.

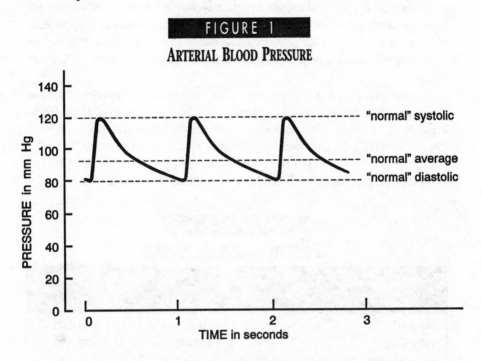

FIGURE 1

ARTERIAL BLOOD PRESSURE

Because the heart normally relaxes for longer than it contracts, the diastolic blood pressure is closer to the average blood pressure than the systolic blood pressure is. Partly for this reason high blood pressure, or hypertension, is usually defined on the basis of diastolic blood pressure.

WHEN IS IT HIGH?

You are said to have hypertension if your diastolic blood pressure is 90 or higher or your systolic pressure is 140 or higher.[2] In the past the diastolic pressure was considered a more reliable indicator and thus used almost solely in deciding treatment. More recent evidence, however, suggests that the systolic pressure may be at least as important,[3] especially in predicting the chance of stroke. The chance of stroke increases greatly when the systolic blood pressure is above 156 mm Hg.[4]

In the United States, a diastolic pressure between 85 and 89 used to be called normal but is now considered "high normal," partly because in 1979, new life insurance company statistics[5] showed that the death rate of people with diastolic pressures of 89 is greater than in people with pressures of 80 (see Figure 2, page 23).

TYPES OF HYPERTENSION

There are two types of high blood pressure—*primary* (also called essential) and *secondary*. Of the 50 to 60 million hypertensives in this country, only about 5% have secondary hypertension, so called because it is actually caused by another identifiable condition, such as kidney disease or an adrenal gland tumor. The remaining 95% suffer from primary hypertension, a condition that has no "parent" disease.

We can now go a step further. Beginning with the 1993 Report of the Joint National Committee on Detection, Evaluation, and Treatment of High Blood Pressure, the severity of hypertension is now divided into four stages: Stage 1 (formerly "mild"), Stage 2 (formerly "moderate"), Stage 3 (formerly "severe"), and Stage 4 (formerly "very severe") cases, depending on both the diastolic and systolic blood pressure of the individual. Table 1 shows the breakdown.

TABLE 1

CLASSIFICATIONS OF BLOOD PRESSURE

CLASSIFICATION OF BLOOD PRESSURE	DIASTOLIC BLOOD PRESSURE (MM HG)	SYSTOLIC BLOOD PRESSURE (MM HG)
Normal*	less than 85	less than 130
High normal	85–89	130–139
Stage 1 (Mild high blood pressure)	90–99	140–159
Stage 2 (Moderate high blood pressure)	100–109	160–179
Stage 3 (Severe high blood pressure)	110–119	180–209
Stage 4 (Very severe high blood pressure)	120 and over	210 and over

*In their 1993 Report, the Joint National Committee on Detection, Evaluation, and Treatment of High Blood Pressure admidts that the "normal" range of blood pressure is not optimal for health. They now define optimal blood pressure as diastolic pressure less than 80 and systolic pressure less than 120. It turns out that 120/80 isn't really normal, or healthy, it's just average for the United States.

And so, if after running tests, your doctor tells you have primary hypertension and your reading is either 130/92 or 145/88, you have a Stage 1 hypertension.

THE DANGER OF ELEVATED BLOOD PRESSURE

But don't let the words "mild" or even "normal" deceive you. Figure 2 illustrates the consequences of having blood pressure above the normal range.

FIGURE 2

DIASTOLIC BLOOD PRESSURE

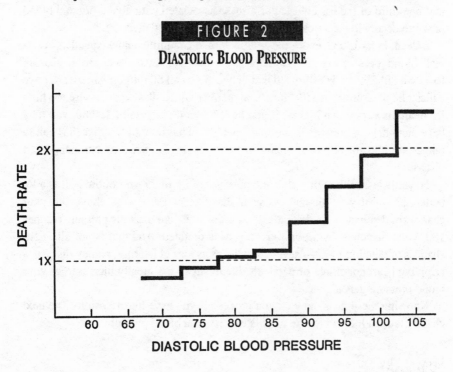

Fig. 2. The effect of diastolic blood pressure on the chance of death. Death rate (read vertically): 1x refers to the "normal" rate of death for men and women (averaged together) with diastolic blood pressures of 78–82 mm Hg. A death rate twice as high is indicated by 2x (based on data in a 1979 large-scale life insurance study).[6] A study of 80,000 people in Bergen, Norway, showed a similar pattern with mortality increasing as diastolic pressures rose above 70 mm Hg.[7] Data from the Society of Actuaries & Association of Life Insurance Medical Directors of America: *Blood Pressure Study 1979.*

Notice that your chances of death actually *decrease* as your diastolic blood pressure drops below the so-called normal value of 80 mm Hg. And with 70, you're even better off than with 75! The fact that a diastolic pressure between 80 and 85, previously considered "normal," is not really normal—or healthy—is further illustrated by the fact that a diastolic pressure of 84 is associated with a substantially greater risk of having either a stroke or coronary heart disease than is a diastolic pressure of 76.[8] Thus, as the Joint National Committee has pointed out, the risks of stroke and of cardiovascular heart disease increase with higher levels of blood pressure *even among those who would usually be considered "normotensive"* [having "normal" blood pressure][9] (emphasis mine). In fact, it is estimated that one-third of the cardiovascular disease associated with above-optimal blood pressure occurs in the so-called "normal" range of blood pressure.[10]

Indeed, in its 1993 Report, the Joint National Committee now considers "optimal" blood pressure to be a systolic pressure less than 120 and a diastolic pressure less than 80! Since it is estimated that between 50 and 60 million Americans have a diastolic pressure above *90,* the actual number with a diastolic pressure too high for health is very much higher. If you have a blood pressure of 120/80, you may have thought your pressure is "normal," but in fact it is definitely above the healthy range required to minimize your chance of having a stroke or coronary heart disease.

Nevertheless, although a diastolic pressure of 80 to 85 isn't optimal, it is a lot better than if it were higher. As your diastolic pressure rises above 90, your chances of death increase dramatically. By the time your diastolic pressure reaches 100, your chance of dying in a given year is doubled. And that is not all: Your chances of developing such severe handicaps as loss of hearing, kidney disease, a crippling heart condition, or paralysis due to stroke are greatly increased as your blood pressure gets higher.

Knowing these facts, how do you proceed if you have hypertension? The next chapter takes a look at the use of pills to treat high blood pressure.

SUMMARY

Almost one out of three American adults eventually develops hypertension as defined by the usual criterion of a diastolic blood pressure of 90 or above.

Although 80 has, until now, been considered "normal," life insurance statistics indicate that as the diastolic pressure rises above 70–74 mm Hg, the chances of death begin to increase. The recognition that a blood pressure of 120/80 is too high is revolutionary, since it means that a huge number of Americans who have thought they are OK actually have a blood pressure too high for optimal health! As the Working Group of the NHBPEP points out:

"Most important, blood pressure-related vascular complications can occur *even prior* to the onset of established [according to Table 1] hypertension since the blood pressure-cardiovascular disease risk relationship is continuous and progressive, *even within the normotensive ["normal"] blood pressure range"* (emphasis mine).

We've known for a long time that hypertension kills or cripples people because it greatly increases the chance of a stroke, heart failure, or kidney disease. Because the chance of death increases dramatically as the diastolic pressure goes above 90, almost doubling at 100 mm Hg, the medical community has understandably focused upon treating those people with a diastolic pressure above 90 or a systolic pressure above 140. As they have rightly pointed out, you cannot afford to ignore having high blood pressure even though you can't feel it.

But the realization that even the classic "normal" blood pressure of 120/80 is too high provides justification for the decision by the Working Group of the NHBPEP to launch a new national campaign to keep blood pressures in the optimal range. The reasons to be optimistic about the possible success of this campaign are explained in Chapters 4, 5, and 6.

CHAPTER 2

Drugs–The Usual Treatment

When we treat high blood pressure, we treat today for what tomorrow may bring.

N. K. Hollenberg[1]

The drugs used to treat hypertension were designed with only one objective in mind—lowering elevated blood pressure with minimal side effects. But we now know that rather than being the primary problem, high blood pressure is a *symptom* of a unhealthy imbalance in the cells and tissues throughout the whole body.

In the old view of hypertension, it was always assumed that the bad things that result from this disorder are entirely due to the mechanical pounding of the elevated blood pressure. This is consistent with a medical worldview that has conceived of the human body as a *mechanism* that consists of parts, as opposed to an organism that is an indivisible entity that must find its own balance. In this "modern" view (often called the "medical model"), if something goes wrong it must be "controlled" for normal function to be restored. After all, machines don't fix (or heal) themselves.

Because this mechanical bias until recently has remained unexamined, and thus unquestioned, it was natural to assume that lowering the blood pressure would eliminate all of the dire consequences of hypertension. The pressure itself was assumed to be the problem.

And since the old view was that hypertension must be inevitable in people who have the wrong genes, there was almost no emphasis upon prevention and a "cure" seemed out of the question. So in view of the dire consequences of hypertension, it's understandable that over the years doctors have tried almost every imaginable approach to lowering elevated blood pressure. As an example of the extremity of such efforts, in the 1950s the worst cases were sometimes treated by an operation called a *sympathectomy,* which removed some of the nerves that normally maintain blood pressure.

Around the same time, however, a totally different, more natural approach was also being tried. Many severe cases of hypertension were cured by a special rice-fruit diet developed by Dr. Walter Kempner[2] of Duke University. But because information summarized in this book did not exist at that time, the Kempner diet, unlike that specified in this book, was unnecessarily very restricted. Moreover, Dr. Kempner didn't know exactly why it worked, and the 1950s was not a time when the medical establishment was inclined to believe that diseases could be treated or cured by changing one's nutrition.

And our whole culture was mesmerized by technology's supposed power over nature, including the idea that we could find a drug that would act like a "magic bullet" to target any health problem. The astonishing success of penicillin and other "miracle" drugs during World War II had prepared both doctors and the public to believe that a drug could be developed for almost anything. So it's understandable that most doctors not only breathed a sigh of relief but were delighted at the appearance, in 1957, of the first drugs that could effectively lower elevated blood pressure. These drugs are called *diuretics* and lower the blood pressure because they cause the kidneys to excrete more sodium and water.

It was very reasonable. Almost no one disagreed: Drugs were the answer! After all, drugs got the blood pressure down, and that in turn should put less stress on the arteries and the heart. And drugs were easy: easier than surgery and easier than anything as flaky as nutrition—which nobody believed in anyway. Just take your pills and things will be all right.

Of course, there were some unpleasant side effects such as weakness, diarrhea, nausea, and loss of sex drive—but everything has its price. And of course, you had to be prepared to take the pills for life. But they *did* get the blood pressure down. More to the point, they seemed to be saving lives, since there were fewer deaths among people with hypertension who were treated with drugs.

To produce ever newer drugs designed to lower blood pressure, a whole industry was spawned. Today this industry takes in several *billion* dollars a year[3] in the United States alone. The use of drugs for treating primary hypertension became the marching order of the day. Until 1984, even the Joint National Committee on Detection, Evaluation, and Treatment of High Blood Pressure, a group sponsored by the National Institutes of Health (NIH), recommended that doctors use drugs to treat everyone with hypertension.[4]

So for the past thirty years, doctors treating patients with high blood pressure have typically prescribed drugs as the first line of defense.

But in the last few years, studies of the long-term results of using antihypertensive drugs have produced mixed results. In spite of repeated studies, the effectiveness of drugs in reducing death due to coronary artery disease has been less than expected.[5] Moreover, in spite of the demonstrated ability of drugs to produce a 34% reduction in death due to strokes, the largest drug study ever done found that drugs had no effect upon overall death rate due to mild hypertension.[6]

Before we discuss these new developments, let's briefly review the types of drugs used, how they are used, what they do, and their side effects.

TYPES OF DRUGS

Until recent years, the drugs doctors prescribed most often were *diuretics,* such as chlorothiazide, which stimulate the elimination of sodium and water through the kidneys. (See Chapter 18 for more on how specific antihypertensive drugs work.)

The other drugs most often prescribed include:

- Beta blockers (such as propranolol)
- Angiotension-converting enzyme inhibitors (ACE-inhibitors)
- Calcium antagonists
- Inhibitors of sympathetic nerve function, such as propranolol and reserpine
- Dilators of blood vessels, such as hydralazine and minoxidil

HOW DRUGS ARE USED

In 1984, the government-supported Joint National Committee recommended that when using drugs to treat primary hypertension, doctors follow the "step-care" procedure, which, until 1988, consisted of four successive steps.[7] This approach consisted of "initiating therapy with a small dosage of an antihypertensive drug, increasing the dose of that drug, and then adding or substituting *one drug after another* in gradually increasing doses as needed until goal blood pressure is achieved, *side effects become intolerable,* or the maximum dose of each drug has been reached" (emphasis mine).

A significant change in the step-care procedure appeared in the 1988 report of the Joint National Committee. In this report,[8] the Joint National Committee added a *new* first step in which nondrug approaches be tried *before* the four drug steps are entered (see Figure 3). Moreover, in the 1988 report, the committee began recommending that when drugs are used, once blood pressure is in the normal range the physician attempt to decrease drug dosage by a "step-down" procedure.

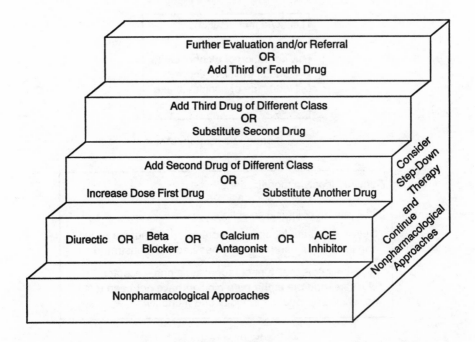

FIGURE 3

REVISED STEP-CARE PROCEDURE

Further Evaluation and/or Referral
OR
Add Third or Fourth Drug

Add Third Drug of Different Class
OR
Substitute Second Drug

Add Second Drug of Different Class
OR
Increase Dose First Drug   Substitute Another Drug

Diurectic OR Beta Blocker OR Calcium Antagonist OR ACE Inhibitor

Nonpharmacological Approaches

Consider Step-Down Therapy and Continue Nonpharmacological Approaches

Fig. 3. The main difference between this 1988 "step-care" procedure and the 1984 version is that a "nonpharmacological," or lifestyle, approach was added as the first step. As the report stated, "For some patients, nonpharmocological therapy should be tried first; if blood pressure goal is not achieved add pharmacological therapy." These lifestyle approaches—sodium restriction, weight control, alcohol restriction, and other cardiovascular risk factors—are to be continued even if drugs are added according to the other four steps. In addition, once blood pressure is "controlled," it is recommended that in conjunction with the "nonpharmacological" approaches, an attempt be made to "step-down" the dosage of drugs and perhaps even discontinue using them provided blood pressure remains low.

The 1993 report of the Joint National Committee (JNC 5) has moved even further in the direction of emphasizing changes in lifestyle. This report replaces the step-care approaches with a "treatment algorithm" as illustrated in Figure 4.

FIGURE 4

TREATMENT ALGORITHM

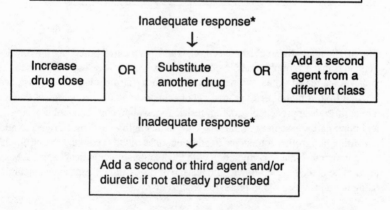

Lifestyle modifications:

Weight reduction
Moderation of alcohol intake
Regular physical activity
Reduction of sodium intake
Smoking cessation

Inadequate response*
↓

Continue lifestyle modifications

Initial pharmacological selection:

Diuretics or beta blockers are preferred because a reduction in morbidity and mortality has been demonstrated

ACE-inhibitors, calcium antagonists, alpha$_1$-receptor blockers, and the alpha-beta blocker have not been tested nor shown to reduce morbidity and mortality

Inadequate response*
↓

| Increase drug dose | OR | Substitute another drug | OR | Add a second agent from a different class |

Inadequate response*
↓

Add a second or third agent and/or diuretic if not already prescribed

Fig. 4. In their 1993 report, the Joint National Committee switched from the step-care strategy to a "treatment algorithm." In this strategy, it is made explicit that if there is an inadequate response to lifestyle modifications, they nevertheless be continued when drugs are begun.

---

*Response means achieved blood pressure goal, or patient is making considerable progress towards this goal.

You will notice that in this new approach, treatment begins with the lifestyle modifications emphasized in this book: weight reduction, moderation of alcohol intake, regular physical activity, reduction of sodium intake, and cessation of smoking. Increasing dietary potassium is also mentioned in the JNC 5 report. The only difference with the program developed in this book is that I emphasize the *relationships* among these various factors, especially between potassium and sodium.

In the 1993 JNC report recommends that "If blood pressure remains at or above 140/90 mm Hg over a three- to six-month period despite vigorous encouragement of lifestyle modifications, antihypertensive medications should be started . . ."[9] You will also notice that the Treatment Algorithm recommends that the physician and patient "continue lifestyle modifications" even after drug treatment is begun.

SIDE EFFECTS OF THESE DRUGS

Besides lowering blood pressure, all antihypertensive drugs can produce undesirable side effects. This is not surprising, since they alter basic body functions not only in the blood vessels but in the nervous system and kidneys as well. Since they alter basic functions, *all* drugs must have several effects. Even if a drug affects only one type of molecule in the body, because all systems in the body are *interconnected* it almost certainly will produce other effects. (In Chapters 4 and 17, these interconnections will be explained to provide a better appreciation that the body is truly an integrated "whole" and not a bunch of parts.) As examples, by limiting the ability of the heart to beat faster, beta blockers reduce the ability of a person to exercise, and (as will be described later) thiazide diuretics produce abnormal changes in the composition of body fluids, including blood cholesterol. So by altering basic bodily functions, drugs affect the ability of the body to adapt to different situations.

Typical side effects of some of the more commonly used antihypertensive drugs include urinary loss of potassium, fatigue, gastric irritation, nausea, vomiting, abdominal cramps, diarrhea, dizziness, headache, rash, weakness, nasal congestion, impotence (loss of sex drive), congestive heart failure, mental depression, short-term memory loss,[10] and in the case of beta blockers, reduction of ability to exercise.[11] In fact, Dr. Randall Zusman of Massachusetts General Hospital has pointed out that this limtation of ability to exercise indicates that "the reduction in blood pressure is associated not with improvement in the function of the cardiovascular system, but rather with a suppression of cardiac function.[12]

Sometimes other drugs are added to treat these side effects.

In addition, antihypertensive drugs may adversely affect other diseases. For example, although beta blockers may improve angina pectoris, certain irregularities of the heartbeat, and migraine headaches, they may worsen asthma and peripheral arterial disease.[13]

How common are complications due to these drugs? In a government-sponsored study of over five thousand patients being treated with drugs for high blood pressure, the percent of patients who had drug treatment discontinued because of side effects during a five-year period ranged from a low of 23% for black women to 41% for white men.[14]

Certain drugs almost always produce some side effects that go unnoticed by the patient because they do not produce symptoms and therefore laboratory tests are required to see them. For example, thiazide diuretics cause increased loss of potassium through the urine to such an extent that in long-term therapy, most patients treated with these drugs will develop lowered plasma potassium concentrations. At least a quarter to a third[15] and perhaps more than 40%[16] of those treated with thiazide diuretics develop serum potassium below the lower limit (3.5 mEq/L)* of the normal level unless potassium-sparing agents are also used. In more than 40% of the cases where diuretics have caused abnormally low serum potassium, an associated decrease in serum magnesium level is also observed.[17] It is recognized that lowered levels of plasma potassium and magnesium predispose people to potentially severe irregularity of the heart beat, including ventricular ectopic beats,† and also to sudden death.[18]

As we will see, a lowered plasma potassium concentration is *already* part of the fundamental problem in people with untreated hypertension.[19] Thus, it is not surprising that there is evidence that although thiazide diuretics lower blood pressure, they can actually result in a worsened outcome for the patient so treated.

In addition, thiazide diuretics (such as chlorothiazide) often increase blood cholesterol and blood triglycerides (a type of fat that is a risk factor for heart attacks),[20] and some beta blockers (such as propranolol) can cause an increase in blood triglycerides (another type of fat that is a risk factor for heart attacks)[21] as well as a decrease in HDL cholesterol (the "good" cholesterol).[22] ACE-inhibitors (such as captopril) and potassium-sparing diuretics can raise serum potassium levels.[23]

The most frequent side effects for each of the commonly used drugs are listed in Table 13 in Chapter 18, Antihypertensive Drugs.

Warning: If you are currently taking a drug for high blood pressure, do not suddenly stop taking it on your own, as this could trigger a heart attack, a stroke, or sudden death. *Any* change in your current medication should be done only in consultation with your physician.

---

*mEq/L is shorthand for milliequivalents per liter.
†"Ectopic beats" means that the initial part of the heartbeat does not begin in the proper location.

THE EVIDENCE IN FAVOR OF USING DRUGS

In the mid-1960s, a Veterans Administration study of 523 men demonstrated that when used for *very severe* cases of hypertension (diastolic pressure greater than 115 mm Hg), drug treatment reduced some complications of hypertension such as stroke.[24] In 1970, the Veterans Administration[25] published a study of 380 men whose diastolic pressures before treatment had ranged between 90 and 114 mm Hg. This study reported that drugs were effective in reducing fatal and nonfatal complications in those patients with diastolic pressures of 105 mm Hg or higher. The complications that were reduced included stroke, heart failure, kidney failure, and worsening of the hypertension. And in the 1970s, a study by the U.S. Public Health Service of 389 patients with hypertension reported that drugs could reduce strokes and prevent the development of more severe hypertension.[26]

These studies involved very small numbers (523, 380, and 389) of people with hypertension and thus were open to criticism on this basis. So in 1979, the first large-scale study of antihypertensive drugs, the Hypertension Detection and Follow-up Program (HDFP), was reported.[27] This study, which followed 10,940 men and women in the United States, reported that patients with mild hypertension (diastolic blood pressure between 90 and 104 mm Hg) who were treated according to the step-care approach had significantly fewer fatalities and serious complications such as stroke than patients treated by physicians practicing "usual" treatment. This study more than any other has been used to justify the widespread treatment of hypertension with drugs.[28]

However, the results of the HDFP study can be misleading, since it did not compare drug treatment to no treatment. Instead, it compared one form of drug treatment (the recommended step-care) combined with restriction of table salt to the usual type of treatment, which most often was based on drugs, given by physicians practicing at the community level. Thus, the conclusion that step-care therapy reduces both cardiovascular and noncardiovascular mortality is valid only when compared to other types of drug therapy (which may or may not have restricted table salt) and cannot be used to judge drug therapy per se.

A later study of 3,427 men and women in Australia (the Australian Therapeutic Trial)[29] did compare the effect of treatment with antihypertensive drugs to the effect of no drug treatment (the latter patients were given "fake," or placebo, pills). This study reported that in people who initially had diastolic blood pressures between 95 and 109 mm Hg, drug treatment resulted in a significant decrease in both fatalities and serious complications such as stroke.

In 1980, a study from Oslo, Norway, reported the result of treating 785 patients with antihypertensive drugs compared to a group receiving no treatment. Several drugs were used, but the two most common were a thiazide diuretic (hydrochlorothiazide) and a beta blocker (propranolol). This study also reported that the drug-treated group had fewer strokes, but a worse outcome in coronary disease. In fact, after ten years of treatment, death due to coronary heart disease was significantly greater in the drug-treated group than in the untreated group. However, no significant effect upon overall rate of death was observed.[30]

Altogether, these studies were seen to justify the assumption that anti-hypertensive drug treatment saves lives and reduces fatal and nonfatal complications of this threat to health. So in spite of the fact that some physicians had begun to worry about the "increasing number of totally unexpected adverse effects,"[31] for the last forty-five years almost all people diagnosed as having primary hypertension have faced the prospect of a lifetime of treatment with drugs.

THE SURPRISING RESULTS OF DRUG TREATMENT

The picture began to change in 1982 when the assumption that drugs provided the answer to hypertension was, for the first time, brought into question. What happened? What triggered this reassessment? The trigger was the completion by the National Institutes of Health of a seven-year study called the Multiple Risk Factor Intervention Trial[32] (MRFIT, or "Mister Fit"), involving 12,866 men who were judged to be at high risk for heart attacks because they smoked, had elevated serum cholesterol, and had high blood pressure. This study, which cost U.S. taxpayers $100 million, compared the effects of an intensive "special intervention" approach to the "usual care" approach of family physicians. The results were totally unexpected.

To the surprise of many scientists and doctors, the MRFIT study found that in people with hypertension characterized by initial diastolic blood pressure between 94 and 99 mm Hg, *even though drugs did lower their blood pressure, there was no evidence this affected the rate of death.* Even more shocking was the finding that for people with borderline hypertension, 90 to 94 mm Hg, aggressive use of drugs according to the step-care program apparently *increased* the rate of death. Only for people with diastolic blood pressure greater than 100 mm Hg—moderate or severe hypertension—was the death rate clearly decreased through the use of drugs. Unfortunately, like the HDFP, the MRFIT study can be misleading, since it too did not compare drug treatment to no treatment. Instead, it compared the results of step-care drug treatment coupled with lifestyle changes (substantial reduction in dietary saturated fat to lower blood cholesterol levels, weight reduction, and counseling to achieve smoking cessation) to the usual treatment of the patient's family physician.

In 1990, a follow-up of the MRFIT study was published for the period 1982 to 1985. This study did demonstrate a significant decrease in deaths in the special intervention group compared to the usual care group. This decrease was primarily due to a 24% decrease in death due to myocardial infarctions,[33] but it is not clear whether step-care drug treatment, lifestyle changes, or drugs used in the "usual care" treatment of the family physicians are responsible for this difference.

Another study in Australia came up with similar findings. This study reported that in people with mild hypertension, those treated with thiazide diuretics had a higher than expected rate of death and a higher than expected incidence of heart attacks.[34] Moreover, the use of drugs to reduce blood pressure also increased the death rate of those subjects in the MRFIT study who had abnormal electrocardiograms (a record of the electrical activity of the heart). Indeed, this latter finding of the MRFIT study prompted an editorial in the *Journal of the American Medical Association* commenting that the implications of these surprising findings are so important as to demand caution and would cause considerable debate and prompt follow-up studies *"since the results fly in the face of current medical dogma and practice"*[35] (emphasis mine).

But the biggest challenge to the idea that drugs are the answer was provided in 1985 by results from a study conducted by the British Medical Research Council. This was the most thorough, the most carefully thought out, and the largest study ever done. Since strokes and coronary events are known to be the most common cause of debilitation and death in patients with mild hypertension, the British study was designed to confirm that drug treatment would indeed reduce these.

In this study over 17,000 hypertensive patients were followed for an average of five and a half years. At the beginning of the study, before treatment, each of these patients had diastolic blood pressure in the range of 90 to 109 mm Hg.

During the study, patients were given pills without knowing whether they were fake (placebo) or contained an antihypertensive drug. The purpose of this strategy, which is called a single-blind study (the physicians know who is receiving the real drugs), is to eliminate any psychological response—or "placebo effect"—to the taking of pills. About half the patients received a real drug—either a thiazide diuretic (bendroflumethiazide) or a beta blocker (propranolol)—and the other half received placebo pills that looked like the real thing.

In those patients receiving a drug, the dose was increased rapidly enough so that within six months the diastolic blood pressure would be below 90 mm Hg. In a few cases, achieving this level of blood pressure required addition of a third drug (methyldopa).

The results were really unexpected. The authors of this study summarized the outcome:

. . . these results provide clear evidence that active treatment was associated with a reduction in stroke rate in this mildly [diastolic pressure initially between 90 and 109 mm Hg] hypertensive population and show no clear overall effect on the incidence of coronary events. *Active treatment had no evident effect on the overall all cause mortality,* but there was a beneficial effect in men and an adverse effect in women" (emphasis mine).

They concluded:

> The trial has shown that if 850 mildly hypertensive patients are given active antihypertensive drugs for one year about one stroke will be prevented. This is an important but an infrequent benefit. Its achievement subjected a substantial percentage of the patients to chronic side effects, mostly but not all minor. Treatment did not appear to save lives or substantially alter the overall risk of coronary heart disease.[36]

When one looks at the actual data in this study, one sees that drug treatment did produce a 45% overall reduction in strokes and a 34% reduction in fatal strokes. However, in this study drugs failed to reduce the number of heart attacks and failed to produce a reduction in the total of all cardiovascular events (stroke, heart attack, ruptured and dissecting aneurysm) taken together. In spite of the decrease in death due to strokes, this study revealed that active drug treatment of patients with initial diastolic pressure of 90 to 109 mm Hg *did not reduce the overall rate of death.* *

Moreover, the fact that drug treatment of hypertensive women was associated with a 25% *increase* in rate of death led the accompanying editorial to wonder whether ". . . it seems justified to conclude that to treat all women with mild hypertension is not worth while."[37]

Especially in view of the less than optimal results of drug treatment, it is important to point out that the study did find evidence that people with hypertension who do not smoke (compared to those who do) had a *much lower rate* of strokes and heart attacks than did those who received drug treatment.[38] In an editorial that accompanied the study, this finding led to the conclusion that "In advising hypertensive patients we must continue to emphasise the great importance of stopping smoking, for this may turn out to be a more important therapeutic manoeuvre than the prescription of blood pressure lowering drugs."[39]

In summary, the British study clearly demonstrates that drug treatment can prevent close to half of the strokes due to hypertension. But in spite of producing a 34% decrease in death due to strokes, the overall result of drug treatment had *no*

---

*Although drugs did not produce any overall reduction in the rate of death among these people with hypertension, this statement hides a difference in response between the sexes. Men treated with drugs did have a 13% *reduction* in mortality. However, women receiving drug treatment had a 25% *increase* in mortality compared to the untreated women. The difference between these two percentages, -13% and +25%, was statistically significant (p=0.05).

effect upon overall rate of death in hypertensive patients whose initial blood pressure was between 90 and 109 mm Hg.*

Another study in 1985 reported the effects of using antihypertensive drug treatment in people over age 60. The European Working Party study,[40] unlike the British MRC study, involved only 840 people and included patients with higher blood pressure; diastolic pressures ranged from 90 to 119 mm Hg and systolic pressures ranged from 160 to 239 mm Hg. This was the first study designed to consider the problem produced by the ability of thiazide diuretics to lower plasma potassium levels. To offset this effect, a potassium-sparing diuretic, triamterene, was added to the thiazide diuretic. In this study of elderly patients with moderately severe hypertension, drug treatment did significantly reduce mortality from coronary artery disease, although the frequency of myocardial infraction was not reduced. Moreover, like the MRC study, this investigation was unable to find clear evidence of an overall lowering of death rate in response to drug treatment.

There have been attempts to uncover evidence that drug treatment does decrease the overall rate of death by pooling together the data from several studies. For example, a paper published in 1990[41] analyzed data pooled from several of the antihypertensive drug studies mentioned above. Based upon the large number of individuals, a total of 37,000 in these combined studies, this analysis confirmed the previously demonstrated conclusion that a decrease of 5 to 6 mm Hg in diastolic blood pressure by drugs is associated with approximately a 35% to 40% reduction in strokes, as well as 20% to 25% reduction in coronary heart disease. This study has been used to support the statement that reducing blood pressure with drugs decreases the incidence of cardiovascular mortality and morbidity. But

---

*One physician I know challenged my statement that the MRC study was so good, claiming it failed to use proper controls. Well, it certainly is the largest. Moreover, it was one of the few to use placebo controls (MRFIT and some others were comparisons of treatment). True, it wasn't double blind, but randomized single blind ("single blind" means only the patients didn't know whether they were getting a drug or a fake pill).

He also pointed out—correctly—that one can never "prove" a null hypothesis; in other words, one can't "prove" that drugs failed to save lives. Nevertheless, the evidence that drugs didn't reduce overall mortality is about as good as you can get. In the MRC study, the mortality rate of those (men and women combined) treated with drugs was 5.9 per 1,000 patient years whereas that of the untreated placebo control group was 5.8 per 1,000 patient years. Not only are those two figures not significantly different; the closeness of those two figures is remarkable!

As for the statement that apparently drug treatment increased the rate of death in women, the difference in rate of death between men and women treated with drugs was just statistically significant ($p=0.05$).

there is a potential flaw in this 1990 study in that 10,940 of the 37,000 people lumped together in this analysis were from the Hypertension Detection and Follow-up Program (HDFP) study. You have already seen that in this study, the group treated with drugs according to step-care *also* had their dietary sodium reduced. This means that the results claimed for drugs could also have been due, at least in part, to reduction in dietary sodium. Thus, including the HDFP study in this analysis seems a bit like comparing apples to oranges. Because of this, some scientists think this undermines its conclusion that antihypertensive drugs decrease cardiovascular mortality and morbidity.

Finally, there is evidence that driving the blood pressure down too far with drugs may in some people actually increase the chances of a heart attack. These more recent analyses of drug studies have indicated that when the reduction of blood pressure is moderate, the chance of heart attacks can be reduced. They found, however, that in those patients whose blood pressure was lowered the most, the incidence of heart attacks increased again. In other words, when the diastolic pressure during treatment is plotted versus the incidence of heart attack, a J-shaped curve[42] is observed. In this curve, the lowest incidence of heart attacks occurred when the diastolic pressure was lowered to the range of 85 to 90 mm Hg. When the pressure during treatment remained above this range, or was lowered *below* this range, the incidence of heart attack was higher. Similar results were reported in another study[43] in which the drug-induced drop in diastolic blood pressure was divided into three groups: small (less than 7 mm Hg), moderate (7 to 17 mm Hg), and large (greater than 17 mm Hg). Again, a striking J- or U-shaped relation was observed between heart attack and reduction of diastolic blood pressure. Those patients with a moderate reduction of diastolic pressure showed the lowest incidence of heart attacks, and those whose pressure drop was smallest *or* largest had approximately three times the frequency of heart attacks.

The most likely explanation for the J-shaped relation is that in those patients who have some narrowing of their coronary arteries, a slightly higher than "normal" blood pressure may be required to ensure adequate flow of blood to the heart muscle. This interpretation is based primarily upon the fact that the majority of people have a lower chance of death if their blood pressure is lower than 85 or even 80 mm Hg.

SUMMARY OF STUDIES

On the basis of several scientific studies, it is safe to conclude that antihypertensive drugs significantly reduce, although they do not eliminate, the excessive rate of strokes and stroke-related death that results from hypertension. And more recent studies suggest that lowering blood pressure with drugs can produce some reduction of the chance of heart attack *provided* steps are taken to prevent low plasma potassium levels. Moreover, in people whose initial diastolic pressure was above approximately 109 mm Hg, the evidence supports the view that drug treatment does reduce the mortality in this group.

On the other hand, in people with a diastolic blood pressure below the 104 to 109 mm Hg range, the evidence that antihypertensive drugs save lives is still subject to debate. Even if treatment with antihypertensive drugs does reduce death, it does not eliminate the excessive rate of death associated with hypertension.

So it is clear that the use of antihypertensive drugs has been a partial success. As the 1993 Report of the Working Group of the National High Blood Pressure Education Program, supported by the National Heart, Lung, and Blood Institute, points out:

> Even those who derive optimal benefit from their antihypertensive treatment are likely to have a higher risk of morbidity [damage such as strokes and heart attacks] and mortality than their untreated "normotensive" counterparts with a similar level of blood pressure.[44]

Thus, the idea that antihypertensive drugs are the ultimate answer to hypertension simply hasn't stood up to scrutiny. Together with other developments discussed in the next few chapters, these findings, along with other scientific advances, have led to a complete rethinking of the treatment and prevention of primary hypertension.

CHANGING RECOMMENDATIONS

The reassessment of the primacy of drug treatment became evident by 1984. In that year, the Joint National Committee issued a Special Report[45] that recommended that drugs not be used, at least initially, if risk factors are absent and the diastolic blood pressure is between 90 and 94 mm Hg. (Risk factors include being overweight, smoking, drinking too much, getting too little exercise, and experiencing emotional stress. These factors are conditions known to greatly increase the chances of having a heart attack or a stroke.)

The 1984 Special Report recommended seven "natural" steps to good health, as alternatives to drugs for people with borderline cases of primary hypertension: Reduce weight if you're obese, reduce your dietary sodium to less than 2 grams per day, reduce your alcohol consumption, reduce your consumption of saturated fats, stop smoking, exercise, and get into some kind of relaxation therapy to minimize stress.

In 1986, the *British Medical Journal* published a review[46] of all of these studies. Their conclusions were that there is "no appreciable benefit to an individual patient from treating a diastolic pressure of less than 100 mm Hg [and] . . . it is probably more important to stop a patient smoking than to treat his mildly raised blood pressure."

That same year, an editorial in the journal *Hypertension* recommended that before drug therapy is begun, the patient be placed on a "three-month observation period during which appropriate nondrug therapy is initiated." This editorial also expressed the view that "nondrug therapy clearly is the preferred approach to the treatment of patients with hypertension."[47]

In their 1988 report,[48] the Joint National Committee not only recommended that nondrug approaches be used if the diastolic blood presure is between 90 and 94 mm Hg and risk factors are absent, they made this explicit by adding a new first step to the previous four. This new first step consists of nondrug approaches. And in a further move toward nondrug approaches, the 1988 report recommended trying a "step down" in drug therapy in those patients with mild hypertension who after beginning drugs have had normal blood pressure for at least one year.

In the 1993 JNC 5 report, the recommendations of the medical establishment continue to move from drugs toward approaches that emphasize changes in lifestyle. Indeed, the 1993 JNC report recommends that for many, if not most, people with Stage 1 and Stage 2 hypertension (which constitute the vast majority), lifestyle changes be tried for three to six months before resorting to drug therapy and continued even if drugs are begun. Moreover, the 1993 report states that even for those patients placed on drug thearapy, once their blood pressure has remained in the "normal" range for one year, "sound patient management should include attempts to decrease the dosage or number of antihypertensive drugs while maintaining lifestyle modification" and goes on to say this:

> "Step-down" therapy (reducing antihypertensive drug therapy in a deliberate, slow, and progressive manner) is especially successful in patients who are also following lifestyle treatment recommendations: a higher percentage maintain normal blood pressure levels with less or no medication."[49]

The scientific evidence summarized in the next few chapters suggests that a nondrug lifestyle approach involving rebalancing the minerals in the diet and other aspects of lifestyle is preferable in most cases of hypertension and can prevent this problem in the vast majority of Americans.

In Part II, you will find the evidence that proper nutrition and moderate exercise will lead to reduction of elevated blood pressure in most people with primary hypertension. More importantly, we will also discuss recent evidence indicating that a nutritional approach can improve your health and decrease the chance of death due to strokes even when blood pressure *doesn't* come down.

SUMMARY

Because of the deadly consequences of hypertension, doctors have made a great effort to lower elevated blood pressure. Beginning in the late 1950s the approach focused almost exclusively upon using drugs—and upon blood pressure.

Hypertension currently costs people in the United States several billion dollars each year—just for the drugs used to treat it. On top of this are the costs due to premature death, prolonged hospitalization, permanent invalidism due to stroke or kidney disease, and decreased productivity due to drug side effects. Nor is it possible to put a price tag on the damage in human terms.

Because they were thought to provide the answer to the deadly consequences of hypertension, the high cost of drugs has been considered justified. The cost of drugs includes not only the financial expense, but the fact that they often sap your energy and sex drive, and that you're stuck with taking pills *for the rest of your life*—every day without fail (with some drugs, skipping even a day or two can cause problems). And some doctors worry about the fact that nobody really knows what effects these drugs may have over a period of twenty to thirty years.

Moreover, because of the financial cost of drug treatment, the frequent side effects of these drugs, and lack of knowledge of alternative approaches, many elderly citizens on fixed incomes simply give up on treatment for their high blood pressure. In fact, even in clinical studies where an especially strong effort was made to get the patients to stay on their pills, 20% to 30% discontinued treatment because of side effects of the drugs.[50] But because drugs seemed the answer and the *only* answer, having hypertension has almost always meant drug treatment.

After forty-five years of using drugs as the main approach, the argument that they are the ultimate answer to hypertension is crumbling under the weight of accumulated experience and recent carefully conducted clinical studies. Moreover, the experience of many practicing physicians has led them to question the wisdom of automatically using drugs, with their frequent side effects, to treat this condition.

At this point, the overall evidence concerning antihypertensive drug treatment can be summarized as follows. In patients with *severe* (Stage 3 and Stage 4) hypertension, drug treatment *does* save lives. But in patients with diastolic pressures between 90 and 104 to 109 mm Hg (Stages 1 and 2, the group which represents the vast majority—around 90%—of people with hypertension[51]), the *only* benefit from drug treatment that is incontestable is an approximate 40% reduction in strokes and in death due to strokes. Although the reduction in strokes must be considered worth the expense and the side effects, it is important to keep in mind that in a large group of patients with diastolic blood pressure between 90 and 94 mm Hg the cost of maintaining good health for this group of patients for one year by using drugs to reduce the deadly consequences of hypertension has been estimated at about $45,000.[52]

But in the majority of people with less than severe hypertension, at least drugs *are* decreasing strokes. Moreover, since 70% to 80% of hemorrhagic strokes are due to hypertension,[53] the fact that the number of deaths due to strokes in the United States has been steadily decreasing, especially beginning in the 1970s,[54] has been used as an argument that drug treatment is a success. This is a point not to be lightly dismissed, since in 1980, in Americans aged 35 to 74, there were 45,357 fewer deaths from stroke than if stroke death rates had remained the same as in 1970.[55] During this same period, the number of Americans receiving drugs for hypertension increased by six million! At the same time that the use of antihypertensive drugs was increasing, stroke-related deaths were decreasing dramatically! So at first glance, it would seem that this indicates that drugs are preventing huge numbers of deaths due to stroke.

But upon closer examination of all the available data, two investigators, who conducted their study while at Harvard University, estimated that only somewhere between 16% and 25% of this reduction in stroke deaths can be attributed to treatment with drugs.[56] This study concluded that "at least three quarters of the decline in stroke mortality in the United States in the period 1970–1980 is due to factors *other than antihypertensive treatment*" (emphasis mine). In New Zealand, where stroke-related deaths have also been declining, an analysis of all the relevant data led to the conclusion that only about 10% of this reduction is due to treating hypertension with drugs.[57]

The authors of these two studies were unable to account for this large reduction in stroke-related deaths that appears to be independent of drug treatment. They did point out that during this same period cigarette smoking had decreased in these countries, and this most likely is a substantial part of the explanation. Indeed, tobacco smoking seems to be second only to hypertension in increasing the risk of stroke.[58] (This applies to both hemorrhagic [due to leakage of blood] and thrombotic [due to clotting of the blood with resultant blockage of arteries] strokes).

During recent years, Americans have been eating more fruits and vegetables—both high-potassium categories of foods. So increasing dietary potassium, and thus the K Factor, may have also played a significant role in this reduction in stroke-related deaths. As we will see in Chapter 6, there is now evidence that increasing dietary potassium equal to the amount in a single banana or potato can produce the *same* reduction in stroke-related death as do drugs!

PART TWO

THE ANSWER: MOVING FROM THE MYTH OF CONTROL TO A BALANCE WITH NATURE

We've seen that the usual approach to high blood pressure is to attempt to control it using drugs. And we've seen that the results have been less than an unqualified success. When a strategy is pursued for over a third of a century without clear evidence of success—indeed, some would say with evidence of failure—perhaps it's time to reexamine the assumptions behind this strategy.

First, let's consider the origin of this word "control" to see if we can better understand its true meaning and the linguistic foundation of its use. According to *The Oxford English Dictionary*, the roots of the word control are CONTRA and ROLL, or COUNTERROLL.* In other words, to "control" means to attempt to move something counter to its natural role—to try to dominate it. For purely mechanical objects, say automobiles, this makes sense because they have no natural role.† Your car does not *by its nature* move from your house to your workplace. For the car to do that, you must *control* it.

Also, you'll recall that the conventional approach to treating hypertension, based on drugs, has assumed that the problems due to hypertension are the result of the mechanical pounding of the elevated blood pressure. This is consistent with the "medical model" that views the human body as a *mechanism* consisting of parts (as opposed to an organism that is an indivisible self-regulating entity that must find its own balance). In this "modern" view, since the human body is viewed as a

---

Contra against, counter (cf. CONTRA) + *rotulus* ROLL. = COUNTER-ROLL 1. a the fact of controlling, or of checking and directing action; the function of power of directing and regulating; domination, command, sway.

†With the advent of computerization, and someday "smart" automobiles, we might be able to argue this point. But during the four centruies of the "modern" period—in which nature has been considered to be purely a machine—only in recent years has the realization dawned that we can have machines that are self-regulating. During the bulk of the modern period, the predominant view that has programmed the subconscious minds of industrialized peoples has been that of a purely mechanical universe. Everything has come to be seen as mechanism. The emphasis upon control is an inevitable result.

machine, if something goes wrong, it seems obvious that we should attempt to control it if normal function is to be restored. After all, machines don't fix (or heal) themselves.

But both assumptions—that the blood pressure is the whole problem and that *we* can control it—have turned out to be shaky indeed. The next chapter will establish that the problem with hypertension involves much more than just elevated blood pressure. And the image of nature in general, and the human body in particular, as being like a machine has crumbled under the impact of recent scientific developments. We have rediscovered, as the older generations of physicians knew, that the human body is a *self-regulating organism*—not a machine composed of a collection of parts. Moreover, we are rediscovering that Walter Cannon* was right: The body has its own wisdom.

Fortunately, at the same time that both assumptions supporting the use of drugs have been found wanting, recent scientific insights have breathed new life into an old approach that because of cultural biases has until recently been ignored.

In the news media it may sound as though all is confusion and controversy, with some specialists saying the amount of sodium in your diet doesn't matter, others claiming that hypertension *is* relieved by decreasing sodium, and still others saying that people with hypertension should eat foods with more calcium, magnesium, or potassium. But seldom commented upon by the press is that in these debates, the focus has begun shifting away from drugs toward nutritional approaches to hypertension.

Also unreported is the new understanding of the biophysics† of the living cell. For the first time, a scientific framework exists within which we can begin to see just *how* high blood pressure can arise. This knowledge at the cellular level is leading to a major shift in our understanding of hypertension that also suggests that many, perhaps most, of its dire consequences derive not so much from the blood pressure as from biophysical imbalances in minerals inside the cell. This shift is also leading us to recognize that unproved assumptions underlay the belief that drugs were the answer to primary hypertension. These and other related developments highlight the need for a complete rethinking of methods of prevention and treatment.

Moreover, our new understanding of the biophysics of the living cell clearly shows that all variables (such as sodium, potassium, magnesium, and calcium) *are*

---

*Cannon was a pioneer of the (then) new science of physiology at the beginning of this century.

†Biophysics is that area of science that looks at the living cell as a whole system. In so doing, biophysics takes into account not only the molecules of the cell, but also electrical forces and fields and how these are all interrelated.

*interrelated.** The living cell is a *multivariable system*—not a machine made up of discrete parts.

Thus, it is impossible to understand hypertension by looking at just one variable at a time. An analogy to the confusion resulting from examining only one variable at a time in a multivariable[†] system would be trying to explain how an airplane flies by looking at just one variable—such as airspeed. Everyone knows that an airplane must maintain at least a certain speed (the stall speed) to remain in the air. But the stall speed depends upon other variables: altitude, payload, angle of attack, and smoothness of the wings. So if several different investigators were to study the stall speed ignoring these other variables, they could only come to a confusing accumulation of apparently incompatible facts. One who studied the airplane at high altitude would argue that its stall speed was, say, 200 miles per hour. Another who studied it at an altitude near sea level would insist that the first was wrong and the stall speed was only 100 miles per hour. Still another, who had studied a plane with ice on its wings, would argue that its stall speed was so high that it couldn't fly at all! This example reminds one of the heated arguments among experts who are looking at only one variable at a time.

NEW SCIENTIFIC INSIGHTS

Fortunately, at the same time we realize that drugs are not the ideal answer for most people with high blood pressure, our new view of primary hypertension offers a better alternative. This new view, which comes from scientific studies of how living cells work as well as from studies of people with hypertension, gives fresh insight into the old idea that both the problem and the answer involve table salt.

This new view of primary hypertension is supported by the convergence of six main lines of evidence, all of which indicate that the real key to primary hypertension is not just sodium, or even just potassium, but the balance between potassium and sodium. We now realize that in the living cell, it is this *balance* between potassium and sodium that influences the levels of magnesium, calcium, and acid inside the cell. And it is the levels of magnesium and especially of calcium and

---

*Irvine Page, a pioneer in hypertension research, emphasized this interconnectedness of several factors in the causation of hypertension. Dr. Page used the metaphor of a mosaic of factors to express this connectedness.

†"Multivariable" refers to a system in which *all* variables interact and thus are essential. Because in our culture we are more familiar with mechanical thinking, I have chosen an airplane as an example. One reviewer took me to task for this, but if the reader will indulge, it does seem to get the point across. Indeed, since an airplane won't work without each "part" functioning, it is, in a sense, a "holistic" system more like a living object than some machines. Besides, I like airplanes.

acid inside the cell that must be properly balanced to maintain the integrity of the living cell and thus prevent the narrowing and weakening of arteries.

Moreover, with this new understanding, we begin to see how such apparently unrelated factors as obesity, lack of exercise, too much dietary fat, too little dietary magnesium and calcium, and improper balance of dietary potassium and sodium can all produce the same result. All these factors lead to an imbalance between potassium and sodium in the body's cells and thus to a calcium imbalance inside cells (in Chapter 4, we'll explain how this imbalance can cause high blood pressure).

What follows is a brief outline of the five lines of evidence, each of which will then be described in greater detail:

1. *Hypertension is more than just high blood pressure.* In part because of recent advances in the biophysics and biochemisry of the living cell, it is now well established that people with hypertension have more than just elevated blood pressure. Whether or not they are treated with drugs, people with hypertension have abnormalities throughout their bodies, including the composition of their blood. These abnormalities include elevated blood insulin, elevated blood cholesterol, and disturbances in carbohydrate metabolism. *All* of these abnormalities are known to predispose to heart attacks *independently* of blood pressure.

2. *The K Factor and the living cell.* It was my own involvement in basic research into how the living cell regulates its levels of sodium, potassium, and calcium that led me, and others, to recognize the importance of the ratio in the diet of potassium (chemical symbol K, from its Latin name *kalium*) to sodium (chemical symbol Na, from the Latin name *natrium*) to hypertension. This ratio is called the K factor. It is now well established that people with hypertension have abnormalities in the balance between potassium and sodium within the cells throughout their body. You'll be provided with a simplified explanation of how the balance between sodium and potassium regulates levels of calcium, magnesium, and acid inside body cells. You'll see that this imbalance within the cell leads to elevated blood pressure and get some idea of how it may result in the abnormalities in the blood, including elevated insulin levels. In the process, you will also see that we are now beginning to understand the frequent connection between diabetes and high blood pressure.

3. *Cultural evidence.* The diet most of us eat is "abnormal" if we compare it to what our ancestors ate. These so-called primitive diets all had a K Factor that was at least ten times higher than in our modern diets. There are several groups of native people in the world today that still eat this "primitive" diet. The diet of almost all vegetarians also has a high K Factor. High blood pressure is very rare among all these people.

4. *Tests of the K Factor approach in human and animal studies.* Consistent with the new understanding of cell biophysics, recent evidence demonstrates that even a slight increase in dietary potassium can significantly decrease deaths due to strokes in people with hypertension! Moreover, experiments with laboratory animals with high blood pressure show that increasing the K Factor in the diet reduces strokes, reduces kidney disease, and restores a normal span of life *even if it doesn't reduce blood pressure.* The importance of these findings can't be emphasized enough. They mean that something other than just elevated blood pressure needs to be corrected, and that increasing the K Factor can do it.

But increasing the dietary K Factor does lower the blood pressure in most cases. Medical studies on people have demonstrated time and again that most cases of primary hypertension can be helped, and often cured, by a combined reduction in dietary sodium *and* an increase in dietary potassium.

5. *The K Factor, weight, and exercise.* You've probably heard that if you have hypertension, the loss of excess weight reduces elevated blood pressure. And recent studies show that regular aerobic exercise can help reduce elevated blood pressure even when there is no loss of weight. We will discuss recent scientific research showing that both obesity and lack of exercise cause abnormal levels of hormones that normally help the body regulate its balance between potassium and sodium.

All lines of evidence taken together point to the conclusion that most people develop hypertension because they eat too little potassium (and, in some people, too little magnesium or calcium) and too much sodium. Lack of exercise and being overweight are the other major factors in causing high blood pressure.

Some other factors, of lesser importance, that can contribute to high blood pressure are discussed in Chapter 8.

CHAPTER 3

Hypertension: More than Just High Blood Pressure!

Blood pressure reduction in hypertensive patients is a surrogate for the real therapeutic goal of reducing the risks consequent to hypertension.

N. K. Hollenberg[1]

We've pointed out that the working definition of *hypertension* is elevated blood pressure. Thus, many have used the terms "hypertension" and "high blood pressure" interchangeably. And everybody knows that the problems that occur in people with hypertension are the result of the constant pounding against the arteries by the elevated blood pressure. So it's obvious that the goal in treating hypertension should be to just get the blood pressure down—right? Wrong!

If, as we used to think, elevated blood pressure were the only problem with people who have hypertension, then the standard approach of using drugs to lower the blood pressure would be just the right thing to do. But we now know that hypertension is a condition in which the elevated blood pressure is *just one of several abnormalities.* In the last couple of years, several physicians[2] doing research on hypertension have come to realize that what we call hypertension is a *syndrome*—a word that means "a related group of symptoms."

Moreover, as will be explained in the next five chapters, the evidence now clearly indicates that hypertension is a consequence of our modern lifestyle—particularly its nutritional imbalances and lack of exercise—and thus is *not* inevitable. How our lifestyle can result in imbalances within the living cell and how those imbalances in turn lead not to just elevated blood pressure but also other abnormalities will be explained in the next chapter.

In 1985 I pointed out[3] that work done in my research group by Dr. Mark Fidelman and Dr. John Munford implied that inside the living cell there is a biophysical common denominator between diabetes and hypertension. The importance of these connections will be brought out here and in the next chapter. In 1986, in our book *The K Factor*,[4] Dr. George Webb and I described additional compelling evidence that primary hypertension is a condition involving *much more* than just elevated blood pressure.

In *The K Factor,* we called attention to the already established facts that people with hypertension have an abnormal balance between potassium and sodium within the cells throughout their body and that they also frequently have an elevated level of the "sugar hormone," insulin. We explained (in the next chapter, this explanation is updated) how biophysics has shown us that in the living cell, *everything* is interconnected. Moreover, we showed why a decrease in the ratio of potassium to sodium almost certainly would lead to other serious abnormalities. We predicted these would include an elevation of calcium inside the cell, probably a change in the level of magnesium, and most likely a change in the amount of acid inside the cell.

Moreover, between 1979 and 1982, Dr. Fidelman, Steve (now Dr.) Seeholzer, and I had shown that elevated levels of insulin decrease the amount of acid inside the living cell. We also showed that this change in acid inside the cell can have profound effects upon metabolism of carbohydrate.[5] In light of these basic findings, it became clear that the elevation in blood pressure is just the tip of the iceberg in hypertension. Our* investigations into the interconnections within the living cell were giving us a clear glimpse that the bulk of the iceberg—the fundamental problem—lay hidden deep within the cell. From that new scientific perspective (including other considerations reviewed in the next five chapters) we argued that to treat only the blood pressure was to miss the point.

We now know a whole lot more. Hypertension indeed turns out to be a whole *group* of abnormalities. The evidence that elevated blood pressure is only part of the problem—*probably not even the most important part*—in primary hypertension is now *irrefutable*. Even in people with borderline hypertension, damage typical of the hypertensive state occurs to body tissues in spite of an only modest elevation of blood pressure.[6] In fact, the conclusion that elevated blood pressure is a symptom of far deeper problems has been confirmed to an extent greater than even we forsaw in 1986. Consider these additional facts that have recently been established:

---

*"Our" refers not only to the scientists working in our laboratory, but also to scientists working in several laboratories around the world.

The prediction that the imbalance between potassium and sodium inside the living cell would lead to elevated calcium levels and change the level of magnesium and of acid inside cells has been confirmed. The full significance of this is developed in the next chapter. In addition, people with hypertension not only have elevated blood levels of the hormone insulin, but not surprisingly—in view of Dr. Fidelman's findings—they also have abnormalities in carbohydrate metabolism. And that's not all: they also have dangerous abnormalities in blood cholesterol levels!

All of these abnormalities predispose to heart attacks *independently* of blood pressure! And it is important to emphasize that all of these changes in blood composition are present *before* any antihypertensive drugs are given.

So there is now a growing consensus that in hypertension, the elevated blood pressure is indeed just the tip of the iceberg. *In people with hypertension, a lot more than blood pressure is out of balance!*

Just what is this new evidence that is revolutionizing our understanding of hypertension?

HYPERTENSION INVOLVES AN ABNORMAL RESPONSE TO INSULIN

Let's first consider the relation I mentioned between diabetes and hypertension. What can this tell us? Insulin-dependent diabetics (IDDM)* are *not* prone to hypertension. But people who have non-insulin-dependent diabetes (NIDDM[†] diabetes is the type that often occurs in overweight adults) are very prone to hypertension. Besides their tendency to hypertension, what's so different about NIDDM diabetics?

You undoubtably know that insulin is the key hormone in diabetes. And as you may know, in IDDM diabetes, which usually occurs in juveniles, there is a decrease in the level of blood insulin.[‡] In contrast, NIDDM diabetics actually have an *elevated* level of blood insulin, their diabetes being due to a tissue *resistance*[§] to the hormone.[7] This may help explain why blood pressure often increases very early after the onset of diabetes.[8] We will see that the blood insulin level may often play a key role in many aspects of hypertension.

In fact, *all* groups that tend to have elevated blood levels of insulin—NIDDM diabetics, obese people, and people who don't exercise[9]—also tend to have

---

*IDDM stands for insulin-dependent diabetes mellitus.
†NIDDM stands for non-insulin-dependent diabetes mellitus.
‡Again, it is actually the plasma insulin level that is relevant. The plasma is that part of the blood that does not contain red and white cells.
§Because the cell is resistant to insulin, the body overcompensates to increase the blood level of insulin in order to overcome this resistance.

primary hypertension. Even more intriguing is the finding that at least in Caucasians,* *non*obese people who have primary hypertension *also* have elevated levels of blood insulin compared to control groups with normal blood pressure.[10] So "insulin resistance"[†] with an elevated level of blood insulin is characteristic of many groups of people who have hypertension.

Why is insulin so important here? Elevated levels of insulin promote the storage of fat in adipose tissue, thus promoting obesity.[‡] More importantly, "insulin resistance" together with elevated levels of insulin is known to increase the production of serum triglycerides,[11] decrease levels of the "good" (HDL)[§] cholesterol, and promote increased levels of total and LDL cholesterol.[12] Moreover, insulin promotes uptake of cholesterol by cells, thus increasing the amount of cholesterol esters and triglycerides in blood vessels. This hormone also increases the thickness of arteries and stimulates the growth of the vascular smooth muscle that constricts arteries.[13] In view of these effects of elevated levels of insulin, it is not surprising that elevated blood levels of insulin are recognized as greatly increasing the risk of coronary artery disease.[14] In fact, "insulin resistance" and the associated high levels of insulin appear to be at the center of a web of interrelated hormonal and metabolic factors that lead to coronary artery disease whether or not blood pressure is elevated.[15] Supporting this view is a 1992 analysis, based upon 11 previous reports, that concludes that high insulin levels play a key role in producing the pathology associated with primary hypertension.[16]

So you can see that "insulin resistance" and the elevated insulin levels that often occur in people with hypertension are of critical importance and cannot be ignored. In the next chapter, you'll see how insulin action at the cell level can compound the problem even further.

HYPERTENSION INCLUDES ABNORMAL CHOLESTEROL LEVELS

In view of what we just said about the ability of insulin to raise serum triglyceride levels and decrease levels of the "good" (HDL) cholesterol, wouldn't one expect to find these changes in people with hypertension? Not surprisingly, recent studies have indeed shown that not only do people with hypertension have elevated blood levels of insulin,[17] they do indeed have elevated blood triglycerides.[18] Moreover,

---

*Apparently this is less true of blacks and not true of Pima Indians.

†Here "insulin resistance" refers only to the effect of insulin upon carbohydrate metabolism.

‡People with extra abdominal fat tend to be insulin resistant and have the associated metabolic disturbances we discuss here. This is why these people are at greater risk for coronary heart disease.

§HDL cholesterol (high-density lipoproteins) help remove cholesterol from tissues.

they also have elevated levels of total LDL (the "bad" cholesterol)[19] and *decreased* blood levels of the "good" cholesterol, HDL.[20] And—*independently of blood pressure—all* of these changes greatly increase the chances of heart attacks.

And guess what? The most frequent consequence of hypertension is cardiovascular disease, including heart attacks. So it's obvious that the elevation of blood insulin and associated abnormal cholesterol levels in people with hypertension may help explain the increased frequency of coronary artery disease and heart attacks in these people.

DO DRUGS HELP THESE OTHER PROBLEMS?

So what does this tell us about treating hypertension with drugs designed only to lower the blood pressure? Does lowering blood pressure with drugs improve the "insulin-resistant" state? Not necessarily. One analysis comparing blood insulin levels in treated and untreated people with hypertension found that simply lowering the blood pressure did not reduce the elevated insulin levels or the degree of "insulin resistance."[21]

You will recall from Chapter 2 that studies of the effectiveness of antihypertensive drugs have reported that in people with borderline hypertension, drug treatment may actually *increase* the rate of death. Most of the drugs used in these studies were either thiazide diuretics or beta blockers. In fact, using thiazide diuretics to treat borderline hypertension apparently doubles the rate of death—with most of these deaths resulting from heart attacks.[22]

It turns out that although both types of these drugs lower blood pressure, they also make many of the other abnormalities in hypertension *worse*.

Treatment with thiazide diuretics[23] impairs carbohydrate metabolism, elevates blood insulin levels, and makes "insulin resistance" worse in people with hypertension. And thiazide diuretics also elevate the total blood cholesterol[24] level, which as everyone now knows increases your chances of having a heart attack. An analysis of data from a study of virtually the whole population of Framingham, Massachusetts, found that in 55-year-old men, although treating hypertension with diuretics reduced blood pressure by 12%, these drugs increased serum cholesterol level by 8% and decreased regulation of blood glucose levels.[25] Thiazide diuretics also lower potassium levels in the blood plasma, which can be very dangerous in people who have an irregular heartbeat. Moreover, as we will see, a low potassium level actually contributes to the problems in hypertension.

At first, it looked as though beta blockers would be a good replacement for the thiazide diuretics. In fact, treatment with beta blockers[26] can make "insulin resistance" worse in people with hypertension. A study in Oslo, Norway, reported that one beta blocker, propranolol, can increase serum triglycerides (by about 24%) and lower HDL cholesterol (the "good" cholesterol) by as much as 13%.[27] Other studies have confirmed the fact that propranolol can not only increase serum triglycerides and lower HDL cholesterol, but can also increase LDL (the "bad" cholesterol).[28] Other beta blockers, including atenolol[29] and oxprenolol, have been shown to increase blood triglyceride levels, and the latter can also lower serum HDL cholesterol[30] (although pindolol and acebutolol do not[31]).

So now you see why I emphasized that these abnormalities in blood levels of insulin and cholesterol are present in people with hypertension *before* they start taking drugs. Thiazide diuretics and some beta blockers produce changes in blood cholesterol and triglyceride levels that can actually accentuate problems *already present* in people with hypertension.

What has been the response to this disturbing news? For one thing, the use of thiazide diuretics is declining. In addition, newer drugs are now being tried that are lipid neutral or beneficial. These include the alpha blocker prazosin, calcium channel blockers, angiotensin-converting enzyme inhibitors (ACE-inhibitors), and clonidine.[32]

As you will see in Chapter 17, the enzyme called angiotensin-converting enzyme (or ACE for short) can play a key role in elevating blood pressure. Thus a class of drugs, the angiotensin-converting enzyme (ACE) inhibitors, was developed with the expectation that they would more specifically address the problem in people with elevated blood pressure. Of the ACE-inhibitors, captopril has been the most studied, with results indicating that this drug has no effect upon total blood cholesterol, triglyceride, or HDL cholesterol levels.[33] Moreover, some* ACE-inhibitors, including captopril, have been reported to decrease insulin resistance in people with hypertension. However, this appears to be associated with increased blood flow, and thus increased rate of delivery of insulin and glucose, in skeletal muscle—the major site of "insulin resistance."[34] (Fat cells also appear to be a site of "insulin resistance.") Thus the improvement in insulin resistance by captopril may be an artifact of increased blood flow and may not reflect a restoration to balance at the level of the cell.[35]

Since calcium must go into the interior of the muscle cells that contract arteries if blood pressure is to rise, a group of drugs was developed to block the calcium channels in the surface of these cells. As expected, these calcium channel blockers do lower blood pressure. Moreover, the calcium channel blockers and central adrenergic inhibitors such as clonidine appear to not affect "insulin resistance."[36] Furthermore, most calcium channel blockers appear to have no effect upon lipid metabolism and blood cholesterol levels,[37] nor upon serum potassium or uric acid levels.[38]

---

*Those ACE-inhibitors containing sulfhydryl groups, such as captopril, appear to reduce insulin resistance, whereas those ACE-inhibitors without sulfhydryl groups apparently have no effect (see Flack and Sowers, 1991).

Among other drugs used to treat hypertension, prazosin actually lowers total LDL (the "bad" cholesterol) in the blood,[39] has been shown to minimize the elevation of blood insulin and appears to decrease "insulin resistance," and decreases both serum triglyceride and cholesterol levels.[40] Similarly, clonidine has been shown to lower LDL cholesterol, total cholesterol, and triglyceride levels while increasing HDL cholesterol levels.[41]

But even if a drug is found that not only lowers blood pressure but also restores normal cholesterol levels, that still misses the point. The problem is not just in the blood but goes deep inside the cells of the whole body. In the next chapter, you'll see that it is now scientifically established beyond reasonable doubt that hypertension involves a biophysical imbalance within the cells of the body and that the problems in the blood are the result of this imbalance.

Moreover, as with the biochemical abnormalities, these biophysical imbalances probably are at least in part related to the abnormal cellular response to insulin and consequent elevated blood insulin levels that are found in all three of these conditions: hypertension, adult onset diabetes (NIDDM), and obesity.

Treating the problems of the blood, whether the blood pressure or the blood cholesterol level, still does not get at the fundamental underlying problem: *an imbalance within the living cell.*

CHAPTER 4

The Action at
the Cell Membrane

The cell membrane is like the surface of the earth, that's where the action is.

Suppose you could place a tiny remote camera inside a body cell of someone with high blood pressure. Amid the complex, swirling patterns of membranes and proteins, amid the dancing molecules and atoms, amid the carefully regulated voltages between different regions of the cell, amid the kaleidoscopic, synchronized movements orchestrated in those special rhythms peculiar to life—what would you see that was different about the cell in a person with primary hypertension? And which body cells would be most involved?

In the answer to these questions lies the key to understanding, and therefore to curing and preventing, high blood pressure. For like all diseases, *hypertension represents a disturbance in the organization and function of body cells.*

In this chapter, I will trace how explorations by myself and others into the ordering of the cell led us to hypertension research and the realization of the importance of the K Factor. I will present the biophysical evidence in simple form. I hope that in following this story, you will appreciate the evidence on the microscopic, cellular level that supports this book's recommendations.

THE ORDER OF THE CELL

My involvement in this story actually began a quarter century ago, when I became active in basic scientific research without any goal other than to understand the fascinating phenomenon called the living cell. At the time, it never entered my mind that this research would lead to insights about hypertension. The motivation was simply curiosity and wonder, without any thought to practical applications.

Amid the dynamic, constantly changing patterns of the cell, there are hints of an underlying order. In fact, the living cell consists of matter that is highly organized, organized to a degree not observed in nonliving things. The big question nagging biophysicists is, How do living cells build up so much order?

Since the cell is part of the physical universe, we know that none of the laws of physics are violated in this cellular order. In particular, we know that this order does not violate the famous Second Law of Thermodynamics, or the "entropy law": The entropy—disorder or chaos—of any closed system must increase as time goes on. (Those of you who are parents are probably familiar with the effects of this law every time you look at your child's room.)

So to rephrase the burning question: How do living cells keep their entropy so low?

We now understand the basic concepts. The entropy decreasing in our body cells is connected to the increasing entropy in another part of the universe: the sun. Of course, the connection is the available energy (some physicists would say neg-entropy) in sunlight, which plants can capture and use to make food, which provides the fuel that our cells can use to order themselves. We are literally tied to our star.

Although there's still a lot to learn, we are beginning to understand some of the details of how the living cell keeps so organized. Back in the late 1940s and 1950s, it was discovered that one mechanism at the cell surface functions to keep sodium outside and potassium inside the cell and thus helps keep the cell organized.

This was something that could be studied. The understanding we have gained about this mechanism during these past forty years led to the insights in this chapter—and to a new view of hypertension.

PUMPS AND BATTERIES

Drawing analogies to familiar, everyday objects when discussing the functions of actions at the cellular level is often useful. Many of the functions in the cell that are important to our discussion closely resemble the functions of ordinary pumps and batteries.

Although it is almost never explained in textbooks, every living cell has its own electrical system. In fact, in each case there is a generator that charges a battery, which in turn provides electricity to run other mechanisms. Of course there are some important differences. Whereas electricity in your car is carried by negative electrons, in the living cell electricity is carried by positive sodium ions (represented by Na^+).* And of course, this means that the cell needs a different kind of

---

*In addition, some cell mechanisms use electrons for purely local energy movement.

electric generator. Instead of an alternator like in your car, the living cell generates the electricity to charge its battery by a mechanism called the sodium-potassium pump.

THE SODIUM-POTASSIUM PUMP

The sodium-potassium pump is a mechanism that several of us began to study back in the 1950s. It moves sodium out of the cell in exchange for potassium moving in (see Figure 5).

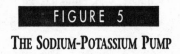

FIGURE 5

THE SODIUM-POTASSIUM PUMP

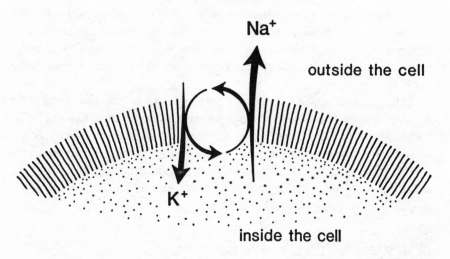

Fig. 5. Na$^+$ is sodium; K$^+$ is potassium.

This ordering—potassium to the inside, sodium to the outside—is similar to the ordering you might use when you put your plates in one cabinet and your glasses in another. In the cell there is a *fundamental relation* between potassium and sodium.

By moving sodium out of the cell and potassium into the cell, the sodium-potassium pump keeps the ratio of potassium to sodium (the K Factor) of the cell high. In fact, this is why almost all natural, unprocessed foods have a high K Factor: Their own cells have a lot more potassium than sodium.

We call this mechanism a pump because it takes energy to run it, since both the sodium and the potassium are being moved "uphill"—that is, from areas of low concentration to areas of high concentration. It's the same general idea with any pump: It takes energy to move water out of a well, and the mechanism we use is a water pump.

The sodium-potassium pump gets its energy from food burned by the cell.*
According to some estimates, as much as *one-third* of the calories we eat are used
to run the sodium-potassium pumps located on the surface membrane surrounding
every single body cell.[1] The sodium-potassium pump in relation to the cell as a
whole is illustrated in Figure 6.

FIGURE 6

THE SODIUM-POTASSIUM PUMP IN THE CELL

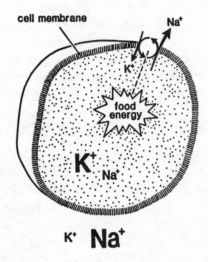

Fig. 6. Large letters indicate a high concentration; small letters indicate a low
concentration.

But instead of calling it a pump, we could have called it a electric generator,
because that's what it is. Besides ordering potassium to the inside and sodium to
the outside of the cell, the sodium-potassium pump produces an electric current. If
you look again at Figures 4 and 5, you will notice that the arrow symbolizing
sodium moving out is longer than the arrow representing potassium going into the
cell. This reflects the fact that the sodium-potassium pump moves more sodium

---

*In metabolizing food, the cell ultimately stores most of the energy in a molecule called
ATP (adenosine triphosphate). It is this molecule, ATP, that provides the direct source of
energy for the sodium-potassium pump, for some other pumps (two we will mention), for
contraction of muscle (when you move your arm—or any group of muscles—the immediate source of energy is ATP), and for several other processes within the cell.

ions (Na$^+$) out of the cell than potassium ions (K$^+$) in.* Since both sodium and potassium ions carry one charge, moving, say, three sodium ions out in exchange for two potassium in results in an excess of one positive electric charge being moved out of the cell. Since the movement of electric charge is, by definition, an electric current, you can see that the sodium-potassium pump generates an electric current that moves from the inside to the outside of the membrane of the surface of the cell.

Incidentally, from this analysis you might also correctly guess that for the sodium-potassium pump to work properly, there must be a sufficient level of potassium outside the cells and in the blood. We'll see that part of the problem in people with hypertension is that their blood potassium level is actually low.

If by now you've guessed that by eating high-K-Factor foods, you prevent high blood pressure at least in part by stimulating the activity of the sodium-potassium pump, which maintains the balance between potassium and sodium in the cell, you're right! The connection is somewhat complicated and some details are still unclear, but we'll oversimplify a bit in this chapter to give the general picture.

THE ROLE OF THE SODIUM-POTASSIUM PUMP IN HYPERTENSION

In the 1960s, a paper by Dr. Ken Zierler of John Hopkins University led me to wonder if insulin might not stimulate the activity of the sodium-potassium pump— something my research group confirmed in the early 1970s.[2] From this fact, our group predicted that the deficient insulin action seen in diabetes should decrease activity of the the sodium-potassium pump. We found evidence to support this hypothesis with tests on diabetic animals.[3]

In fact, together with Dr. John Munford, Tom Pillsworth, and others in our group, we showed that the level of sodium inside muscle cells is increased in animals when they become diabetic.[4] In Chapter 7, I'll explain how the effect of insulin on the sodium-potassium pump may play a part in causing hypertension in overweight people.

One day in the early 1980s, I received a phone call from Dr. Henry Overbeck of the University of Alabama School of Medicine, who was studying hypertension. He was interested in what we knew about ways to increase the activity of the sodium-potassium pump. Henry mentioned evidence that people with primary

---

*In textbooks, it is claimed that when three sodium ions are moved out, two potassium ions are moved in. Actually, the ratio is not fixed at 3 to 2 but can vary. However, in general, this pump moves more sodium ions out than potassium in.

hypertension have a hormone, a chemical substance, in their blood that decreases activity of the sodium-potassium pumps in the tiny muscle cells surrounding their blood vessels. (I'll explain how this works later in this chapter.)

I replied that if this view was correct, his own work indicated that diabetics would tend to have hypertension. "Well, they do!" he replied. From that moment, and thanks to Dr. Overbeck, I became fascinated with the problem of hypertension.

In the intervening years, the evidence for such a hormone in the blood that decreases activity of the sodium-potassium pumps has become virtually indisputable. This substance produces the same type of inhibition of the sodium-potassium pump as does the heart medication digitalis. In fact, both its structure and the effects it produces are virtually indistinguishable from a specific form of digitalis-like compound called ouabain.[5] Since this hormone is a digitalis-like substance and since it is produced endogenously (within the body), it is called the endogenous digitalis-like substance—or EDLS for short.

The normal role of this hormone, EDLS, is to help the body rid itself of excess sodium. Either increasing dietary sodium (which would be equivalent to decreasing the K Factor), or giving steroid hormones that cause retention of sodium, increases EDLS levels in the blood. The increased level of EDLS then causes the kidneys to excrete more sodium in the urine.*

We will be able to discuss the role of EDLS, and related substances, after we discuss the "sodium battery" and the calcium pump.

THE "SODIUM BATTERY"

Like the electrical system in your car, the electricity generated in the cell is stored in a battery. But in the case of the cell, we are dealing with a different kind of a battery. As we've just discussed, the electricity in the cell is carried by sodium ions (Na^+).

As discussed above, in the process of its work of keeping potassium in the cell and sodium out, the sodium-potassium pump produces a positive[†] electrical current from the inside to the outside of the cell. This current produces a voltage, which is shown by the plus and minus signs in Figure 7.

---

*See Chapter 17 for more detail and documentation.
[†]Benjamin Franklin defined all electric current as positive in the direction of movement of the positive charge.

FIGURE 7

THE CELL MEMBRANE VOLTAGE

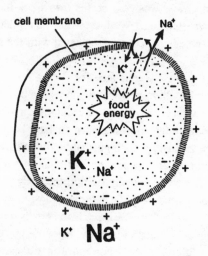

Fig. 7. The cell membrane voltage is due to the difference in electric charge between the outside (positive) and the inside (negative) of the cell membrane. This voltage is due to activity of the sodium-potassium pump.

In a single, tiny muscle cell, the cell membrane voltage is almost a tenth of a volt. This may not sound like much, but this voltage is over such a small distance that it is equivalent to about 200,000 volts over 1 inch! Moreover, if one takes into account the size of the current produced by the sodium-potassium pump together with the voltage of the "sodium battery" in each cell, then each cell in your body produces about as much electrical energy for its weight as a nuclear power plant produces for its (obviously far larger!) weight.

The exact causes of this voltage are beyond the scope of this book, but as already explained, the voltage is partly due to the fact that the sodium-potassium pump moves more sodium out than potassium in, and also partly due to the fact that the cell membrane is leakier to potassium than to sodium. If the sodium-potassium pump is slowed, after a while the concentrations of sodium and potassium inside the cell will come closer to the concentrations outside, and the membrane voltage will become much smaller.

Because the sodium-potassium pump keeps potassium inside the cell and sodium outside, sodium is much more concentrated outside the cell than inside. This difference in concentration results in a tendency (called a chemical potential) for sodium to move into the cell. In addition, sodium is positively charged, whereas the inside of the cell is negatively charged. Because opposite charges attract each other, the positive charge of the sodium gives it a tendency to move into the negatively charged cell interior. This tendency is called the electrical potential for sodium. The combined effect of the electrical potential and the difference in the chemical concentrations (the chemical potential) of sodium on the two sides of the membrane is called the electrochemical potential for sodium.

Because of this electrochemical potential, the cell membrane itself acts like a battery—that is, a device that produces a voltage that can drive electric current. We shall call this potential energy of sodium in relation to the cell the "sodium battery" (see Figure 8).

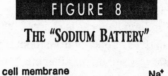

FIGURE 8

THE "SODIUM BATTERY"

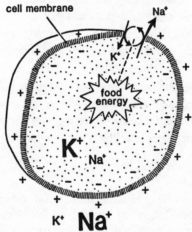

Fig. 8. The "sodium battery" is due to the cell membrane voltage and to the lower concentration of sodium inside the cell than outside. Both act to drive an electric current carried by Na$^+$ into the cell.

In a flashlight battery or car battery the electric current is carried by negatively charged particles called electrons. In the cell membrane "sodium battery," though, the electric current is carried by positively charged sodium atoms (or sodium ions).

The potential in the "sodium battery" is capable of performing work, just as the potential available in a car battery is. The "electric generator" that charges the sodium battery and makes all that potential for work is the sodium-potassium pump.

Since the Nobel Prize-winning work of Alan Hodgkin and Andrew Huxley in 1952, it has been known that the potential produced by the sodium-potassium pump and stored in the "sodium battery" plays a key role in the transmission of signals along nerves. But the "sodium battery" can play many other roles, some of which have had an impact on our technology, and on our language.*

But the "sodium battery" also plays a role in hypertension. You will see how discharge of this battery, due to failure of the sodium-potassium pump to charge it properly, can lead to elevated blood pressure and other problems that occur in hypertension.

THE CALCIUM PUMP

We have seen how the "sodium battery" is charged by the action of the sodium-potassium pump, which derives its energy from food. But, again like the battery in your car, the "sodium battery" itself drives other mechanisms, including one that is very important to hypertension: the calcium pump.

How can one pump drive another? The connection is the "sodium battery." Remember, the electrochemical potential of the "sodium battery" comes from the stored energy of all that sodium pushed outside the cell by the sodium-potassium pump but "wanting" to come back in because of its natural electrical tendency. One type† of calcium pump acts by letting some of the sodium back into the cell; the energy that is released thereby drives calcium out of the cell (see Figure 8). This type of calcium pump is called a sodium-calcium (or Na^+/Ca^{++}) exchange pump.

---

*One of the unique roles the electrochemical potential plays is illustrated by the electric eel. Do you know how electric eels generate all that electricity? You guessed it: the sodium-potassium pump and the "sodium battery" have something to do with it. In fact, my colleague Dr. George Webb did some research on how this works. In the electric eel, thousands of special cells are lined up so their "sodium batteries" all point in one direction. All these batteries together act like one big battery. And with each cell able to produce about a tenth of a volt, it can really add up—to 600 volts!

In terms of technology, consider the Italian physicist Volta, who invented the electric battery in 1799 and got his idea for the battery after studying how the cells in electric fish are stacked up to produce their electricity. Today your car battery has six cells stacked together to make a total of 12 volts, 2 volts from each cell.

Our language reflects such experiments. For instance, in 1791, another Italian scientist, Galvani, first demonstrated that electricity causes muscle to contract. From this comes our colloquialism "galvanize into action."

†There are other types of calcium pumps that, like the sodium-potassium pump, get their energy from ATP produced by metabolism.

FIGURE 9

THE SODIUM-POWERED CALCIUM PUMP

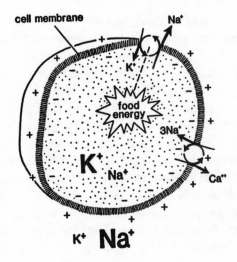

Fig. 9. Calcium is represented by its chemical symbol, Ca^{++}, potassium by K^+, and sodium by Na^+.

This calcium pump operates by a very simple device. Imagine a wheel with nets to hold rocks; three small rocks are placed on one side and one large rock (weighing a bit less than the total of the three small rocks) is placed in a net on the other. The effect of gravity on the three small rocks is greater than on the one large one, so the wheel uses the energy of the three small rocks going down to lift the one large one. Similarly, as illustrated in Figure 8, this type of calcium pump picks up three sodium atoms (each carrying one positive charge) at a time. The effect of the "sodium battery" on these three sodium ions (atoms with excess charge are called ions) into the cell is greater than on the one calcium ion (which carries two positive charges), so the energy of three sodium ions going into the cell drives the one calcium out. This type of calcium pump exists in the surface membrane of nerves, skeletal muscle, and smooth muscle from arteries.[6]

Let's look at this calcium situation more closely. The dissolved calcium inside a healthy living cell should be kept more than 10,000 times lower than outside. Keeping the calcium low is especially important in a muscle cell, because even a small rise in the calcium inside will cause the muscle to contract. The muscles that allow us to move and to maintain our posture can relax completely when the internal calcium level is very low, or they can contract (shorten) when the internal calcium is raised because of the action of nerve signals sent to the muscle cells from our brain.

The tiny muscle cells that surround blood vessels and help control blood pressure work the same way, except that they generally don't relax completely: They maintain some degree of tension or "tone," which in turn depends on the internal level of calcium. The big difference in the levels of calcium inside and outside muscle cells, plus the negative charge inside these cells, causes a strong tendency for the positive calcium to leak into the cell. Therefore, it takes energy to keep the level of calcium inside the cell from rising too high.

This situation is somewhat like being in a leaky boat. How do you keep the water (calcium) inside the boat (cell) from rising? Well, there are two things you can do: You can bail or pump the water back out—or you can plug up the leaks. A smart sailor would do both.

And the cell is "smart." It does both. It has tiny pumps (the calcium pump we're discussing here) in the surface membrane that bail or pump the calcium back out. And it keeps the membrane itself from getting too leaky to calcium so the calcium doesn't get back in.

The fully charged "sodium battery" takes care of both tasks. We have already discussed how it provides energy to the calcium pump. But it also helps keep the membrane from becoming leaky to calcium. It turns out that there are atom-sized "holes" in the cell membrane, through which calcium can leak. But these holes close when the membrane voltage is high enough—that is, when the "sodium battery" is fully charged.

When the membrane voltage is slightly discharged these holes open, letting in calcium, which in the muscle cells of blood vessels causes them to contract and narrow the blood vessel. The blood vessel muscle cells are slightly discharged most of the time, so that calcium is constantly leaking in to provide a continuous muscle tension. The relation between calcium, narrowing of blood vessels, strokes, and blood pressure will be discussed toward the end of this chapter.

THE ACID PUMP

The "sodium battery" is important not only for providing the energy to keep the level of calcium ions in your cells at a healthy level, and thus keeping your blood pressure from getting too high. It is also important in maintaining the proper level of acid (hydrogen ions: H^+) inside the cell. In order to do this, acid (H^+) has to be moved out of the cell. Maintaining the proper level of acid inside the cell is important because hydrogen ions (H⁺) affect many metabolic processes—especially those involving energy.[7]

The "sodium battery" not only powers the calcium pump; it also drives an acid (H⁺) pump* called the sodium-hydrogen (or Na⁺/H⁺) exchange pump (see Figure 10). This particular acid pump exists in every type of body cell,[8] and as you are about to see, it plays a vital role in regulation of cell function.

FIGURE 10

THE SODIUM-POWERED AMINO ACID AND H⁺ PUMPS

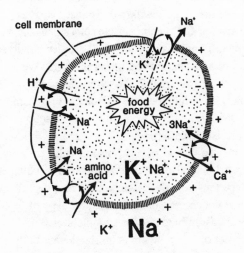

Fig. 10. In addition to providing the energy for the Na⁺/H⁺ exchange pump to move acid out of the cell, the "sodium battery" also provides energy to drive an amino acid pump. The amino acid pump moves type A amino acids into the cell.

Notice that this acid (H⁺) pump works by letting sodium move in while moving H⁺ out. The principle is the same as with the Na⁺/Ca⁺⁺ exchange pump. The energy for moving the acid "uphill" (out of the cell) comes from the "sodium battery."

---

*Like the sodium-potassium pump and some calcium pumps, there are also types of (H⁺) pumps that get their energy directly from the ATP produced by metabolism.

So if the sodium-potassium pump slows (from a low-K-Factor diet) and therefore the "sodium battery" runs down, all things being equal, acid will tend to accumulate in the cell. But as we'll see, other things are seldom equal.

WHY TALK ABOUT THE NA⁺/CA⁺⁺ EXCHANGE PUMP AND THE NA⁺/H⁺ EXCHANGE PUMP IN A BOOK ON HYPERTENSION?

First of all, don't forget that the problem in hypertension is more than just elevated blood pressure. It's important to keep in mind that, as we discussed in the last chapter, blood insulin levels are elevated in people with hypertension.

We've seen that a decrease in charge of the "sodium battery" might be expected to result in increased levels of Ca^{++} inside the body's cells. But what could be the significance of these increased levels? As we just discussed, the most obvious is that an increased level of Ca^{++} inside muscle cells makes them contract more. This means that the smooth muscles of your small arteries would squeeze down, thus narrowing the artery and thus raising blood pressure. We would also expect an increase in the level of Ca^{++} inside the sympathetic nerves that regulate blood vessel contraction. This would increase the release of transmitting hormones such as epinephrine (adrenalin), thus causing further contraction of the smooth muscle cells of the small resistance arteries.[9]

Moreover, increased levels of Ca^{++} inside cells may increase growth and division of cells, and may also increase production of collagen* in those tissues affected by the hypertensive state.[10] Calcium can also disturb protein manufacture, affecting the rate at which proteins are made, the type of proteins that are made, and the way they are assembled into larger structures.[11]

But another aspect of this problem is more relevant to the fact that high blood pressure is a *symptom* of other problems, including "insulin resistance" and elevated blood levels of insulin. Increased levels of calcium (Ca^{++}) inside cells decrease their ability to remove glucose from the blood in response to insulin.[12] In other words, increased levels of Ca^{++} inside body cells results in what is called "insulin resistance."

Reminiscent of the relation between potassium and sodium, inside the living cell there often is a reciprocal relation between the levels of free Ca^{++} and Mg^{++}. Dr. Resnick and co-workers at Cornell University Medical School have found that

---

*Collagen is a tough structural protein that produces stiffness around some cells and forms the basic protein in cartilage and tendons. If the amount of collagen increases in arteries, it makes them more stiff. Increased collagen probably explains why people who have had hypertension for some time have arteries that are stiffer than usual.

not only is "insulin resistance" increased by elevation of the level of Ca^{++} inside the cell, it is definitely correlated with a decrease in the level of Mg^{++} inside red blood cells.[13] Moreover, a decreased level of Mg^{++} inside cells may lead to a further decrease in the activity of the sodium-potassium pump, which will lower the charge on the "sodium battery," leading to decreased activity of the Na^+/Ca^{++} exchange pump and thus further compounding the problem.

So it's clear that decreased activity of the Na^+/Ca^{++} exchange pump could lead to "insulin resistance" and associated increased blood insulin levels. But how likely is this to occur?

A diet with a low K-Factor should result in an increase in the level of EDLS in the blood plasma.* The increase in this substance will decrease activity of the sodium-potassium pumps in cells throughout the body. Since a low-K-Factor diet will also tend to decrease the level of potassium in the blood plasma, (see Chapter 15), this will further tend to decrease the activity of the sodium-potassium pump[†] thus leading to a decrease in the charge of the "sodium battery"[‡] with a resulting increase in blood pressure.[14]

Inhibition of the sodium-potassium pump by elevated EDLS and low serum potassium levels would increase the level of sodium inside the cell and decrease the voltage (electrical potential) across the cell membrane. My colleague Dr. George Webb and one of his students have found that in skeletal muscle of hypertensive rats,[15] this indeed is the case. Compared to rats with normal blood pressure, the level of sodium inside skeletal muscle cells from rats with hypertension was increased by 40% and the voltage of their membranes decreased by 3%.

Although these differences may look small, Drs. Mordecai Blaustein and John Hamlyn of the University of Maryland School of Medicine have calculated that as little as a 5% increase in sodium inside the cell would be sufficient to elevate the level of Ca^{++} by at least 15% to 20%,[16] which in turn could cause as much as a 50%

---

*But, you object, the experiments have demonstrated that EDLS increases in response to increased dietary sodium. How do we know that a low K Factor will cause EDLS to rise? Good question, so let's examine that a bit. First, increasing dietary sodium while keeping dietary potassium constant (as was done in these experiments) obviously decreases the ratio of dietary potassium to sodium, i.e., decreases the K Factor. In addition, in Chapter 15 you can see that increasing dietary sodium tends to cause the body to lose potassium, thereby producing an effect similar to decreasing dietary potassium. With sodium and potassium in the body, increasing one almost always decreases the other.

†If you wonder why the elevated blood levels of insulin don't prevent this decreased activity of the sodium-potassium pump, see Chapter 17.

‡Remember that a highly charged "sodium battery" requires both a high membrane voltage and a low level of sodium inside the cell.

increase in resting tension of the arterioles.[17] With changes such as those found by Dr. Webb, the increase in Ca^{++} inside the cell could possibly reach as much as 200%, although almost certainly it would be somewhat less.

Direct measurement using nuclear magnetic resonance (NMR) shows that the level of free Ca^{++} inside cells does indeed increase in hypertension. Dr. Jelicks and Dr. Raj Gupta[18] of the Albert Einstein Medical School have found that the level of sodium inside cells of arteries from hypertensive rats was 117% higher than in rats with normal blood pressure. Moreover, as first predicted by Drs. Blaustein and Hamlyn, the calcium level inside the cells of these arteries is indeed elevated—by 84%—a very significant change! With Dr. Terry Dowd, Dr. Gupta[19] has also used NMR to demonstrate that the level of calcium inside cells of kidneys from rats with hypertension is elevated by 64%.

The finding that sodium, and therefore almost certainly Ca^{++}, is increased in skeletal muscle of animals with hypertension implies that this tissue, which makes up the largest tissue mass of the body, will be resistant to the effect of insulin upon carbohydrate uptake. Since this would be blunting the major means of removal of carbohydrate from the blood, it would tend to cause an elevation of blood glucose levels and a consequent elevation of blood insulin.

"INSULIN RESISTANCE" DOES NOT MEAN LACK OF INSULIN RESPONSE

Before proceeding, I should emphasize that "insulin resistance" refers *only* to a decreased ability of insulin to stimulate glucose uptake and metabolism by cells. This does *not* mean that other systems are unresponsive to this hormone. Quite the contrary is true. As far back as 1964, Dr. Ken Zierler of Johns Hopkins School of Medicine provided evidence that the effect of insulin upon glucose metabolism involves different mechanisms than are involved in this hormone's effect upon transport of potassium.[20] Consistent with this, in people with hypertension whose glucose uptake *is* resistant to insulin, the ability of this hormone to stimulate potassium uptake by cells is unimpaired.[21,22] Moreover, insulin retains the ability to increase sodium retention by the kidney in spite of "insulin resistance" to glucose uptake.[23,24] And in spite of "insulin resistance" involving glucose uptake in hypertension, this hormone retains its ability to inhibit the breakdown of fat molecules in fat cells.[25]

HOW MIGHT ELEVATED INSULIN PLAY A ROLE IN HYPERTENSION?

First, elevated levels of insulin increase the production of triglycerides and of LDL cholesterol. But the elevated insulin levels are probably related to another abnormality in hypertension that has only been discovered since *The K Factor* was published.

ACTIVITY OF THE NA⁺/H⁺ EXCHANGE PUMP IS INCREASED IN HYPERTENSION

Several investigators have provided evidence that in people with hypertension, the Na^+/H^+ exchange pump is more active in *several* types of body cells. Specifically, in humans this acid pump has been studied in those cells that can be readily removed from the body without harm—namely, blood cells. The finding was that in humans with hypertension, the activity of this acid pump is elevated in their blood platelets[26] and in their white blood cells.[27]

In experimental animals, where investigators can remove any type of cell from the body, hypertension is associated with increased activity of the Na^+/H^+ exchange pump in white blood cells,[28] kidney cells,[29] the small resistance arteries* that control blood pressure,[30] and even skeletal muscle.[31] Not only is an increase in Na^+/H^+ exchange associated with hypertension, but the expectation that this results in less acid (a higher pH) inside body cells has been confirmed in cells of the small resistance arteries,[32] in white blood cells,[33] and in blood platelets.[34]

Two findings clearly suggest a causal link. The increase in diastolic blood pressure is proportional to the increased activity of the Na^+/H^+ exchange pump.[35] Moreover, the increased Na^+/H^+ exchange in the small arteries becomes elevated at the same time that the blood pressure starts to rise and the structure of these arteries starts to change.[36]

Since muscle makes up the largest mass of tissue in the body, all of this evidence points toward the conclusion that the syndrome we call hypertension involves something wrong with the vast majority of cells of the body. O.K., so activity of the Na^+/H^+ exchange pump *is* increased throughout[37] the body—so what?

WHY WOULD INCREASED ACTIVITY OF THE NA⁺/H⁺ EXCHANGE PUMP BE IMPORTANT?

What's important is that the Na^+/H^+ exchange pump plays an important role in promoting the growth and division of cells. As explained earlier, stimulation of the Na^+/H^+ exchange pump reduces acid (H^+) inside the cell; the scientific (and more

---

*Resistance arteries, or arterioles, are discussed later in this chapter. They are the narrow arteries that provide the resistance to blood flow that raises blood pressure.

accurate and more convenient) way of saying this is that increased activity of this pump raises the pH inside the cell. An elevated pH inside the cell promotes protein synthesis[38] and appears to be necessary for cell growth* and for manufacture of new DNA and subsequent cell division.[39] As a demonstration of this, when activity of the Na^+/H^+ exchange pump is inhibited by a specific drug (amiloride), the rate of growth of smooth muscle cells from blood vessels is dramatically decreased.[40]

Not only can an increase in pH affect protein manufacture, as we've already seen, a change in calcium inside the cell can also affect the rate at which proteins are made, and both pH and calcium can have dramatic effects on the type of proteins that are made or the way they are assembled into larger structures.[41]

BUT WHY IS ACTIVITY OF THE NA$^+$/H$^+$ EXCHANGE INCREASED IN HYPERTENSION?

Looking through the literature, one finds occasional statements like this: Now that we know activity of the Na^+/H^+ exchange pump is elevated, the next step is to look for the gene that causes increased activity of the Na^+/H^+ exchange pump. I suspect this tendency to focus on only one of the possible explanations reflects the mechanical, deterministic metaphors of the "medical model." Maybe our genes, which we can't change,† aren't the place to look for the answer.

REGULATION OF THE NA$^+$/H$^+$ EXCHANGE PUMP BY INSULIN

More than once in my life, I have looked at 2 and 2 without recognizing that it adds up to 4. One of these times was when my colleague Dr. Webb and I finished our book, *The K Factor,* in late 1985.[42] In that book, we pointed out that people with hypertension frequently have elevated blood levels of insulin. That's the first "2."

The second "2" was the fact *first discovered by my own research group* during the late 1970s and early 1980s that insulin stimulates the Na^+/H^+ exchange pump.[43] I didn't even mention our finding in *The K Factor!* Our early experiments

---

Caveat: Someone who has done research in this field, as I have, realizes all too well that the true situation is much more complex than that outlined here. Only scientists who have spent their lives looking at these systems can truly appreciate what a fantastically interconnected system the cell actually is. A spider's web is the best analogy I can think of. If you touch one part of the web, every other part moves also. But whereas the spider's web is a two-dimensional network, the living cell is a multidimensional network. Where the different regions of a spider's web move a bit when one part is touched, different regions of the living cell can go through complete transformations as a result of an initial change in just one particular part. The cell is a miraculous phenomenon indeed.

†Not yet, at least. Some molecular biologists are working on it!

demonstrating insulin stimulation of the Na^+/H^+ exchange pump were on skeletal muscle from frogs and rats. Since then, this action of insulin on the Na^+/H^+ exchange pump has been demonstrated in liver cells, diaphragm muscle from rats, 3T3 tissue culture cells, fibroblasts from the lungs of hamsters, fibroblasts from humans,[44] and tissue cultures of muscle cells.[45]

Now that we've got 2 plus 2, I'll show you how the first 2 (elevated blood insulin levels) and the second 2 (insulin stimulation of the Na^+/H^+ exchange pump) add up to a 4 that may well hold part of the key to hypertension. In people with hypertension, the elevated levels of blood insulin (that's the first 2) and the fact that insulin stimulates the Na^+/H^+ exchange pump (that's the second 2) should result in increased activity of this pump in almost all body cells of these people (that's 4!).

As we've already discussed, this indeed is the case! While it is true that we don't yet know for sure that the increased activity of the Na^+/H^+ exchange pump observed in hypertension is the direct result of elevated insulin levels, the existing evidence suggests that insulin accounts for at least part of the increase. For example, insulin acts to increase the "set point"[46] of this pump, and in blood platelets from humans with hypertension, the set point of this pump is elevated as compared to platelets from people with normal blood pressure.[47]

Since insulin does stimulate the Na^+/H^+ exchange pump, it should help stimulate proliferation of the smooth muscle cells in arteries. In fact, insulin does increase the number of smooth muscle cells.[48] As just one example of this, constant injection of insulin into the main artery of one leg of a diabetic dog causes an increase in the smooth muscle of the artery on that side only.[49] The possibility that the "muscle-bound" condition of small arteries may be due at least in part to insulin stimulation of Na^+/H^+ exchange[50] shows where I didn't add 2 and 2!

Angiotensin II (a hormone often increased in hypertension; see Chapter 17) also stimulates Na^+/H^+ exchange[51] with a resulting increase in pH[52] in tissue cultures of smooth muscle cells from rat arteries. In fact, in tissue culture this hormone has been shown to increase the growth of smooth muscle cells from arteries.[53]

So both insulin and angiotensin II are prime candidates for causing the observed thickening of arteries.

HOW DO THESE PUMPS AND BATTERIES RELATE TO HIGH BLOOD PRESSURE?

Before we go further with the new scientific insights connecting potassium, sodium, and calcium to hypertension, let's briefly review what produces blood pressure in the first place and how it is controlled.

As explained in Chapter 1, your blood pressure is created by your heart pumping blood into your large arteries. If the blood could easily flow through these large arteries, nourish the cells, and return through large veins, not very much pressure would be created. But the large arteries branch out into more than 100,000 very tiny resistance arteries, or arterioles, as they're called. Because of their very small size (less than one one-hundredth of an inch in diameter), these arterioles produce a resistance to the flow of blood out of the large arteries. Thus, blood pressure is due to the heart pushing blood against the resistance of the arterioles.

The situation is very much like yet another water pump (the heart), this one pushing water (blood) into a garden hose (arteries). Either increasing the pumping or narrowing the nozzle (arterioles) on the end of the hose (arteries) will increase the water pressure (blood pressure) in the hose (arteries) (see Figure 11).

FIGURE 11

THE PUMP, HOSE, AND NOZZLE SYSTEM

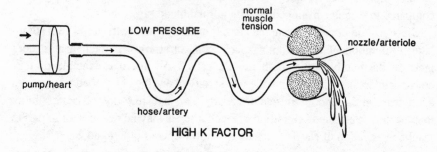

HIGH K FACTOR

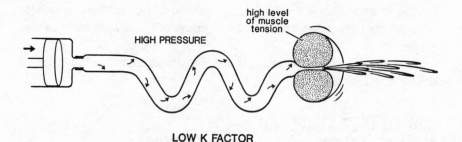

LOW K FACTOR

Because the arterioles are located at the end, or periphery, of the arterial system, the resistance they produce is called peripheral resistance. Since the arterioles can either constrict or relax, they can either increase or decrease the peripheral resistance to blood flow.

The signals that tell the muscles in the walls of the arterioles whether to constrict or to relax are carried by hormones in the blood, or by nerves. But it is ultimately the level of calcium inside the muscle cells that determines the degree of contraction or tension and therefore the diameter of the arterioles (nozzle).

Several studies have shown that in primary hypertension, at least initially, the elevated blood pressure is due to an increase in peripheral resistance rather than to an increase in the volume of blood pumped by the heart.* In the early stages of primary hypertension, the increased peripheral resistance is due to increased contraction of the tiny muscle cells surrounding the arterioles—that is, increased muscle tension. Therefore, to decrease blood pressure, we have to allow these tiny muscle cells to relax their grip on the arterioles. Figure 12 shows cross sections of a relaxed and a contracted arteriole.

FIGURE 12

CROSS SECTIONS OF ARTERIOLES

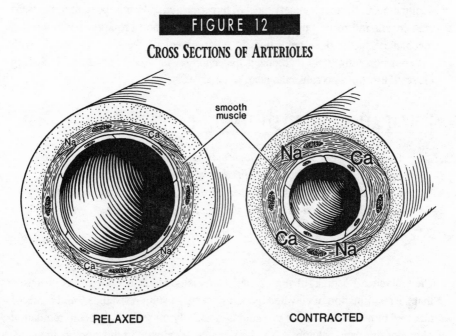

RELAXED   CONTRACTED

We used to think that the restriction to blood flow through these arteries was entirely due to their muscles contracting too much. But as we discussed above, the muscles in the walls of these arteries become "muscle-bound" in people with hypertension. This in turn squeezes the inside of the artery through which blood flows to an even narrower opening, thus increasing resistance.

---

*In Chapter 17, you will see evidence that an increase in blood pumped by the heart secondary to an elevated blood volume must be present for blood pressure to remain elevated over prolonged time.

Remember that elevated insulin levels not only can increase the growth and number of the smooth muscle cells of human arteries but can also increase the amount of collagen in them. The increased collagen resembles scar tissue and results in these blood vessels becoming more rigid.

So if the hypertension is severe and has been present for several years, scar-type tissue (due to collagen) may form in the arterioles, which can make it impossible for them to relax, *regardless of what kind of treatment is given.* In other words, a point can be reached at which some of the damage due to hypertension is *irreversible.* That's why it's so important to detect and treat hypertension *before* too much damage is done.

People with hypertension also frequently develop an enlargement of the left side of the heart. An obvious explanation for this is the well-known fact that making any muscle work harder leads to an increase in size of that muscle. So for a long time, in the mechanical model of hypertension, this enlargement of the heart was considered to be purely due to the elevated blood pressure. Although this mechanical factor does contribute to enlargement of the heart in people with hypertension, now it is recognized that *changes in blood hormones,* including elevated insulin, also cause the heart to enlarge.[54]

HOW IT ALL BEGINS TO FIT TOGETHER

Under different genetic and/or environmental [lifestyle] influences, hypertension or diabetes may predominate clinically, each associated with a predisposition to the other on an intracellular ionic basis [an imbalance between potassium, sodium, calcium, magnesium, and acid inside the cell].

Dr. Lawrence Resnick[55]

Dr. Lawrence Resnick, of the Cornell University Medical Center, has proposed that the combination of elevated blood pressure, "insulin resistance," and levels of elevated blood insulin is due to a common underlying cellular defect in regulation of magnesium and calcium.[56] The perspective developed in this book is in agreement with Dr. Resnick's proposal. But the view proposed here goes further to include an abnormal level of acid as well and views all of these changes as being the result of a cellular imbalance between potassium and sodium.

As we saw in the last chapter, hypertension is a *syndrome,* and this implies that much more is wrong than elevated blood pressure. In addition to the elevated blood pressure, people with hypertension also tend to have elevated levels of blood insulin, high blood glucose levels, increased plasma VLDL (very low density lipoprotein) triglyceride (hypertriglyceridemia), and depressed HDL cholesterol levels.[57] We've just documented that elevated levels of insulin can cause increased thickness of arteries—very likely through stimulation of Na^+/H^+ exchange. It's likely that angiotensin 2 plays a similar role. We also know that at least in the short term, an elevated level of insulin can stimulate the sodium-potassium pumps in the kidney,* and this tends to cause the kidney to retain sodium in the body.[58] The elevated insulin levels also increase the activity of the sympathetic nerves, which makes blood pressure go up.[59] Again, this may involve the sodium-potassium pump, helping regulate the amount of chemical transmitter (noradrenaline) that carries signals from sympathetic nerves to the small blood vessels (arterioles), telling them to contract. We will explain how all this leads to increased blood pressure.

But elevated insulin levels lead not only to an increase in the smooth muscle cells of arteries but also to elevated triglyceride levels[60] and increased production of LDL cholesterol. This fact, plus the finding that elevation of insulin levels results in an increase in cholesterol deposits in the arteries of pigs and dogs,[61] reinforces the hypothesis that much of the coronary artery disease associated with hypertension is due to elevation of this hormone (and perhaps angiotensin II) more than to elevated blood pressure.

One of the hidden problems of being overweight is that it causes blood insulin levels to rise. Lack of exercise also tends to result in an elevation of blood insulin.[62] In fact, *even people with high blood pressure who are not overweight seem to have an increase in blood insulin.*[63] People with NIDDM diabetes, the type that usually begins in adults who are overweight, also tend to get hypertension. Though NIDDM diabetics suffer from a resistance to the action of insulin on their muscle and fat cells, they actually have elevated blood levels of insulin.[64] It now appears that all groups with primary hypertension may have elevated insulin levels.

Not only do people with obesity, adult (NIDDM) diabetes, and hypertension all have elevated insulin levels, they also share many unfortunate consequences: increased rate of coronary disease and heart attack, increased chance of kidney

---

*In 1982 (Moore, R. D., Effects of insulin upon ion transport, *Biochim. Biophys. Acta* 737:1–49, 1983) I pointed out that the effects of insulin upon the various membrane pumps in the cell are so complex and interrelated that it is inevitable that our current attempts to decipher this mystery will necessarily be approximate. Nevertheless, a pattern has begun to emerge. The elevated level of Ca^{++} inside body cells leads to an state of insulin resistance that includes elevated levels of blood insulin. The elevated blood insulin levels would be expected to cause the stimulation of the Na^+/H^+ exchange pump that we have already seen exists. This, of course, produces an increase in pH (decrease of acid) inside the cells. As we have seen, an increase in pH and of calcium promotes both growth and division of cells—removing at least part of the mystery of why the arteries of people with hypertension become "muscle-bound."

disease, and increased chance of stroke. Considerations such as these had led Dr. Eleuterio Ferrannini, of the Institute of Clinical Physiology, Pisa, Italy, to propose the specific hypothesis that "primary hypertension is an insulin-resistant state."[65] Dr. Gerald Reaven of Stanford University has also proposed a similar view.[66]

In any case, hypertension, non-insulin-dependent diabetes mellitus (NIDDM), and the abnormal metabolism associated with obesity appear to be variations on the theme of insulin resistance. In these conditions, the rise of blood pressure is correlated with the elevation of blood insulin level.[67] This strongly suggests, but does not prove, that the increased insulin levels play a role in the development of high blood pressure.

But what could produce this theme? For a clue, let's return to our original approach of looking at the living cell. From all I've just been saying, it may have sounded as though the elevated blood insulin level is the whole problem. No, as I've already indicated, the problem with hypertension goes far deeper than just the properties of blood—whether blood pressure, blood insulin levels, or blood cholesterol levels. It goes right down to the living cell. In fact, we will see that the evidence strongly points toward the conclusion that the basic problem in hypertension is fundamentally an elevated level of sodium and depressed level of potassium within the living cell.

THE KEY PROBLEM: AN IMBALANCE IN THE RATIO OF POTASSIUM TO SODIUM (THE K-FACTOR)

From what you've seen above, you may have already inferred that since the sodium-potassium pump exchanges potassium for sodium, there must be a reciprocal relation between potassium and sodium inside the cell. Some might be skeptical that a reciprocal relation between sodium and potassium inside the cell must always hold. There is, however, another consideration that puts a *lock* on this argument. For purely *physical* reasons (connected with the law of osmotic equilibrium*), inside the cell the sum of sodium plus potassium *must* be constant. This means that sodium can go up *only* if potassium goes down; likewise, if potassium

---

*Sodium and potassium represent over 98% of the positive ions inside the cell. Thus, half of the osmotic pressure inside the cell is essentially due to the sum of the sodium and potassium concentrations (or "activities," to be more precise). Since water moves with ease through the cell's plasma membrane, the inside of the cell must always be in osmotic equilibrium with the outside. Since the osmotic pressure of the blood is regulated by the kidneys to be virtually constant, osmotic equilibrium requires that the osmotic pressure of the inside the cell must also be constant. Thus, the sum of sodium and potassium concentrations inside the cell must be constant in order to prevent the cell from either shrinking or swelling.

goes up, sodium *must* go down. So potassium and sodium are unalterably linked together like two children on a teeter-totter. You can't change one without changing the other.

Thus, in the perspective of cell biophysics, it makes no sense to talk about either sodium or potassium alone—these two substances *always* affect each other in a reciprocal relation. Hence their ratio, the K Factor, reflects the state of the living cell more completely than either sodium or potassium alone. This is the clincher for the K Factor concept: It is not only a simplifying concept but a much more scientifically valid measure of the state of health of the living cell—and therefore of the whole body.

Reflecting the action in the cell, potassium and sodium always work in a reciprocal manner in the whole body (as explained in Chapter 15). This means that increased consumption of potassium will drive sodium out of the body through the kidneys. Thus, potassium has been called "nature's diuretic."

Several research groups have found that human beings with hypertension have elevated levels of sodium in their red blood and white blood cells. A study by Dr. E. Ambrosioni and his colleagues in Bologna, Italy, found that many young people with borderline* hypertension have elevated levels of sodium inside their white blood cells. In people who were definitely hypertensive, the sodium level was significantly[†] elevated. In the people with definite hypertension, the elevated levels of sodium were associated with decreased levels of potassium inside their white cells. This is an example of the fact that elevation of sodium inside our body cells must always be accompanied by a decrease in the potassium level.

In Dr. Ambrosioni's study, when the levels of potassium and sodium inside white blood cells from all of the people (those with normal, those with borderline, and those with definitely elevated blood pressure) were compared, the *one* variable best related to blood pressure was the *ratio* of potassium to sodium. In other words, as the potassium/sodium ratio (which is what we call the K Factor) is decreased, the blood pressure rises.[68] In those who began the study with normal blood pressure and also normal levels of sodium (and therefore a normal K Factor) in their white blood cells, *not one* developed hypertension over the next five years.

What's the common demoninator in all this? You'll recall that the changes in calcium, magnesium, and acid inside cells are largely the result of an increase in sodium in these cells. And remember that when sodium inside a cell goes up, that means that potassium must go down.

---

*In this study, diagnosis of elevated blood pressure was based upon measurement on three different occasions. "Borderline" was defined when at least one of the three measurements showed a diastolic pressure above 90 mm Hg and at least one was below that level.

[†]There was less than one chance in a thousand that the measurement of this elevation was due to chance.

Thus, we have traced the *original problem* back to an imbalance between potassium and sodium within the body, which, in turn, can be caused by (among other things) a deficiency in the K Factor of the diet. Remember that in the cell when potassium goes down, sodium *must* go up.

In Chapter 15 we'll see that people with hypertension have a deficiency in body potassium. This alone may cause "insulin resistance." Although you have already seen the cellular mechanisms that could result in "insulin resistance," the experimental evidence on this is suggestive. The "insulin resistance" produced by thiazide diuretics can be partially corrected by giving the patient additional potassium.[69] In fact, "insulin resistance" occurs in several disease states that are characterized by depletion of potassium from the body.[70] So the fundamental problem may go back to a deficiency of potassium with a consequent decrease in the K Factor in the living cell!*

FROM K FACTOR TO BLOOD PRESSURE AND/OR STROKE: THE CAUSAL CHAIN

You have seen hints that a low-K-Factor diet will slow the sodium-potassium pump. But just how could this work?

When too much sodium is retained in the body, the brain releases a hormone (endogenous digitalis-like substance, or EDLS) that slows the exchange of potassium for sodium by the sodium-potassium pumps in the small arteries. (This is described further in Chapter 17.) Since dietary potassium tends to decrease the amount of sodium in the body, a low ratio of potassium to sodium in the diet, or a low K Factor, will tend to elevate this substance, thus leading to slowing of the sodium-potassium pumps in the body. Several studies indicate that EDLS is elevated in many people with primary hypertension.

But there is another way in which a low-K-Factor diet may slow the sodium-potassium pumps. Because potassium is pumped into cells, there has to be enough potassium on the outside of the cell in order for the sodium-potassium pump to work well, moving the potassium from the outside to the inside. If the potassium ions in the blood (and outside the cells, number 1 in Figure 13) are few and far between, they won't bump into the sodium-potassium pumps as often. This means that the pumps will slow down (number 2 in Fig. 13). In fact, the speed of the sodium-potassium pump depends on the level of blood (serum) potassium. There is evidence that in the normal range of plasma potassium, the level of potassium has a significant effect upon the sodium-potassium pump's speed.[71]

---

*The experiments needed at this point are to put animals on a low-K-Factor diet and see if they develop not only elevated blood pressure (this has already been demonstrated) but also "insulin resistance."

As we have seen, people with hypertension consume too little potassium compared to sodium (i.e., have a low dietary K Factor). This results in a decreased effectiveness of their sodium-potassium pumps, which in turn decreases the ratio of potassium to sodium within their cells. Remember that a decrease in sodium inside our body cells *must* be accompanied by an increase in the potassium level.

Therefore, a low level of sodium inside the cells of your body not only indicates that the sodium-potassium pump must be active, it virtually assures you that the cells will have a high level of potassium to sodium. So your body must have a proper balance of potassium to sodium—in other words, a high K Factor.

But if your body has a low K Factor, this in turn decreases the charge on the "sodium battery" of your cells, which results in an increased level of calcium ions inside the cell.

An overabundance of calcium inside the cell, in turn, can be caused by either a slow calcium pump (pushing less calcium out of the cell) or holes in the cellular membrane allowing calcium to leak back inside the cell. Either of these can result from a "sodium battery" that is run down. And either slow sodium-potassium pumps or a membrane leaky to sodium will allow the "sodium battery" to run down. This causal chain is diagrammed in Figure 13.

FIGURE 13

THE K FACTOR AND CELLULAR CALCIUM

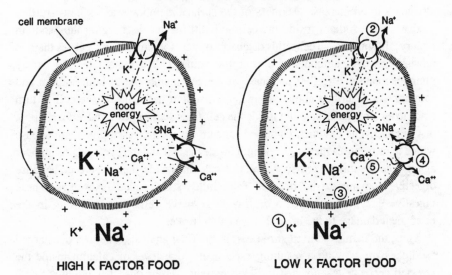

HIGH K FACTOR FOOD   LOW K FACTOR FOOD

Fig. 13. Key to numbers: 1, potassium ions outside cell; 2, sodium-potassium pump; 3, "sodium battery"; 4, calcium pump; 5, calcium ions inside cell. These numbers show the causal chain of events leading from a low-K-Factor diet to a higher level of calcium inside the cell and thus to high blood pressure. See text for detailed discussion.

The increase in calcium level causes "insulin resistance," with an associated increase in blood insulin level. The abnormally elevated blood insulin is at least part of the cause of several problems: high blood LDL cholesterol levels, low HDL cholesterol levels, and development of abnormal ("muscle-bound") structure of arterioles, and perhaps increased blood volume. The "muscle bound" arteries in turn may increase peripheral resistance. But increased peripheral resistance may also be the result of excessive tension, or contraction, of the muscle cells encircling the arteriole walls. And we know that muscular contractions are caused by an increase of calcium inside the cell. So the elevated calcium levels inside cells will tend to lead to elevated blood pressure.

But how about strokes? We've already seen evidence that reducing blood pressure drugs to the "normal" range only prevents about 40% of strokes and death due to strokes. Moreover, in the next chapter you will see that extra dietary potassium can produce the same reduction in death due to strokes *even when the blood pressure isn't changed.* So clearly something more than blood pressure is involved in strokes. The elevated calcium levels inside cells provides a key to understanding this.

It is now pretty well established that much of the brain damage due to strokes is from an increase in calcium inside nerve cells.[72] The mechanism for this is that if blood flow to a part of the brain is decreased too much, the resulting deficiency of oxygen ultimately leads to a decreased activity of sodium-potassium pumps and thus to a decreased charge of the "sodium battery." In nerve cells, this discharge also leads to an increase leakiness of the surface membrane to sodium—further increasing the sodium inside the cell and still further discharging the "sodium battery." In some nerve cells, this discharge of the "sodium battery" causes them to release excessive amounts of a neurotransmitter called glutamate. But excess glutamate causes a further leakiness of the cell membrane to both sodium and calcium. As described above, an increased sodium level inside the cell in turn leads to an increase in calcium inside the cell. This starts a positive feedback loop, or viscious cycle, in which increased calcium causes increased glutamate release which in turn causes increased calcium inside the cell and the cycle begins all over again. The resulting excessive levels of calcium inside these nerve cells cause digestive enzymes to be released from little "sacs" called lysosomes. These digestive enzymes proceed to destroy these nerve cells, thus resulting in the permanent damage to the brain that we call a stroke.

Thus, the damage due to strokes is, in the final analysis, due to a discharged "sodium battery" with a resulting excessively high level of calcium inside the affected nerve cells—not just to blood pressure. From this, it is obvious that a deficiency of the K Factor would make a stroke more likely.

Thus the whole chain of events leading to hypertension begins with inhibition of the sodium-potassium pumps as a result of too much sodium and too little potassium. This inhibition is partly due to the presence of a digitalis-like hormone,

EDLS, but it probably is also partly due to the decreased plasma potassium levels seen in these people. Thus, restoring a normal level of plasma potassium through dietary means should help reduce the inhibition of the sodium-potassium pumps and allow the "sodium battery" of the body cells to recharge, resulting, among other things, in a drop in blood pressure.

So you can see that either adding too much sodium to your body (by eating too much of it) or taking away potassium (by eating too little) could slow the sodium-potassium pumps' charging of the "sodium batteries" (number 3 in Figure 13), which then slows down the calcium pumps (number 4) and increases membrane leakiness to calcium, which increases calcium inside the cells (number 5), which increases muscle tension, peripheral resistance, and finally blood pressure (recall Figures 11 and 12).

Superimposed on all this are inherited differences in other hormone systems that regulate the sodium-potassium pumps and in the leakiness of our cell membranes (which makes the pumps work faster just to keep up). Thus, because of our inheritance, some of us are more likely to develop high blood pressure when we eat a low-K-Factor diet than are others of us. But in Chapter 5 you'll see that if you eat foods with a high K Factor, it's unlikely you'll get hypertension, regardless of your inheritance.

In the final analysis, to keep the calcium low inside the tiny muscle cells so your arterioles can relax, your body must have a normal balance between potassium and sodium: The sodium batteries must be charged.

Is Calcium Bad?

From what we have said so far, you might expect that extra dietary calcium would be bad for hypertension. If calcium builds up in the cell, we get too much muscle tension, too much peripheral resistance, and too much blood pressure.

But in Chapter 6 you will see how Dr. Addison demonstrated that a high-calcium diet helped control blood pressure. How can this be?

When we look at the cell a little closer, this isn't so surprising. A charged sodium battery is not the only thing that prevents leakiness in the cell wall. Paradoxically, the very presence of lots of calcium outside the cell membrane (remember, 10,000 times more calcium outside than inside), pressuring to get in, helps keep the membrane tight and thus slows the leak of calcium into the cell. If the amount of calcium in the blood drops very much, the membrane becomes leaky. As a result, the calcium level inside the cell actually goes up. To keep the calcium low inside, you've got to keep it high outside! Surprising at first sight, but true.

So either a low K Factor or a low amount of dietary calcium can cause hypertension. (Too much calcium in the diet can also contribute to hypertension—either too little or too much is bad.)

HOW ABOUT MAGNESIUM?

How does magnesium help? Magnesium in the blood outside the cell, like calcium, helps stabilize the cell membrane by helping to keep it tight and to prevent leaks. Not only that, magnesium is necessary for the sodium-potassium pump to operate properly. In fact, sufficient magnesium is essential for the cells of the body to maintain normal levels of potassium.[73] So it should not be surprising that sufficient magnesium must be present to keep the "sodium battery" charged.

In Chapter 8, you will see evidence that too little magnesium in the diet can also help cause high blood pressure.

Increasing the K Factor (which helps the sodium-potassium pumps and so charges the "sodium battery") decreases strokes (due to either blowout or obstruction of arteries) even when the blood pressure doesn't come down, as we describe in Chapter 6. In addition, in 1985 a research group in Australia[74] reported that even in people with normal blood pressure, people who eat high levels of sodium, or a *low K Factor,* develop increased stiffness of their arteries. This indicates that a high K Factor is necessary for strong, pliable arteries, built from the proper protein. Conversely, it's not surprising that a deficiency of the K Factor seems to lead to weak arteries from insufficient or improper protein (see Figure 14).

FIGURE 14

A STRONG AND A WEAK ARTERY

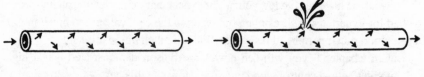

HIGH K FACTOR FOOD   **LOW K FACTOR FOOD**

You've got to have those "sodium batteries" charged up. Otherwise, not only will the blood pressure tend to go up, but the cells of your arteries (and probably elsewhere) may tend to be weakened. And since drugs aren't designed to help keep the "sodium batteries" charged (the thiazide diuretics can even run them down), it's not surprising that while they may lower blood pressure, they often fail to prevent strokes or death.

TESTING THE MODEL

What we have presented in this chapter is oversimplified. Many details remain to be worked out and confirmed. Nevertheless, several predictions necessarily follow from the model presented here. Demonstrating that any one of these predictions is wrong would invalidate, or disprove, the model or at least require it to be modified. Among the predictions that have been confirmed by scientific studies are these:

Prediction 1: The potassium in body cells (and therefore total body potassium) will be decreased in people with primary hypertension.
Confirmation: In fact, Scandinavian scientists have shown that in people with untreated primary hypertension, the total amount of potassium in their bodies is significantly decreased.[75] Moreover, in rats with hypertension, the level of potassium inside the cells of their arteries is significantly decreased.[76]

Prediction 2: The potassium level in the blood plasma of people with hypertension should tend to be decreased.
Confirmation: Chapter 15 presents evidence that shows that people with hypertension generally have a slightly lower level of potassium in their blood plasma.

Prediction 3: The sodium inside the cells of the body should be increased in people with primary hypertension.
Confirmation: The white blood cell is an easily studied cell with many sodium-potassium pumps. Many studies have shown, apparently without exception, that there is an elevated level of sodium in white blood cells from people with hypertension compared to people with normal blood pressure.[77]

Prediction 4: Increasing the level of potassium in the blood should cause the small resistance arteries to relax.
Confirmation: Raising plasma potassium from 3.6 mEq/L to 6 mEq/L produces a significant relaxation of the small arteries with a resulting drop in blood pressure.[78]

Prediction 5: Inhibiting the sodium-potassium pump in the small resistance arteries should block this relaxing effect of potassium.
Confirmation: Inhibiting the sodium-potassium pump with a specific inhibitor blocks the relaxing action of potassium on these small arteries.[79]

Prediction 6: Because NIDDM diabetics have "insulin resistance" and elevated blood levels of insulin, they should have similar changes in activity of their Na^+/H^+ and Ca^{++} pumps and thus be much more likely to develop high blood pressure.
Confirmation: Having diabetes mellitus greatly increases a person's chances of developing high blood pressure.[80]

Prediction 7: Inside the cells of people with hypertension, there should be an increase in pH (a decrease in acid).
Confirmation: Above, we pointed out that in animals with hypertension, the interior of the the cells of their small arteries,[81] of their white blood cells,[82] and of their blood platelets,[83] the pH is indeed elevated.

Prediction 8: Giving adequate potassium compared to sodium in the diet should help lower elevated blood pressure.

Confirmation: Chapter 6 documents studies that show that increasing the ratio of potassium to sodium, the K Factor, in the diet can restore blood pressure toward normal in people with hypertension.

Prediction 9: Giving adequate potassium compared to sodium in the diet should help reduce the complications of hypertension.

Confirmation: Chapters 5 and 6 present evidence that a proper dietary K Factor not only lowers blood pressure but also reduces strokes and may prolong life.

All in all, the evidence for the following statement is very strong:

The real problem isn't just blood pressure, it's deeper than that and involves an imbalance between potassium and sodium, and also calcium, within the living cell. Drugs don't get at that problem; the K Factor approach does.

SUMMARY

In light of this newer perspective, hypertension is seen to be due to an imbalance in the living cell. This imbalance is the consequence of a diet too high in sodium chloride and/or too low in potassium. As a result of this imbalance, the sodium-potassium pumps tend to slow, allowing the "sodium battery" to run down not only in blood vessels, but in cells *throughout the body.*

The abnormalities throughout the body include both a decreased activity of the Na^+/Ca^{++} exchange pumps and increased activity of the Na^+/H^+ exchange pumps. These changes are probably related to the elevation of blood insulin levels that often occurs in people with hypertension. Moreover, increased blood insulin levels lead to increased blood levels of triglycerides and higher cholesterol levels. The fact that so many changes occur in body cells emphasizes the fact that in hypertension, elevated blood pressure is just *one result* of an imbalance inside the living cell. Elevated blood pressure is a sign that the whole body is out of balance.

But is this imbalance a purely inherited, and thus inevitable, problem, or could it be due to some aspect of the way we live? People with hypertension have a deficiency in body potassium, and as we just saw, this alone may cause "insulin resistance."

Thus it should not be surprising to find that either an excess of sodium or a deficiency of potassium in the diet can contribute to high blood pressure.

On the other hand, extra potassium can help stimulate the sodium-potassium pump and recharge the "sodium battery"! A fully charged "sodium battery" helps keep cell calcium levels low, thus relaxing arterioles, normalizing insulin action, and keeping the blood pressure low. The "battery" also helps promote the manufacture of proteins by the cells. A discharged "sodium battery" might also explain a decreased strength of artery walls in people or animals with hypertension.

One might say that in the body, sodium and potassium balance each other. As an approximation, sodium and potassium may be seen as representing opposing forces. As such, they must be kept in a kind of balance if you are to function the way nature intended.

One "pushes" where the other "pulls." One is the yin and the other yang. To have a complete effect, both must be changed.

That's why the term "K Factor" is useful: It's a measure of the balance between potassium and sodium.

CHAPTER 5

High Blood Pressure Is Not Inevitable: Cultural Evidence

> *. . . a blood pressure in the . . . optimal range of less than 120 mm Hg and less than 80 mm Hg . . . is the norm in unacculturated [native] societies where age-related changes in blood pressure are uncommon.*
>
> Working Group Report on
> Primary Prevention of Hypertension, 1993[1]

We used to think that high blood pressure just happened. Later we realized that primary hypertension tends to occur in those with an inherited, or genetic, tendency. Now our new understanding of the biophysics of the living cell suggests that a lifestyle-generated* imbalance between potassium (K) and sodium (Na) in the living cell produces other cellular imbalances that lead to hypertension. Can we find evidence to support this thesis by looking at people with different lifestyles?

Studies of population groups living today in different places around the world indicate that high blood pressure is *not* a necessary part of the human condition. Anthropologists have studied blood pressure in over thirty groups of indigenous people, including African hunter-gatherers and aboriginals in Australia and in South America. *None* of these groups has been afflicted with high blood pressure until they adopt a modern lifestyle. Hospital records in Africa illustrate that in the

---

*True, there is an inherited tendency that makes some of us less able to tolerate the effects of a nutritional imbalance and other lifestyle mistakes. But you will see that if we correct our mistakes of lifestyle, regardless of our genes, the vast majority of us won't get hypertension.

early part of this century high blood pressure just wasn't observed in such "primitive" areas. But after adopting a modern lifestyle, including the use of salt and processed foods, these same records show that hypertension began to occur in these people.[2] So the lack of high blood pressure in these native groups before eating such processed and salted foods is not due to an inherited resistance to high blood pressure. Because no exceptions to this have been found, anthropologists who have looked into the matter are agreed that *hypertension is a cultural disease*—a disease of *lifestyle*. In other words, hypertension is *not* inevitable, and since it is due to mistakes of lifestyle, it is preventable and should be curable.

But what aspect of our modern culture leads to high blood pressure? The evidence shows that most cases of high blood pressure are produced by modern methods of food preparation, by obesity, and by insufficient exercise.

THE STONE AGE DIET

The first "diet" for low blood pressure was eaten thousands of years ago. Studies of the tools the Stone Age people used to obtain their food and the location of their living sites suggest that about one-third of their diet was meat from wild animals and the other two-thirds was from plants. This indicates that they ate foods that were low in sodium and very high in potassium. As will be demonstrated in the chapters to come, such a diet would have prevented hypertension. Of course, we don't know what their blood pressure actually was. But examination of their bones gives us reason to believe that if they escaped childhood diseases and didn't meet an unhappy fate with a wild beast, many of our ancient ancestors lived at least into their fifties, a point where bones no longer reliably indicate age.[3]

THE STONE AGE DIET TODAY

It turns out that in spite of "civilization," there are a few places left in the world where aboriginal people are still eating the diet of our ancient ancestors. In every such group that has been studied, *no more than 1%* of the people have high blood pressure. *Even though 5% to 10%* commonly live to their sixties or seventies, those individuals do not develop hypertension.[4]

Contrast this to the United States, where about 30% of the adults have high blood pressure. The percentage is even higher in U.S. black adults. Also, the incidence of high blood pressure increases with age in the United States. This is not true of those groups still eating the diet of our ancestors.

Following is a list of some of the low-blood-pressure groups of aboriginal people that have been studied around the world. All of these groups have diets high in potassium and low in sodium.

Aita people, Solomon Islands[5]
Australian aborigines[6]
Botswana natives[7]
Carajas Indians, Brazil[8]
Cuna Indians, Panama[9]
Eskimos, Greenland[10]
Kenya natives[11]
Melanesians, northern Cook Islands[12]
Natives, New Guinea[13]
South African natives[14]
Tarahumara Indians, northern Mexico[15]
Ugandan natives[16]
West China natives[17]
Yanomamo Indians, Brazil[18]

Not only do these groups of aboriginal people have almost no hypertension, but they also seldom have strokes, heart attacks, or diabetes.

FIGURE 15

MAP SHOWING LOCATIONS OF THESE INDIGENOUS PEOPLES

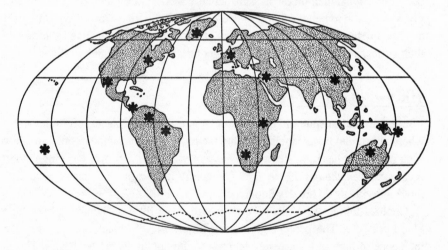

Fig. 15. The map illustrates the distribution of known groups who do not have hypertension. The random distribution reveals that whether or not you are likely to get hypertension doesn't depend upon where you live, whether you are in an aboriginal or modern culture, or what race you are. The only common denominator among these groups is that they all have a high dietary K Factor.

Nathan Pritikin, founder of the Pritikin Program for health, was among the first to realize the importance of the observations that aboriginal peoples do not experience hypertension. Pritikin was especially impressed by the fifty thousand Tarahumara Indians who live in the Sierra Madre mountains of northern Mexico, near the border of the United States. Pritikin noticed their unusual health and stamina (they run up to 200 miles in their games of kickball, which last several days). He also noticed that scientists had been unable to find any evidence that these people ever die from heart disease.[19] These Indians eat primarily corn and beans, supplemented with squash and chili peppers. Pritikin focused upon the fact that their diet has a very low fat content (about a fourth of that of the average person in the United States), is low in cholesterol, and is also high in fiber. We would add the important fact that their diet is high in potassium and low in sodium.[20]

When people from such primitive groups move to modern cities and begin eating processed foods, which are lower in potassium and higher in sodium than the unprocessed foods they had been eating, they then develop high blood pressure with the same frequency as modern folk.[21]

Many attempts have been made to explain away these observations. Some have suggested that these groups don't have high blood pressure because they all inherit a resistance to it. But these people are so diverse geographically and racially[22] (see Figure 15) that it is almost inconceivable that they all have a genetic resistance to high blood pressure whereas Europeans, Americans, and Japanese do not.[23]* More significantly, when either children or adults in native cultures adopt a diet and lifestyle characteristic of industrialized cultures, their blood pressure rises and they do develop hypertension.[24] When these people *have* adopted a modern lifestyle, they actually tend to have *more* hypertension than Europeans and Americans. Based upon this and other evidence, it is fairly certain that approximately 25% of these "primitive" people are genetically susceptible to hypertension.[25]

If anything, one could argue that there has been some genetic adaptation of Europeans and Americans that makes them slightly less prone to the harmful effects of a Western lifestyle than the "primitive" people, who are probably more genetically similar to our ancient ancestors.[26]

It has also been argued that these "primitive" people have low blood pressure because they are comparatively thin. But many of the Cuna Indians of Panama are moderately obese; they do, however, eat a high-K-factor diet, and less than 1% of the adults have high blood pressure.[27] In addition, members of the primitive

---

*One could argue that these groups develop resistance because of genetic mutations. But since genetic mutations occur randomly, one would then expect those people who don't have hypertension to be distributed randomly, and equally, throughout the world, including Europe, America, and Japan.

Qash'qai tribe of nomads in southern Iran are thin, but they eat a low-K-Factor diet and have as much high blood pressure as do people in the United States.[28]

It has even been argued that high blood pressure is caused by stress. The very word *hypertension* suggests tension or stress. So some might wonder if these primitive people escape hypertension because of the simple, idyllic life they supposedly live. But neighboring villages of Brazil's Yanomamo Indians and other tribes in the Amazon rain forest practice a "politics of brinkmanship" that results in humiliation, loss of property and women, and constant warfare, with between 30% and 42% of adult males dying in battle.[29] Although stress is difficult, if not impossible, to measure, it seems reasonable to assume these people have more than their share. Yet in spite of living with daily fear, they have no high blood pressure.[30]

THE CLINCHER:
Even in industrialized cities, being
a vegetarian virtually eliminates hypertension.

This statement should be placed in *flashing neon lights!* The simple fact that being a vegetarian prevents hypertension clearly tells us that—regardless of our genetic heritage—something about *nutrition* is at the root of this problem.

What is the evidence for this? Even in the United States and other "advanced" industrialized countries, there are groups in which hypertension is rare,* strokes and heart disease are uncommon, and the blood pressure does not tend to rise with age. These include

> Vegetarians in Boston, Massachusetts[31]
> Trappist monks in Holland and Belgium[32]
> Seventh-Day Adventists in Australia[33]
> Vegetarians in Tel Aviv, Israel[34]

So clearly it's not whether you live in an aboriginal culture versus an industrialized culture that affects whether you get hypertension.

The groups listed above in industrialized countries who are free of hypertension are all vegetarians.† And not only do vegetarians not have hypertension, their

---

*Usually 1% to 2% versus 30% to 40% for nonvegetarians in these countries.

†Here the term "vegetarian" is used in the more general sense of those who get the majority of their calories from fruits and unboiled vegetables. Whether or not dairy products are consumed is not important in this specific context. Thus, the term "vegetarian" would include not only those who consume lactovegetarian and macrobiotic diets (provided they do not include high levels of sodium-containing sauces), but also those who eat a purely vegetarian diet as well as those who consume small amounts of meat, fish, or poultry. The key is that all these groups get most of their calories from fruits and unboiled vegetables.

average blood pressure is much lower than the average (or so-called normal) pressure of Americans in general. As opposed to the "normal" 120/80, the group of vegetarians in Boston,[35] whose ages ranged from 16 to 29 years, was 106/60 mm Hg.* In fact, out of these 210 vegetarians, *not one* had a diastolic pressure greater than 86 mm Hg!

All well and good, you might say; it looks as though being a vegetarian protects you from getting hypertension, or at least elevated blood pressure. But what about people who already have hypertension? Well, when modern city people who have the usual incidence of hypertension adopt a vegetarian diet, their incidence of hypertension drops to that of aboriginal people.[36] And you will remember that when people from such "primitive" groups move to modern cities and begin eating processed foods, they then develop high blood pressure with the same frequency as modern folk.[37]

Since we have already shown that hypertension involves not only elevated blood pressure, but also abnormal cholesterol levels, we must ask if being a vegetarian not only decreases the chance of having high blood pressure, but also other elements of hypertension such as abnormal cholesterol levels.

Actually, it is fairly well known that vegetarians have lower levels of total blood cholesterol. For example, a comparison of Seventh-Day Adventists, who are mostly vegetarian, with other citizens in Sydney, Australia, found that the Adventists had significantly lower blood cholesterol levels.[38]

A comparison of Trappist monks with Benedictine monks is especially revealing. Both groups have the same religion, live in monasteries, perform daily prayers, and in many other ways have similar lifestyles. But the Trappists (who are strict vegetarians except for consuming dairy products) were found to have significantly lower blood cholesterol than the Benedictine monks (who are meat eaters with a diet typical of industrialized people). By age 50 and over, the blood cholesterol of the Benedictines averaged about 250 "points" (mg/100 ml)—a value typical of groups in industrialized countries—but that of the vegetarian Trappists averaged only about 200.[39] Of course, this might be expected in view of the lower level of saturated fats and no cholesterol in purely vegetarian diets. However, because of their relatively high consumption of dairy products, the

---

*This value is closer to the level that life-insurance companies find is associated with the *lowest* rate of death. Indeed, any diastolic pressure above around 74 mm Hg is associated with a greater risk of death. Thus, the "normal" of 120/80 is just the average for Americans and isn't truly healthy or normal, but in fact indicates an unnecessary risk of death. Given these facts, we see that the traditional definition of hypertension as being a diastolic blood pressure greater than 90 is purely arbitrary. According to the data of insurance companies, the vast majority of Americans have blood pressure that is too high for optimum health and longevity.

Trappists consumed 85% as much saturated fatty acids and 39% as much dietary cholesterol as did the Benedictines. The main difference in the two diets was that the Trappists consumed 2.3 to 2.6 times as much peas, beans, and vegetables and 3.6 to 5 times as much fruit as did the Benedictines.

We'll see that the extra fruits and vegetables provide the key.

THE K FACTOR

As we have seen, all around the world aboriginal people who eat the "Stone Age diet" have an extremely low incidence of hypertension when compared with modern Western societies. And even *within* today's modern societies, we find that vegetarians have an almost nonexistent incidence of hypertension. So something common to both the Stone Age diet and a vegetarian diet clearly prevents most cases of high blood pressure.

So, we have to ask, just what *is* this key factor common to a vegetarian and a Stone Age diet that prevents hypertension?

Perhaps it's eating meat that causes hypertension; after all, aren't aboriginal peoples also vegetarians? Well, no they're not. We've already pointed out that Stone Age people probably obtained about a third of their calories from meat. After all, they are called *hunter*-gatherers. And although most native peoples today do consume a large amount of plant food, almost all of them eat meat. Moreover, adding protein[40] or animal products including meat and eggs[41] to the diet of vegetarians does not increase their blood pressure. In addition, increasing the ratio of saturated to unsaturated fatty acids in the diet of vegetarians does not raise their blood pressure.[42]

So the difference between vegetarian and meat-containing diets in affecting blood pressure apparently doesn't seem to be due to the extra protein or to the high amount of saturated fatty acids in meat as compared to plant foods. The study of vegetarians in Tel Aviv also considered the question of just what it is about a vegetarian diet that prevents hypertension. One possibility considered is the decreased obesity typical of vegetarians. But this study found that *regardless* of obesity, vegetarians have lower blood pressure than nonvegetarians. Moreover, the vegetarians in their study had just as positive a family history of hypertension as did the nonvegetarians. And it wasn't just the fact that vegetarian diets are inherently low in sodium; indeed, evidently because of their use of table salt, the vegetarians in Tel Aviv were consuming almost the same amount of sodium as were the nonvegetarians.

Thus these findings have led several investigators to conclude that the effectiveness of vegetarian diets in lowering blood pressure isn't primarily due to eliminating unhealthy substances in the meat, or in decreasing table salt; it must be due to something "good" in the fruits and vegetables. But what could be so special about fruits and vegetables?

What *is* good about fruits and vegetables is the *balance* of minerals; that is, compared to sodium, fruits and vegetables are loaded with both potassium and magnesium—having K Factors typically between around 25 and 150 with some fruits up to as high as 400 (see Table 4 in the Workbook, Part Four). In fact, what the Tel Aviv study *did* find[43] was that the diet of vegetarians had a significantly higher ratio of potassium to sodium; that is, the vegetarians were eating a diet with a higher K Factor. Moreover, *within* the vegetarian group, those who had the highest dietary K Factor had, on the average, both systolic and diastolic blood pressure that was significantly lower than in the other vegetarians!

So the only consistent explanation seems to be that both the Stone Age diet that all aboriginals have in common and vegetarian diets are very low in sodium and high in potassium. This explanation is also consistent with the results of our study of how the living cell requires a proper balance between potassium and sodium.

It is the central premise of this book that a diet with an adequate K Factor is the key for you, too, to prevent or reverse your own hypertension.

Recall that the reason the ratio of dietary potassium to sodium is called the K Factor is that K is the chemical symbol for potassium. If a food has the same amount (by weight) of potassium as sodium, its K Factor is 1; if it has more potassium than sodium, its K Factor is greater than 1; if there's twice as much potassium as sodium, the K Factor is 2; if there's three times as much, the K Factor is 3, and so on. On the other hand, if the food has more sodium than potassium, the K Factor is less than 1; if there's twice as much sodium as potassium, the K Factor is 0.5; if there's three times as much, the K Factor is 0.33, and so on. The K Factor of the diet of our ancient ancestors was probably in the range of 16.[44]

In the next chapter, you will see how a diet with a high K Factor—the kind of diet eaten by our "primitive" cousins and our Stone Age ancestors—can help you get rid of any hypertension problem you have.

COMPARING THE K FACTOR IN DIFFERENT ETHNIC DIETS

By looking at several different populations living in the world today, we can see the relation between the frequency of hypertension and the level of the K Factor in their food.

TABLE 2

FREQUENCY OF HYPERTENSION IN VARIOUS POPULATIONS

K FACTOR*	PERCENT WITH HYPERTENSION	POPULATION
20	less than 1	Yanomamo Indians, Brazil[45]
4.9	less than 1	!Kung people, northern Botswana[46]
1.41†	2	Vegetarians in Tel Aviv[47]
1.04	26	Nonvegetarians in Tel Aviv[48]
0.39	27	blacks and whites in Evans County, Georgia[49]
0.36	33	residents of Northern Japan[50]

Modern Americans and Japanese are eating diets with less than 3% of the K Factor of the diet of our ancient ancestors and the Yanomamo Indians!

Although this table alone is not conclusive, notice that once the K Factor drops below a range of between 1 and 2, the frequency of hypertension goes way up. It appears that about two-thirds of us inherit a resistance to hypertension regardless of what we eat. The other third will end up with hypertension if we eat foods with a lower K Factor—especially if we don't get any regular exercise. In some people, calcium and especially magnesium may be very important, but the simplest single measure that correlates with high blood pressure appears to be the K Factor.

In the United States, blacks are twice as likely to get hypertension as are whites and five to seven times as likely to get severe hypertension.[51] In fact, in spite of a third of a century of treatment with drugs, hypertension continues to be the most serious health problem in U.S. blacks.[52] Some specialists have suggested that severity of hypertension in blacks is genetic, and others have suggested that it is because blacks eat more salt than whites. But in one study, black men actually had about one-quarter less sodium in their diet than whites even though they had more

---

*The dietary K Factor was estimated by measuring the amount of sodium and potassium in the urine of these people. Since most of the dietary sodium and potassium is excreted in the urine under normal conditions, the ratio of urinary potassium to sodium is a good approximation of the dietary K Factor.

†In the Tel Aviv study, the value 1.41 was significantly higher than the value 1.04 with a p value of 0.005, which indicates that we can be 99.5% confident that the difference is not due to chance. In this study, they actually reported their data as the ratio of sodium to potassium. Here it is reported as the reciprocal of that, which is the ratio of potassium to sodium, or the K Factor.

high blood pressure.[53] However, because of deficient potassium, the food they ate *did* have a much lower K Factor than the food eaten by the whites. At least three other studies have also found that a lower dietary K Factor is associated with higher blood pressure in U.S. blacks.[54]

Dr. Louis Tobian of the University of Minnesota School of Medicine has pointed out that whereas primitive hunter-gatherers eat about 8 grams of potassium in their daily diets, in the United States white males eat less than 3 grams and black males in the southeastern United States eat only about 1.5 grams of potassium each day.[55] Based upon studies that will be described in Chapter 6 he suggests this is responsible for the fact that these blacks are eighteen times more likely to have hypertensive kidney failure than are whites. These same blacks have a higher stroke rate than any other geographic or ethnic group in the United States.[56] People in Alabama, Mississippi, and Georgia have the highest rate of death from strokes in the United States and also the lowest dietary intake of potassium in this country.[57]

Dr. Tobian also points out that people in Scotland consume only about 1.8 grams of potassium per day and have a substantially greater rate of cardiovascular disease than people of Southern England, France, or Italy, where higher amounts of potassium are consumed. The people of Tibet consume only about 0.8 grams of potassium a day and have an exceedingly high incidence of strokes, much higher than that found in China or in Japan, where the dietary potassium consumption is about 1.8 grams per day—not much different than for U.S. blacks. In China and Japan strokes have long been considered the leading cause of death and occur with much greater frequency than in most Western populations.[58]

Moreover, in 1987, a study of 2,008 men and women in the People's Republic of China was published showing that those with a higher dietary K Factor (as reflected in the potassium/sodium ratio in their urine) had significantly lower blood pressure.[59] Similarly, Dr. Tobian cites a report from Norway that found an almost perfect correlation between a higher urinary potassium/sodium ratio and lower diastolic blood pressure. Studies in Rancho Bernardo, California, on the island of St. Lucia in the Caribbean, and in Honolulu have also found a clear correlation between higher dietary K Factor and lower blood pressure

YOU DON'T HAVE TO EAT A STONE AGE DIET OR BE A VEGETARIAN TO AVOID HYPERTENSION

As already discussed, vegetarian groups consistently have lower average blood pressures than matched control groups.[60] For example, hypertension hits over a quarter of the people living in Tel Aviv. Yet only 2% of the vegetarians living in that city have hypertension.[61] Other than the way they eat, these vegetarians have a lifestyle almost identical to that of the nonvegetarians. And remember the evidence that the principal distinction of a vegetarian diet in preventing hypertension seems to be its high K Factor, relative to nonvegetarian fare.

But you don't have to be a vegetarian or live away from modern civilization to avoid hypertension. Fortunately, it's simpler than that. However, everything does point to the way you eat and to exercise as being the critical factors.

In Japan, high blood pressure is even more common than in the United States. In 1959, researchers compared two northern Japanese villages.[62] Both villages had similar sodium intakes but different blood pressures. The group with the lower blood pressure was found to consume much more dietary potassium.

As a test of this explanation, the researchers had the hypertensive persons eat about six apples, which are high in potassium, each day. This resulted in a significant drop in their blood pressure. (Perhaps we should change the old adage to "Six apples a day keeps the doctor away.") However, as will be described in Chapter 15, eating even two or three apples each day has a definite tendency to decrease blood pressure.

A 1985 study of eight thousand Japanese men living in Hawaii found that those who ate more potassium and calcium had significantly lower blood pressure than those who didn't.[63]

WHAT IS AN ACCEPTABLE K FACTOR?

Four lines of evidence indicate that to prevent hypertension, the K Factor should be at least 4.

The first line of evidence comes from Table 2, which suggests that hypertension is uncommon (about 1%) when the K Factor is above approximately 1.4. In the next chapter, we'll discuss medical studies in which the K Factor approach was consistently successful in lowering blood pressure when the value was 3 or above and show data from animal studies that indicate that 2 may or may not be high enough. Finally, the K Factor of human milk might also provide a guideline, since that recipe evolved over millions of years to provide optimal nutrition for human infants. That value, about 3.5,[64] reinforces a tentative choice of a K Factor of at least 4.

However, keep in mind that our ancestors ate a diet with a much higher K Factor. Therefore, because of the arguments made above, not only is a K Factor of well above 4 in your diet recommended to prevent hypertension, it is well within the range to which our bodies are accustomed. A K Factor of 4 requires eating four times as much potassium as sodium, which is about the proportion occurring naturally in your body. Remember, the ratio between the amount of potassium and the amount of sodium you eat is more important than the absolute amounts. It's the balance that counts. Chapter 10 contains specific recommendations for obtaining the proper level of K Factor.

SUMMARY

The idea that people get primary hypertension only if they have a genetic weakness led to a sense of inevitability. But studies by anthropologists around the world make it clear that hypertension is not an inevitable part of the human condition. Rather, it is clear that even in those with the genetic tendency, hypertension is due to the way they live—that is, to lifestyle. The psychological stress of modern civilization is *not* the main culprit. Evidence from studies of various population groups suggests that proper nutrition and exercise can keep blood pressure from getting too high.

The food our ancient ancestors ate and, for the most part, the food eaten by primitive populations and by vegetarians today has a much higher ratio of potassium to sodium (that is, a higher K Factor) than the rest of us are getting. The primitive groups eating this diet today have a very low incidence of hypertension, and we can assume the same was true of our ancestors. This isn't surprising, since our ancestors had adapted to the diet over millions of years.

We have inherited that adaptation. Our bodies are designed for the Stone Age diet and for exercise. Since our bodies are used to, and tuned for, the type of balance in that "primitive" diet, it's not surprising that when we use technology to upset the balance in our food, we run into trouble. Eating food with an artificially low K Factor puts stresses on our body that not only can lead to high blood pressure but may (as discussed in Chapter 4) lead to other problems as well.

CHAPTER 6

Working with the Wisdom of the Body:

An Adequate K Factor Lowers Blood Pressure and Prolongs Life

The wisdom of nature, honed by thousands of years of physiologic adaptations to a naturally high potassium intake should not be lightly dismissed.

Norman M. Kaplan, M.D., and C. Venkata S. Ram, M.D.[1]

Now you've seen some of the evidence that eating food with a high K Factor—a high ratio of potassium to sodium—can prevent hypertension. But what if you already have high blood pressure? Can increasing the K Factor bring it back to normal? More importantly, can increasing the dietary K Factor improve some of the other aspects of hypertension such as blood cholesterol? And *most* importantly, does increasing the dietary K Factor result in fewer strokes or heart attacks in people with hypertension?

So before we get into the effect upon blood pressure of increasing the dietary K Factor, let's get right down to cases. What about strokes and heart attacks?

Of all the things we have learned in the last few years, one thing stands out in importance above all others:

Eating food with more potassium and less sodium (increasing the dietary K Factor) can protect against crippling strokes and premature death, **even when it doesn't decrease blood pressure.**

100

You will recall that the one clear benefit of antihypertensive drug treatment is an approximately 40% reduction in death due to strokes. This was achieved at the cost of many dollars as well as unpleasant side effects.

From the analysis of population studies and of vegetarians, one might suspect there would be fewer strokes if people with hypertension raised their dietary K Factor. Also, from our discussion of the role of membranes and the "sodium battery" in the living cell, one would expect to find that increasing dietary K Factor would reduce the chance of strokes.

But how much potassium might it take to confer that benefit? Based upon the analysis in the two previous chapters, I would have predicted that increasing the dietary K Factor by the amount of potassium in, say, a couple of bananas would be insufficient to produce a detectable effect upon blood pressure. Of course, I've already made the point that blood pressure isn't the only, or—in the view developed in this book—even the main, problem. Nevertheless, if you had asked me how much of an increase it would take, even I would never have *guessed* that increasing daily dietary potassium by an amount as small as that contained in one banana could produce a significant reduction in strokes.

But that is exactly what Kay-Tee Khaw and Dr. Elizabeth Barrett-Connor[2] found when they studied the effect of dietary composition upon rate of death of 859 men and women in Rancho Bernardo, California, for an average of twelve years.* As I would have expected, they found that a daily increase of only 390 mg potassium intake was not enough to lower blood pressure. However, this small increase *was* associated with a statistically significant[†] decrease in stroke-related death! As a matter of comparison, 390 mg potassium is a little less than that in a medium banana (about 440 mg), and the same as that in half a medium potato (391 mg)! But even more striking, the reduction in stroke-related death associated with this small—and obviously easy to achieve—increase in dietary potassium was not small. It was 40%—the same percentage decrease as has been observed when drugs are used to get the blood pressure down to "normal" levels.

WOW!

As you will see, increasing dietary potassium, and thus the K Factor, by a larger amount can indeed lower the blood pressure also. The fact that it takes less of an increase to lower stroke-related deaths than to reduce blood pressure is extremely important for at least two reasons.

---

*In the April 14, 1988, issue of the *New England Journal of Medicine,* a letter to the editor from Dr. Chun N. Lee and co-workers of the Kuakini Medical Center of Honolulu compared his results to those of Khaw and Barrett-Connor. In a sixteen-year study of 7,591 Japanese men, increased potassium intake did not lower strokes due to hemorrhage but did lower strokes due to blood clots.

[†]At $p < .001$, which means that there was less than one chance in a thousand that this conclusion is due to chance effects.

First, from a practical aspect the importance is obvious: since it's so easy to increase the K Factor enough to produce a 40% reduction in strokes, moderately higher increases—which also lower the blood pressure—hold definite promise of reducing stroke rates still further. In fact, the study by Kay-Tee Khaw and Dr. Elizabeth Barrett-Connor suggests that. That study found that in women consuming more than 2,600 mg potassium per day (about the amount in three and a third potatoes) there were no stroke-related deaths at all. In men, there were no stroke-related deaths when potassium consumption was greater than 2,964 mg per day.

Second, this finding reinforces the conclusion that blood pressure is not the key problem in hypertension. If it were, it would be *impossible* to reduce strokes without lowering blood pressure.

THE K FACTOR PROTECTS AGAINST STROKES IN ANIMALS

Dr. Louis Tobian at the University of Minnesota Medical School has been one of the main pioneers in establishing that increasing the K Factor by giving potassium not only can lower blood pressure but also can protect against the damaging consequences of hypertension, including strokes, kidney disease, and enlargement of the heart.

At the 1983 meeting of the American Association for the Advancement of Science, Dr. Tobian reported on experiments that confirm that *even when blood pressure is not lowered,* increasing dietary potassium decreases the chance of death and restores a normal life span to hypertensive rats.[3]

In a more detailed study, the Minnesota group showed that increasing dietary potassium could nearly eliminate strokes in two species of hypertensive rats. In one species (stroke prone, spontaneously hypertensive rats) placed on a diet with a sodium level[4] similar to a Japanese diet,* within seventeen weeks, 83% had died. During this same period in another group of identical rats on an identical diet—but with enough extra potassium to moderately lower their blood pressure—only 2% had died. The odds that this dramatic reduction in death by added dietary potassium was *not* due to chance was estimated to be 99.9999%—about as close to certainty as we can get in science! In two subgroups of these rats who had virtually the same blood pressure, those receiving the extra potassium experienced a reduction in mortality from 64% to 9%. Clearly strokes are due to something more than blood pressure.

In another species of hypertensive rat (Dahl salt-sensitive rat), adding potassium to the diet over a nine-week period resulted in a reduction of mortality from 55% to 4%. Again, when the effect of the lower blood pressure due to potassium was subtracted out, the effect of the extra potassium still reduced mortality from 38% to 5%.[5] Rats not receiving extra potassium often suffered partial paralysis

---

*The Japanese consume a very high level of sodium in their diet—up to 13 grams per day.

before death. Moreover, autopsy revealed that 40% of the rats not receiving extra potassium had cerebral hemorrhages, whereas no cerebral hemorrage occurred in the rats receiving the extra potassium. Thus the reduced rate of death in rats receiving extra potassium was most likely due to a decrease in strokes.

This study not only confirms the ability of potassium to lower blood pressure but establishes the fact—at least in these two species of experimental animals— that a large part of the stroke-protecting action of potassium is *independent* of its ability to lower blood pressure. This reinforces the observation in hypertensive human beings that potassium can reduce death due to strokes independently of lowering blood pressure.[6]

The ability of extra dietary potassium to decrease death rates in hypertensive rats independently of blood pressure change has also been observed by Dr. John Smeda.[7]

WHAT ABOUT BLOOD CHOLESTEROL AND CHOLESTEROL DESPOSITS IN ARTERIES?

If the analysis in the previous chapter of how the the living cell and its "sodium battery" are involved in hypertension is correct, increasing the dietary K Factor should decrease insulin levels and thereby might improve blood cholesterol levels. In 1990, a group led by Dr. P. S. Patki of the School of Ayurvedic Medicine near Bombay, India, reported that increasing the dietary K Factor by simply adding potassium (4.4 grams of potassium chloride) does indeed lower blood cholesterol.[8] The patients (eight men and twenty-nine women) in this study all began with mild (diastolic pressure less than 110 mm Hg) hypertension with an average diastolic pressure of 100.4 mm Hg. Since sodium intake was not decreased, the increase in dietary potassium produced only a modest increase in their dietary K Factor— from a low of 0.5 (which, as you have seen, is typical of hypertension) to a value of about 0.8. Nevertheless, over an eight-week period, even this modest increase in dietary K Factor resulted not only in a significant drop of 13.1 mm Hg in diastolic (and about the same drop in systolic) blood pressure, but also in a statistically significant reduction of 19% in serum cholesterol! And this was without any change in dietary fat or cholesterol.* This same group also found that adding 1.9

---

*This study used a design called "double blind, placebo controlled, crossover." This means that all patients took pills, some containing the extra potassium and some being fake (or "placebo") with only an inert filler. "Double blind" means that neither the patients nor the doctors knew, at the time, whether a given patient was taking a placebo or a potassium-containing pill. "Crossover" means that after 8 weeks (plus a 2-week "wash-out" period), the pills of each patient were switched from placebo to potassium-containing or vice versa. In addition to these two types of pills, for 8 weeks each patient received pills containing the same amount of potassium *plus* magnesium. The total length of the study was 32 weeks.

grams of magnesium chloride per day, whether with or without supplemental potassium, had no significant effect upon blood pressure or upon blood cholesterol.

O.K., so potassium can decrease blood cholesterol; how about the bottom line? How about coronary artery disease and cholesterol deposits? In humans there haven't been any studies published yet on these relationships. But in experimental animals, the results are encouraging indeed. Dr. Tobian and his research group studied the effect of increasing dietary potassium on cholesterol in rats.[9] Two groups of rats were given a cholesterol-promoting diet containing large amounts of cholesterol, coconut oil, and sodium chloride.* In the first group the potassium level of the diet was normal, and in the second group the potassium was 4.2 times higher. The extra dietary potassium resulted in a lowering of blood pressure by 4 mm Hg and a lowering of blood cholesterol from 229 to 214 points.† But the exciting result was that although extra potassium lowered the blood cholesterol only 7%, it decreased the amount of cholesterol deposits in the arteries by 64%!

So its entirely possible that the 19% reduction in blood cholesterol produced by a modest elevation of dietary K Factor in humans may be accompanied by a very significant decrease in cholesterol deposits *independently* of changes in dietary fat.‡

THE K FACTOR ALSO PROTECTS AGAINST THESE CONDITIONS:
KIDNEY DISEASE

Dr. Tobian's work went further and also showed that the increased dietary potassium also protects the rats against kidney damage. In particular, he showed that potassium prevented the ruptures of the small arteries in the kidneys that occurred in the rats not receiving potassium.[10]

"MUSCLE-BOUND" HEART

Cardiac hypertrophy (an abnormal increase in the muscle mass of the heart) is a common consequence of hypertension and can make the heart more susceptible to problems such as abnormal rhythms. Since in hypertension the heart must work harder to pump blood against the elevated blood pressure, one would expect that as with any muscle that is worked harder, its muscle mass would increase. Until a couple of years ago, I too had thought that this consequence of hypertension was purely due to the elevated blood pressure. Indeed, some blood-pressure-lowering drugs have been shown to prevent or reverse cardiac hypertrophy.[11]

---

*The amounts were, respectively, 4%, 15%, and 7%.
†"Points" is shorthand for milligrams per 100 milliliters, or mg/dL.
‡Which nevertheless should be kept low—especially saturated fats.

But so can potassium! Dr. Tobian's group has reported that independently of change in blood pressure, the hearts of hypertensive rats given supplemental potassium were only about 87% as large as those without the extra potassium.[12]

THE PROTECTIVE PROPERTIES OF A HIGH K FACTOR ARE NOT RECENT NEWS

In 1962, Dr. W. Priddle called attention to the protective properties of a high dietary K Factor. In commenting on his experience of treating people with hypertension using a high-K-Factor nutritional program over a period of thirty years, Dr. Priddle stated:

> Although admittedly, in a considerable percentage of cases, there appeared to be little influence on the blood pressure levels, we were impressed with the low incidence of complications and the improved survival rate. From these clinical observations, we felt that in many cases perhaps the tempo of the disease was decreased in spite of the stationary or slowly increasing blood pressure readings.[13]

In some things, there is no substitute for experience and observation. Physicians of Dr. Priddle's generation had been trained to look at more than numbers—they had been trained to observe the whole person and to have faith in their intuition.* Such physicians are often able to sense the presence of the many subtle changes that can occur in someone who, in spite of normal laboratory measurements, nevertheless is experiencing a progression of the disease. Thus, they can be aware that in two groups of patients who *both* have the same measurement on one test, one group may have a lower "incidence of complications" and experience a decreased "tempo of the disease."

Dr. Priddle's observations of the protective effect of potassium on his patients has also been borne out in animal experiments. As far back as 1956, Dr. David Gordon and Dr. Douglas Drury reported that giving extra potassium to hypertensive rabbits *prevented internal bleeding* due to ruptures in the small arteries in their intestines.[14] Two years later, in Nashville, Tennessee, Dr. George Meneely and his colleague Con Ball were experimenting with laboratory rats, making them hypertensive with a diet high in sodium chloride (table salt).[15] Scientific papers are

---

*As an example, by the early 1950s astute cardiologists had concluded that intoxication by the heart drug digitalis can be lessened by giving potassium. It was a couple of years later that scientific evidence appeared to confirm their judgment. This evidence came from studies, such as those discussed in Chapter 4, that showed that digitalis works by inhibiting the sodium-potassium pump and that potassium can "compete" with digitalis to lessen its inhibition of this vital pump.

usually pretty dry, but these two pioneers managed to slip a little "tongue-in-cheek" past the editor. After the usual technical summary, they concluded, "Salt is rough on rats"—which should hardly be surprising to you by now.

But their study also came up with some results that are astonishing indeed—and set the stage for Dr. Tobian's work: When the dietary K Factor was increased by the addition of potassium chloride while sodium chloride was kept constant, the average life span of the hypertensive rats was *increased by 50%, even when the elevated blood pressure didn't go down!* These two researchers pointed out that the extra life span conferred on these rats by potassium was equivalent to twenty to twenty-four years for a human!

Incidentally, it was probably these two scientists who, in 1958, first suggested the use of the dietary potassium-to-sodium ratio, now called the K Factor, as an indicator of the likelihood that a person will develop hypertension.

By 1972, a scientist who provided the basis for much of our present understanding about sodium, potassium, and hypertension, Dr. Lewis Dahl, and his co-workers confirmed the conclusions of the Meneely-Ball study: Blood pressure was lowered by increasing the K Factor in the food of a group of rats that had become hypertensive on a high-sodium diet. And, more significantly, the rats on a high-K-Factor diet *lived much longer* than the others.[16]

This study also showed that not only is the K Factor, or ratio of potassium to sodium, important, but the absolute amounts of sodium and potassium also affect blood pressure. When the K Factor was kept constant, increasing the amount of both sodium and potassium threefold resulted in significant rises in blood pressure. This result highlights the fact that *you must not only increase the potassium in your diet but also minimize the amount of sodium.*

At the other extreme, the effect of too little potassium cannot be totally countered *just* by decreasing sodium. This, plus the fact that most Americans are getting only about 17% to 33% of optimal dietary potassium,[17] may explain why many studies have failed to demonstrate a decrease in blood pressure upon lowering dietary sodium.

Again, the key to hypertension *is not just one variable.* Over the range of potassium and sodium in our diets, the *balance* between them is the important thing.

HOW ABOUT BLOOD PRESSURE?

You've seen that increasing the dietary K Factor with amounts of potassium too small to affect blood pressure can nevertheless reduce strokes and probably prolong life. But can increasing the dietary K Factor also lower the blood pressure in people with hypertension? To answer this question, several studies have already been conducted on modern people who had been eating food with a low K Factor and had developed high blood pressure. The experimenters had them change to a diet with a high K Factor. If you already have high blood pressure, these studies should be of great interest to you because, although it's too late now to change what you ate in your youth, you can change what you eat now.

By 1986, there had been at least twelve reports of treating people with hypertension by increasing the dietary K Factor. All told, a few thousand patients have been treated this way, with success rates of lowering blood pressure varying from 67% to 100%!

THE BACKGROUND: BEFORE THE 1980s

Treating hypertension by reducing sodium intake and increasing potassium intake is hardly a new idea. In 2600 B.C., the emperor Su Wen[18] described in gruesome detail how too much sodium in the diet can cause a stroke: "If too much salt is used in food the pulse hardens . . . the corresponding illness makes the tongue curl up and the patient unable to speak."

Another ancient medical text—a physician's prescription book from Sumeria (c. 2000 B.C.)—mentions that potassium should be included in the diet.[19] But the most complete evidence about the K Factor began to accumulate at the very beginning of this century. And now there is lots of it.

THE AMBARD-BEAUJARD REPORT (1904)

One of the earliest modern medical studies of a high-K-Factor diet for treating hypertension was conducted and summarized in a report way back in 1904 by two French physicians, Ambard and Beaujard.[20] These two doctors increased the K Factor by decreasing the amount of table salt (sodium chloride) and raising the amount of potassium-rich foods in the diet of their patients. They succeeded in lowering the blood pressure in five out of eight of these patients.

THE ADDISON STUDY (1928)

The first study in which the K Factor was increased by giving potassium salts was conducted in the 1920s by a Toronto physician, W. L. T. Addison. The results of this study were reported in the *Journal of the Canadian Medical Association* in 1928.[21] Addison got his inspiration from a paper written in Paris by a researcher named Blume, who had discovered that potassium displaces sodium in the body to cause diuresis—that is, increased excretion of water and sodium through the kidneys.

In 1924, Addison had reported that giving calcium reduced the blood pressure in many of his hypertensive patients.[22] A possible reason for this was given in Chapter 4. Dr. Lawrence Resnick,[23] of Cornell University Medical College in New York City, as well as other investigators,[24] has confirmed the ability of calcium to lower blood pressure in certain patients with hypertension. In those patients whom calcium didn't help, Addison found that giving them potassium salts often brought their blood pressure down, frequently back to normal.

In 1928, he reported the results of treating five hypertensive patients with potassium chloride or potassium citrate.[25] To increase potassium intake, he also put all five patients on a low-salt, meatless diet that emphasized fish once daily, vegetables, fruits, cereals, and milk. In each of the five patients, giving extra potassium lowered the blood pressure.

The most dramatic case was that of a sixty-four-year-old man whose blood pressure was initially 182/128. After he had taken large amounts of calcium chloride each day, his blood pressure decreased to 165/117 and stayed there for several months. When this man was then given 7.8 grams of potassium citrate (840 mg potassium) each day instead of the calcium chloride, his blood pressure decreased to 140/88. In each of the five patients, substitution of sodium chloride for the potassium salt resulted in return of the blood pressures to the previously elevated levels, which were then lowered again by a return to the potassium salt.

Addison's success is illustrated in Figure 16, a graph of the blood pressure of one of his patients. On day 1, this patient had a blood pressure of 162/98 and was given potassium chloride (KCl). By day 5, his blood pressure was down to 150/82. He was then given table salt, sodium chloride (NaCl), and by day 9, his blood pressure was up to 186/118. Then he was given potassium bromide (KBr); in two days, his blood pressure was down to 144/104. Then he was given sodium bromide (NaBr), which, in another two days, brought his blood pressure back up to 172/116. Finally, he was given potassium citrate; in three days his blood pressure was down to 134/78.

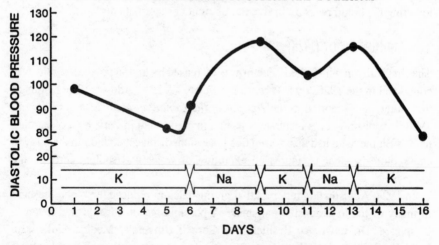

FIGURE 16

RESPONSE OF BLOOD PRESSURE TO SODIUM AND POTASSIUM

Fig. 16. Representative example of five case studies presented by Addison.[21] Supplemental potassium or sodium salts were given daily as indicated. Notice the opposite effects of sodium and potassium on blood pressure.

Addison clearly demonstrated the fact that sodium makes blood pressure go up and calcium or potassium can make it go down. By giving either calcium or potassium, he was able to lower the blood pressure in 70% of his hypertension patients.[26]

In this landmark paper, Dr. Addison concluded: "One has forced on one the concept that the prevalence of arterial hypertension on this continent is in large part due to a potash [potassium] poor diet, and an excessive use of salt [sodium chloride] as a condiment, and as a preservative of meat." In other words, Dr. Addison was maintaining that the prevalence of hypertension is due to a low dietary K Factor. *His conclusions were published in 1928!*

PRIDDLE AND MCQUARRIE (1930S)

Studies by Dr. W. Priddle in 1931[27] and by Dr. McQuarrie and associates in 1936[28] also indicated that a high potassium intake lowers blood pressure in people with hypertension. Dr. Priddle achieved 100% success in reducing the blood pressure of forty-five hypertensive patients by giving them potassium citrate combined with a low-sodium diet.

THE KEMPNER DIET (1940S)

In the 1940s, Dr. Walter Kempner popularized a rice-fruit diet that succeeded in lowering the blood pressure by at least 20 mm Hg in two-thirds of his hypertensive patients, with most of the remaining third having at least a partial reduction of blood pressure toward normal.[29] This diet emphasized fruits and vegetables.

By 1972, Dr. Lewis Dahl had recognized what he considered the indisputable effectiveness of Kempner's rice-fruit diet and concluded that it was often useful in treating even severe cases of hypertension.[30] This conclusion was based not only upon Dr. Kempner's reports but also upon Dr. Dahl's own observations of several physicans who were themselves incapacitated by progressive hypertensive heart disease and were able to return to practice after several months on the Kempner diet.

Although it was not stressed at the time, the Kempner rice-fruit diet is in reality a low-sodium (about 160 mg per day)/high-potassium diet. In fact, the K Factor in this diet can be as high as 20.[31] Unfortunately, most Americans found the recipes used in this diet too tasteless. (But don't you worry. In Chapter 10 you will find a long list of tasty foods that can help you easily achieve a high K Factor.)

THE PRITIKIN EXPERIENCE (1960S-1985)

In the previous chapter, we discussed Nathan Pritikin's observations of the Tarahumara Indians of northern Mexico, who eat corn, beans, squash, and chili peppers (a remarkably high-K Factor diet). For at least twenty years, Pritikin and his followers had people follow a program that included a similar diet, along with moderate exercise. Pritikin's Longevity Centers treated over ten thousand people. Of those who had hypertension, 85% were off drugs and had normal blood pressure within 4 weeks on this diet-exercise program.[32]

RECENT CONTROLLED MEDICAL STUDIES

Although the results of the early medical studies of increasing the K Factor in the diet were dramatic, they were not designed so that they could be analyzed with statistics. More recently, however, medical studies have been conducted in which people given high-K-Factor diets were compared with control groups of hypertensives eating their usual diet. The results could then be statistically analyzed.

These studies have demonstrated that lowering sodium chloride does lower blood pressure and that raising dietary potassium lowers it still further. Some of these scientifically controlled studies are described in more detail in Chapter 15.

THE AUSTRALIAN EXPERIMENT (1982)

If you are already taking pills for high blood pressure and would rather not, a scientifically controlled study conducted by Dr. Trevor Beard and others will be of special interest.[33] In Australia, ninety volunteers were all taking medicine that had brought their blood pressure under control. The volunteers were randomly assigned to each of two groups. One group followed a special high-potassium, low-sodium diet; the other didn't. Everything else was the same in both groups, and the doctors and nurses didn't know who was in which group.

Before the study, most of the volunteers were eating food with a K Factor of less than 1; that is, they were eating more sodium than potassium. The forty-five volunteers who changed their diet (under the advice of a nutritionist) ended up eating over six times as much potassium as sodium, or a diet with a K Factor greater than 6.

In the high-K-Factor diet group, four out of every five of the volunteers were able to reduce their dose of blood pressure medicine, and one out of every three was completely able to stop taking any drugs by the end of the 12-week study! In the control group, less than one out of ten was able to stop taking medicine. The reason the control group showed any improvement at all is that the extra blood pressure measurements and attention to health associated with participating in the study had a beneficial effect. This is why a control group is necessary.

Notice that this was done under their doctors' supervision. *Warning:* Don't try to do this without your doctor's supervision. Stopping some kinds of medicines suddenly can be **lethal!**

A 1991 study from the University of Naples has shown that increasing the dietary K Factor* by increased consumption of natural, unprocessed foods (legumes, fruit, and vegetables) high in potassium can allow a *more than 50% reduction* in antihypertensive drug dosage in 81% of patients,[34] thus minimizing side effects. Moreover, at least a third (38% of the total receiving increased dietary potassium) of these developed normal blood pressure *even when all drugs were discontinued.* Based upon their results, these investigators concluded: "Increasing dietary potassium intake from foods is a feasible and effective measure to reduce antihypertensive drug treatment."

THE LONDON EXPERIMENTS (1982)

How are we to know if the people on the high-K-Factor diet were cured because of their faith in the diet? Two studies, by Dr. Graham MacGregor and his co-workers in London, took care of this problem, since the volunteers did not even know which group they were in.[35]

Everybody ate a similar diet, supplemented with pills. In the first experiment both groups ate a low-sodium diet that dropped their blood pressure.[36] To test that this drop was not due to something else in the diet, one group was then given sodium chloride pills, while the other group received look-alike, blank (placebo) pills. In the second experiment, one group received potassium pills, while the control group received placebos.[37] The potassium pills increased the dietary K Factor from 0.75 to about 1.20. Until the studies were over, nobody (except the drug company that provided the pills) knew which was which. Statistical analysis of the results showed beyond any reasonable doubt that reducing sodium or increasing potassium in the diet each produces a partial reduction of blood pressure in people with hypertension.

Dr. MacGregor and his co-workers pointed out that the increase in potassium intake could be achieved with a potassium-based salt substitute (such as is commonly found in grocery stores in the United States) and an increase in vegetable and fruit consumption. They stated: "Moderate dietary sodium restriction with dietary potassium supplementation may obviate or reduce the need for drug treatment in some patients with mild to moderate hypertension." They ended their report with this statement:

> Dietary alteration of sodium and potassium intake may obviate the
> need for drug treatment in many patients with essential hypertension

---

*From Table 1 of their paper, which shows values of urinary potassium and sodium excretion, one can estimate that the K Factor was increased from approximately 0.57 to about 0.8. Compensating for this modest increase is the fact that it was maintained for one year.

and it might also improve the efficacy of drugs in those patients in whom dietary measures alone are insufficient. Education of the population at risk of hypertension to conform with a more suitable ratio of sodium to potassium in their diet may reduce the prevalence of hypertension and the high cost of drug treatment. The cooperation of the food industry in labeling the approximate sodium content of their foods and in using potassium rather than sodium based additives would help people comply with such an alteration in diet."

A Japanese Study (1981)

A Japanese group reached almost the same conclusion as the MacGregor studies: "A high-potassium diet has a beneficial effect on blood pressure in patients with mild or moderate essential hypertension, particularly in patients on a high sodium diet."[38] The same group also pointed out that an increase in the daily intake of potassium by about 2.34 grams (which increased the dietary K Factor from 0.44 to 1.15) could be achieved with a potassium-based salt substitute and a moderate increase in fresh fruit and vegetable consumption.

A PERSONAL EXAMPLE

The validity of the conclusions of this chapter is demonstrated by the personal experience of my colleague, Dr. George Webb. In late 1983, George discovered he had hypertension with a blood pressure of about 160/100. By switching to food with a high K Factor (about 4), George has brought his own blood pressure down to about 115/75. During this whole time, George (who was already thin) has not changed his exercise habits nor his weight.

Actually George changed his dietary K Factor in two stages: First he went on a low-sodium diet without changing the amount of potassium; he succeeded in getting his pressure down to about 140/90. For the next six months, it didn't go lower than this. Then, while staying on the same sodium intake, George started increasing his potassium consumption (through natural, unprocessed foods) until he had achieved a dietary K Factor of about 5. Within a few weeks, his pressure was down to about 135/80, and during the next year and a half, it was usually as low as 130/75. This demonstrates that while lowering sodium is very beneficial, raising potassium is equally important. *You've got to do both!*

During the past six years, George's diastolic pressure has remained around the same while the systolic has continued to drop to around 115 mm Hg—for a healthy blood pressure of 115/75—demonstrating once again that the full effect of a proper dietary K Factor takes some time. *You've got to stick with it.*

Incidentally, a blood pressure of 115/75 is about the same as those native populations who eat the diet of our ancient ancestors.

OTHER EVIDENCE

In another "meta-analysis" of several studies, a strong correlation was found between increasing the dietary K Factor (as reflected in measurements of the urine) and the degree of fall in blood pressure.[39]

In 1988, a cooperative study, called the Intersalt study, of over ten thousand men and women aged 20–59 was published. This study found that dietary K Factor (as reflected by the urinary potassium-to-sodium ratio) is even more consistently related to blood pressure than is dietary sodium.[40]

Another way to demonstrate the effect of dietary K Factor upon blood pressure would be not to increase it but decrease it still further. In 1992, it was reported that in twelve people (seven blacks and five whites) with hypertension, reducing their dietary K Factor from its original value of 1.36 to 0.23 resulted in a statistically significant increase in the systolic blood pressure by an average of 7 mm Hg and in the diastolic blood pressure by an average of 4 mm Hg.[41] The connection between a decrease in dietary K Factor and an increase in blood pressure levels has also been demonstrated in men who do not have hypertension.[42]

BUT WHAT ABOUT NEGATIVE REPORTS?

Because the studies mentioned above have finally focused attention upon potassium and the K Factor, in recent years there have been several attempts to confirm or refute the effectiveness of increasing dietary K Factor by additional potassium or decreased sodium.

In the summer of 1984, a widely publicized report appeared that illustrates one type of error that can prevent the importance of the K Factor from being observed. This study claimed that there is no relationship between blood pressure and sodium in the U.S. population.[43] This conclusion was reached by using a statistical program to examine computer tapes that contained information about a large, government-sponsored survey of diet and blood pressure. This study did show that people who ate more potassium—fresh fruits and steamed vegetables—had lower blood pressure. But in the March 15, 1985, issue of the *Journal of the American Medical Association,* Dr. Harvey Gruchow and co-workers[44] reanalyzed the computer tapes used for this report. This new analysis utilized a powerful ("multivariant") statistical technique to analyze the same data and found that people in the United States who eat more sodium *do* indeed have higher blood pressure, while confirming that those who eat more potassium have lower blood pressure.

Then came several attempts to use "controlled studies" to test the effectiveness of increasing the dietary K Factor by either increasing potassium, decreasing sodium, or both. As explained in Chapter 2, in controlled studies patients are divided into two groups, one of which gets a real pill and the other a fake, or placebo, pill. Thus, in the controlled studies of increasing the dietary K Factor, the increase has almost always been achieved by giving pills containing potassium.

Some of these studies have reported that increasing the dietary K Factor using potassium-containing pills, especially if dietary sodium is already low, does *not* lower blood pressure. As we will see, the failure of these studies to show the effectiveness of increasing dietary K Factor is easily explainable. The most common reason for not seeing an effect is that the K Factor was increased either by an insufficient amount, or for an insuffficient time.

What is the basis for maintaining that the K Factor must be increased by not only an adequate amount, but for an adequate time?

You will recall from the previous chapter that four lines of evidence indicate that to prevent hypertension, the K Factor should be at least 4. In Chapter 17, a more thorough discussion shows that there is a "gray" area in which the K Factor may, or may not, be adequate to lower blood pressure. The gray area of the K Factor is roughly between 0.6 and 4—a K Factor above that range provides a very high probability that blood pressure will be lowered, whereas a K Factor below that range almost guarantees that blood pressure will be elevated. But between 0.6 and around 4, the result will vary depending upon other variables. For example, in some people raising a low K Factor to, say, 0.9 or 1.4 may be enough to reduce elevated blood pressure, and in other people it won't.

In addition, after changing the dietary K Factor, it takes the body a while to respond. After all, the bodily changes associated with hypertension take years to develop, so it stands to reason that they won't be reversed in a couple of days—or even a couple of weeks. Remember the example of Dr. Webb: In his case, although the initial drop in blood pressure occurred within a few weeks, and even though he had increased his dietary K Factor to about 5, it took approximately six years to get the full effect upon blood pressure. Several people who read *The K Factor: Reversing and Preventing High Blood Pressure Without Drugs* sent in their personal record of increasing the dietary K Factor and its effect upon blood pressure. In general, it took a few weeks for elevated blood pressure to begin to drop, and especially in people who had hypertension for a long time, it sometimes took a couple of months even to begin to see measureable results.

A 1985 study conducted in Bonn, Germany, illustrates both the gray area and the time threshold. As we might expect, in this study of young (21–39 years) white people (mostly men) with mild hypertension,[45] the initial dietary K Factor averaged about 0.55. In this study, the K Factor was increased by adding extra potassium, in pills, to the usual food eaten by people with hypertension. When the K Factor was increased to 2.12 for one week, there was a very small drop in blood pressure that was not significant. When the dietary K Factor was increased to 17, again for one week, there was a larger drop in blood pressure that did not quite reach statistical significance.

In a second set of experiments, the dietary K Factor was increased to only 1.4. After two weeks, the blood pressure dropped only slightly. But after four and eight weeks, there was a statistically significant drop of 10.5 mm Hg in diastolic and of 14.8 mm Hg in systolic blood pressure. When the potassium-containing pills were replaced by placebo pills, the diastolic pressures in this group went up again.[46]

This study also found that the magnitude of the blood-pressure lowering effect is greater in patients with higher blood pressure levels, and also demonstrated that increasing the K Factor was even more effective in blacks than in whites.

But the Bonn study is especially important because it emphasizes that even when the increase in the dietary K Factor is adequate, enough time must be allowed for the increase to affect blood pressure. In this case one or two weeks was insufficient. In general, even in young people it generally takes at least three or four weeks to begin to observe an effect upon blood pressure of increasing the dietary K Factor. Indeed, inspection of the data in this study suggests that had the extra potassium been continued beyond eight weeks, the blood pressure might have decreased further.

Moreover, the Bonn study also demonstrates that even when the K Factor remains in the gray area, provided the relative change is enough (in this case an increase of about 150%) and provided enough time is allowed, the blood pressure may decrease.

In 1991, a combined analysis[47] (called a meta-analysis) of eighteen different studies (including the one just discussed) confirmed the conclusions that the effect of increasing dietary K Factor becomes more pronounced with time. Inspection of Table 1 of this meta-analysis shows that when the K Factor was increased from below 0.6 (the bottom of the gray area), and provided the increase was more than 100%, a drop in blood pressure would be observed within six to eight weeks even though the K Factor remained within the gray area (below 3).

We have one very clear example of the effectiveness of increasing the dietary K Factor from below 0.6 (the lower limit of the gray area) to within this area provided that the time was adequate. The Working Group Report of the National High Blood Pressure Education Program (NHBPEP)[48] points out that an analysis[49] of the Intersalt data show that a change in the K Factor from 0.56 to 1.7 would be associated with a 3.4 mm Hg decrease in the average level of systolic blood pressure. The significance here is that the data of the Intersalt study are not based upon *changes* in diet, but upon what different people had been eating all along—presumably for years. Therefore, time was not even a factor in concluding that when the dietary K Factor is increased by almost threefold (200%) there is an effect upon blood pressure even though the final value is within the gray area.

A study that demonstrates the effectiveness of increasing the dietary K Factor from below 0.6 (the lower limit of the gray area) in a practical amount of time comes from London, England. This study demonstrated that increasing the dietary

K Factor from about 0.42 to 1.74 (a 300% increase) produced a significant blood pressure reduction in people with hypertension within six to twelve weeks.[50]

Another study that helps us appreciate just how much time is required was conducted in Naples, Italy, and published in 1987.[51] In this study of 37 patients with hypertension, the initial dietary K Factor (as reflected by urinary potassium and sodium) averaged 0.54—below the gray area and typical of people who have hypertension. The amount of potassium added to the diet (in capsules) was not large, just enough to elevate the K Factor to a value, 0.8, just within the gray area. Nevertheless, within three to six weeks, the blood pressure had begun to significantly decrease. Moreover, this decrease continued throughout the fifteen weeks of elevated dietary K Factor, becoming most significant by the fifteenth week.

So we see that in order for an increase in the dietary K Factor to affect blood pressure, two conditions must be met:

1. The increase must be enough—preferably to 4 or above, although smaller increases within the gray area may work if given enough time. For an increase from below to within the gray to be effective, the existing evidence (summarized in the meta-analysis) suggests the increase must be more than twofold (an increase of more than 100%). If the initial K Factor is already within the gray area, the increase would probably have to be even greater for its effect upon blood pressure to be noticeable.
2. Enough time must be allowed. Even with a sizeable increase in the dietary K Factor, a noticeable drop in blood pressure cannot be expected for at least two to four weeks and usually a couple of months.

Failure to satisfy these two conditions will virtually guarantee that the blood pressure will not decrease. Recall too that the degree of drop in blood pressure generally will depend upon its initial value.

An example of a study that allowed insufficient time is one of the first negative reports, a 1984 study from Australia.[52] This study maintained that moderate restriction of sodium *or* addition of dietary potassium had "variable effects" (that were very small and not statistically significant) on diastolic pressure in people with mild primary (essential) hypertension.

Several specialists have quoted this study as indicating that potassium is ineffective in treating primary hypertension. However, when the total picture is considered, an entirely different conclusion emerges. In the Australian study, the extra potassium was given for only four weeks. You have seen that four weeks may not be enough time to ensure a response to increased dietary potassium.

Moreover, in this study the dietary K Factor was not elevated to a level—at least 4—that would ensure a decrease in blood pressure. For example, because the amount of sodium was so high (over 4 grams per day) when potassium was added, the K Factor still was only 1.58. When sodium was restricted, potassium was also decreased, and the K Factor was only 1.16.

So both the magnitude of increase of the K Factor and the time were borderline in this study. Thus, the results do *not* refute the claim that increasing the dietary K Factor can lower blood pressure. Rather, they are totally consistent with the conclusion of Chapters 5 and 17 that the K Factor must be above 4 to ensure lower blood pressure.

As an example of the effectiveness of increasing the K Factor both for an inadequate time and by an inadequate magnitude, in 1985 a study reported that when sodium intake had already been restricted in twenty people with hypertension who were not taking drugs, adding potassium tablets for one month had no effect upon blood pressure.[53] An inspection of their data, however, shows that the sodium restriction itself had increased the K Factor to about 1.8 and that the potassium subsequently added was only enough to increase the K Factor to 2.5, only a 38% increase—and for only one month.

Another study corrected for the inadequate time but was primarily designed not to see how increasing the K Factor would reduce blood pressure but to enable patients to discontinue taking antihypertensive drugs. In this study,[54] published in 1991, all patients had received antihypertensive drug treatment for at least three and a half years. The study, which involved 287 men, concluded that addition of potassium capsules does not reduce the need for antihypertensive drugs in people who have already been placed on a low-sodium diet. In this study (in which the patients continued taking antihypertensive drugs while dietary changes were begun), the initiation of reduced dietary sodium had increased the K Factor to about 0.80; subsequent addition of potassium capsules produced a further increase to about 1.6. This change, which certainly was for a long enough time, produced only a 1% drop in both systolic and diastolic blood pressure, not enough to be significant. However, you will recall from the 1991 meta-analysis study that within the gray area, the dietary K Factor must be more than doubled if any lowering of blood pressure is to be expected.* Moreover, the interpretation of this 1991 study is complicated by the fact that the patients were taking antihypertensive drugs while the dietary changes were carried out.

Lack of appreciation of these principles has led to the design of several studies

---

*The increase from 0.8 to 1.6, which is a doubling, does not satisfy the conclusion that the K Factor must be more than doubled if the final value is within the gray area. Moreover, that conclusion is based upon cases where the K Factor was initially below the gray area. In this study, the initial K Factor was already well above the lower limit, about 0.6, of the gray area, which would suggest that some antihypertensive benefit was already present. Therefore, the relative increase required to observe an effect would be expected to be even higher.

in which the increase in the K Factor was either too small or of too short a duration for any positive result to be expected.

As you will see in Chapter 10, it is quite easy to adjust your eating habits to get a K Factor of at least 4. By eating ample fruits and vegetables it is not too difficult to achieve a dietary K Factor closer to 16, a value achieved by our ancient ancestors.

SUMMARY

Increasing the dietary K Factor reduces blood pressure, provided the increase is of sufficient magnitude and for enough time. Keep in mind that the full effect upon blood pressure may take at least several weeks to a few months. Moreover, to ensure the desired effect, the dietary K Factor should be increased to 4 or above (something quite easy if you follow the nutritional recommendations in Chapter 10).

The general conclusion here really isn't new; as far back as 1976, Drs. Menleey and Battarbee stated:

> The efficacy of a prophylactic/therapeutic low sodium-high potassium [high K Factor] diet should be weighed against the uncertain hazards of a lifetime of pill taking.[55]

THE BOTTOM LINE

It's all well and good to say that a high K Factor can restore your blood pressure to normal levels. But don't forget that even when the blood pressure remains unchanged, increasing the dietary K Factor in humans has been shown to decrease strokes and decrease blood cholesterol, and in experimental animals to decrease cholesterol deposits in arteries and to increase the length of life.

The real question in any treatment of hypertension is, Will it protect you from death and crippling consequences, such as paralyzing strokes? There is very good reason to believe that the K Factor approach *can* protect you from death and crippling consequences. Moreover, the evidence suggests that the K Factor approach can provide some protection even if the blood pressure doesn't return to normal! And that's the bottom line.

CHAPTER 7

Variations on a Theme: The Importance of Fitness

The more obese and sedentary an individual, the greater the degree of insulin resistance, regardless of genetic influences.

Gerald Reaven, M. D.[1]

It has long been recognized that obesity, non-insulin-dependent diabetes (NIDDM diabetes), and hypertension all share many unfortunate consequences: increased rate of coronary disease and heart attack, increased chance of kidney disease, and increase in the chance of stroke. Moreover, being overweight greatly increases your chances of developing primary hypertension and of developing adult onset (NIDDM) diabetes. And having NIDDM diabetes greatly increases your chance of getting hypertension.

In Chapter 3, I pointed out that abnormal cellular response to insulin and consequent elevated blood insulin levels are found in *all three* of these conditions: hypertension, NIDDM diabetes, and obesity.

Moreover, as the above quote indicates, lack of exercise also leads to "insulin resistance" with consequent increased insulin levels. The probable relation of elevated insulin levels to abnormal cholesterol levels in people with hypertension was also discussed in Chapters 3 and 4. By now it should come as no surprise that the other two conditions with elevated insulin levels, obesity and NIDDM diabetes, also are accompanied by unhealthy cholesterol levels.

Clearly, these similarities suggest a common theme underlying these three conditions. Dr. Gerald Reaven,[2] of Stanford University School of Medicine, has proposed that all three of these conditions are variation of one syndrome, which he calls *Syndrome X*. This syndrome includes resistance to insulin-stimulated glucose uptake ("insulin resistance"), high blood sugar, high blood levels of insulin, increased blood levels of VLDL triglyceride (hypertriglyceridemia), depressed blood levels of HDL cholesterol, and high blood pressure.

WHAT COULD EXCESS WEIGHT, INSUFFICIENT EXERCISE, AND EATING FOOD WITH A LOW K FACTOR HAVE IN COMMON WITH SYNDROME X AND HYPERTENSION?

At first sight it must seem, even to most professionals, that obesity and lack of exercise are one thing and a deficient K Factor is another. That's easy to understand, because only in the last few years have scientific articles begun to appear that suggest possible connections linking the K Factor, losing weight, and getting exercise. As expected from our earlier text, one connection often appears to involve insulin.

As was discussed in Chapter 3, *all* groups that tend to have elevated blood levels of insulin—NIDDM diabetics, obese people,* and people who don't exercise[3]—also tend to have primary hypertension. In fact, as already mentioned, among Caucasians[†] even people with high blood pressure who are not overweight seem to have an increase in blood insulin levels.[4] So it now appears that elevated insulin levels often play a role in primary hypertension.

You will recall from Chapter 4 that insulin helps regulate the activity of the sodium-potassium pump.[5] By helping to control the sodium potassium pump, insulin helps maintain the balance of potassium to sodium in body cells—a balance *critical* to normal functioning of the living cell and to the prevention of hypertension.

Incidentally, there is a useful tip-off that you may have an "insulin resistant" state including low HDL and high triglycerides. People who have obesity primarily in the abdomen tend to have elevated insulin levels.[6]

OBESITY

As already indicated, being overweight increases your chances of getting hypertension. And if you already have hypertension, being overweight can make it more difficult to get your blood pressure down than it would be for someone whose weight is normal.

In obesity, the elevated blood insulin partly compensates for a decreased ability of muscle and fat cells to respond to insulin. But the kidneys may respond to these

---

*One of the hidden problems of being overweight is that it causes your blood insulin levels to rise. *Lack of exercise also tends to result in an elevation of blood insulin.*
†Apparently this is less true of blacks and not true of Pima Indians.

elevated insulin levels by speeding up their sodium-potassium pumps to pump sodium from the newly formed urine (kidney ultrafiltrate) back into the blood. So if you're overweight, your body may tend to retain the sodium you eat instead of excreting it as it should. This can upset the balance between potassium and sodium in body cells, leading to a decrease in energy of the "sodium battery" and an increase in calcium inside the tiny muscle cells of the arterioles, causing your blood pressure to go up.

Again, we see that a balance between potassium and sodium in the cell is a key to hypertension.

EXERCISE

Regardless of body weight, people who fail to get regular exercise tend to have higher blood pressure. Here again, insulin may play a role. When people who have regularly participated in vigorous exercise become physically inactive, within only ten days their sensitivity to insulin decreases by about 23%.[7] Both the effectiveness of exercise and its transience are emphasized by the finding that in obese people who have "insulin resistance," a *single* bout of intense exercise can reduce "insulin resistance"—but for only twelve to fourteen hours.[8]

Moreover, in a group of 11 untrained volunteers, fasting blood levels of insulin (that is, levels measured after a twelve-hour stretch without eating) were 71% higher than the insulin levels in eleven volunteers who who were similar except for participating in endurance training at least five times per week. Moreover, the lower blood insulin levels in the group involved in exercise training was associated with decreases in "insulin resistance" as compared to their more sedentary companions.[9] These findings all highlight the necessity of exercising on a *regular* basis.

So being fit tunes up not only your muscles but also the body's mechanisms that regulate the balance between potassium and sodium. So stay tuned up, and tune in to what you eat and how you prepare it. If you'll just give your body a chance, it'll keep your blood pressure—and blood vessels—in good shape.

TABLE SUGAR CAN RAISE BLOOD PRESSURE

Overfeeding sucrose (table sugar) stimulates the sympathetic nervous system in rats[10] with hypertension, elevating the blood pressure still further. Overfeeding the same amount of calories in the form of fat had no effect on either sympathetic activity or blood pressure. In rats with normal blood pressure, overfeeding sucrose produced the same effects, but less dramatically. This effect of sugar is probably due to the resulting increase in blood insulin level, since in experiments where blood glucose is kept unchanged, elevating insulin levels increases sympathetic activity and blood pressure.[11]

FASTING

At the other extreme, another even more dramatic way to illustrate the connection between insulin and hypertension is fasting. In obese people on a "protein-sparing," or partial, fast, elevated blood pressure will almost always decrease toward normal within less than a week. That's because fasting is one way to lower quickly but temporarily the levels of blood insulin and other hormones that regulate the body's ability to keep a proper balance between potassium and sodium. These changes, especially the lower insulin levels, allow the kidneys to get rid of excess body sodium and water. Incidentally, that's why the first pounds lost on a very low-calorie diet are mostly not fat, but water. Fasting also decreases the activity of the sympathetic nervous system,[12] presumably secondary to the decreased insulin levels.[13]

I strongly recommend against a total fast, because after the first day, your body begins to burn up your muscle and other protein. Don't try even a partial fast without your doctor's supervision.

CAN LOSING WEIGHT OR COMMENCING REGULAR EXERCISE REDUCE THE ELEVATED BLOOD PRESSURE, INSULIN LEVELS, AND CHOLESTEROL IN PEOPLE WITH HYPERTENSION?

The compensatory increase in insulin level that occurs in response to "insulin resistance" is closely associated with high triglycerides and low HDL cholesterol. Furthermore, when the conditions that bring about "insulin resistance" are corrected, there is an appropriate change in both triglycerides and HDL that suggests a causal relation.

LOSING WEIGHT

Losing even half of the excess pounds can reduce blood pressure significantly. In two studies,[14] dietary reduction of weight in obese people with hypertension lowered diastolic blood pressure to normal levels in *three out of every four even though no drugs were used!* In fact, losing excess weight has been reported to lower elevated blood pressure even more effectively than drug treatment with beta blockers.[15]

Moreover, losing those excess pounds of fat tends to get the insulin level back to where it should be. (Losing muscle *doesn't* help—that's one reason very-low-calorie diets aren't recommended for weight loss.) As we've seen, when fat loss happens the cells in your body can become better balanced, with the result that both blood pressure and blood cholesterol levels become more healthy.

COMMENCING REGULAR EXERCISE

In most individuals with primary hypertension, initiation of endurance-exercise training can decrease their systolic and diastolic blood pressures by about 10 mm Hg.[16] By 1989, at least 25 studies had been published that examined the effect of exercise upon blood pressure in people with hypertension. Perhaps because some of these studies either did not have controls or had other design limitations, until recently there was a reluctance to accept exercise as a reliable means of lowering elevated blood pressure. However, at least six studies have now been published that avoid such errors, with the result that the effectiveness of exercise in lowering blood pressure in people with essential hypertension is now well documented.[17]

Moreover, the effect of exercise upon elevated blood pressure is not limited by age.[18] As a demonstration of this, endurance training resulted in modest (4–8 mm Hg) reductions in blood pressure in 70- to 79-year-old men and women who had moderate hypertension.[19]

Regular exercise programs have been shown to reduce blood pressure even when no weight loss occurs.[20] This works both in people with hypertension who are obese and in those with normal body weight. When twenty-seven obese, hypertensive women were given a six-month course of physical training, there was a significant decrease in blood pressure in all of them. This decrease in blood pressure toward normal was correlated not with change in body fat but with the degree of reduction of elevated serum insulin and also with the reduction of serum triglycerides.[21] Increased physical activity can also produce a substantial reduction of blood pressure in hypertensives of normal body weight.[22]

One of the first, and most dramatic, studies to document the ability of aerobic exercise to lower elevated blood pressure in many patients was conducted at the University of Florida by Dr. Robert Cade and his co-workers.[23] All of the 105 patients who completed the exercise program started with a diastolic blood pressure of over 90 mm Hg. Roughly half (47) were receiving antihypertensive drugs, and the other half were not. No attempt was made to alter the diet or to restrict dietary sodium.

The exercise program began with each patient walking one mile each day and progressed, at a rate tailored individually, until each patient was running two miles every day. Within three months after reaching two miles per day, 101 of the 105 patients had significant drops in blood pressure. Of the four whose blood pressure failed to respond, one had kidney disease and the others had reduced kidney function due to longstanding high blood pressure.

Of those receiving antihypertensive therapy, roughly half were able to discontinue all drugs and yet achieve lower blood pressure than when they started. Most of those who were still receiving drugs were able to decrease the amount. The decrease in blood pressure was not due to weight changes, since the decrease was as great in those patients who gained weight as in those who lost weight during the study.

Of seven patients who entered the study with severe hypertension (diastolic pressure greater than 115 mm Hg), blood pressure became normal in two and decreased to borderline hypertension in two others. The most dramatic response was seen in a 34-year-old woman who entered the study with primary hypertension and blood pressure of 160/120. After she had run two miles a day for three months, her blood pressure remained an excellent 110/74 without any drugs!

This study has been criticized because of lack of controls to eliminate other factors, such as time or other lifestyle factors. However, fifteen of the patients *themselves* served as "controls." These fifteen were persuaded to stop exercising after three months. After three more months of sedentary life, the average diastolic blood pressure of this group rose from the postexercise value of 82 mm to 100 mm Hg. Several other studies have also indicated that exercise can lower blood pressure without change in weight. Drs. John Martin and Pat Dubbert at the Veterans Administration Hospital in Jackson, Mississippi, conducted a classic controlled study involving nineteen people with primary hypertension. They reported that ten weeks of aerobic exercise for thirty minutes three to four days each week produces a significant drop in blood pressure.[24] This drop in blood pressure was not accompanied by any significant change in body fat.

Not only does regular exercise lower blood pressure, it protects against "insulin resistance." A study at the University of Vermont School of Medicine demonstrated that only twelve weeks of physical training was enough to produce a significant decrease in insulin resistance in overweight volunteers as compared to a paired group on the same low-calorie diet.[25]

But can initiation of an aerobic exercise program reduce already elevated insulin levels? Yes. Even when it doesn't cause weight loss, studies[26] have shown that regular exercise decreases the blood level of insulin and changes the levels of other hormones related to potassium and sodium balance. Moreover, in people with hypertension who entered training programs, the fall in blood pressure occurred only in those who initially had elevated blood insulin levels. Supporting this connection was the observation that the fall in blood pressure was greatest in those who experienced the greatest fall in their insulin levels, *not* in those who lost the most weight.[27] Not only can this drop in blood insulin help explain why a long-term exercise program can decrease blood pressure, it is consistent with the conclusion, developed in Chapter 3, that hypertension involves *more* than elevated blood pressure.

When combined with exercise, weight loss can be especially effective. A large-scale study, the Chicago Prevention Evaluation Program, has demonstrated the effectiveness of increased physical activity together with dietary restriction in reducing blood pressure. The subjects were advised to engage in "modest" light exercise at least three times per week and to reduce caloric intake by 30%. This program produced an average weight loss of 11.7 pounds, which was sustained over five years. In the sixty-seven middle-aged hypertensives who were not receiving antihypertensive medication, systolic blood pressure was reduced by an average of 13.3 mm Hg and diastolic by an average of 9.7 mm Hg.[28]

So there isn't much doubt that getting regular exercise is an important step (pun intended) in keeping your blood pressure, blood cholesterol, and blood insulin levels normal and that if you are overweight, it is essential to get rid of some of those excess pounds of fat.

WEIGHT LOSS, EXERCISE, AND INCREASING THE K FACTOR—WHY DO ALL THREE?

If you lose weight, exercise regularly, and increase your K Factor, you will not only get the maximum reduction in your blood pressure, but you will produce the best "tune up," or balance, in your body's cells. In practice, the different elements of the K Factor program all tie together. The K Factor eating approach not only helps your blood pressure by increasing the K Factor but, by cutting down the fat you eat, also helps you lose pounds. The K Factor and exercise approach helps your blood pressure *and* it helps you keep the weight off. So in practice, the steps are related. They work together. And from what we have discussed about the workings of the living cell, this is not just a coincidence.

SUMMARY

There is evidence that increasing the K Factor in the diet (increasing potassium and decreasing sodium), losing excess pounds of fat, and getting regular exercise are in many ways *doing the same things* inside the body. They all work together to normalize the balance in your body's cells. Although some effects involve the sympathetic nervous system and others involve the kidneys, evidence keeps appearing that indicates that changes in the sodium potassium pump and related cell mechanisms are part of the mechanism whereby either exercise or weight loss can restore elevated blood pressure toward normal.

All groups with primary hypertension have elevated blood levels of insulin. Not only does this tend to cause the kidneys to retain sodium in the body, the elevated insulin levels produce changes inside the body's cells that impair normal metabolism of carbohydrate and of cholesterol and triglycerides. All these changes predispose one to heart problems *independently* of blood pressure elevation. Both weight loss and exercise help lower these insulin levels, and most likely this is part of the mechanism whereby these activities help reduce elevated blood pressure.

Another way of looking at this is that our body's ability to adapt to suboptimal levels of dietary K Factor depends upon how well we take care of ourselves. Normally, a dietary K Factor over 3 or 5 will prevent hypertension, whereas a value below about 0.6 will almost always cause hypertension in those susceptible to it and will probably cause at least some degree of blood pressure elevation in the rest of us. However, when we literally get out of shape by overeating and/or by too little exercise, our body gets out of balance* and thus loses some of its ability to adapt to a low K Factor.

Although many details remain to be worked out, a common theme appears: to cure your high blood pressure without drugs, you need to keep the K Factor in your food at an adequate level *and* eliminate factors, such as obesity and lack of exercise, that prevent the body from maintaining a normal balance between potassium and sodium.

So eating food with a high K Factor, exercising, and maintaining normal body weight to keep insulin levels normal all help maintain the normal balance in your body's cells.

---

*As just one example, elevated insulin levels can interfere with normal excretion of sodium by the kidneys.

CHAPTER 8

Other Factors that Influence Blood Pressure

THE KEY FACTORS

In this book, we emphasize the three key factors for naturally preventing or curing primary hypertension:

- Nutrition, especially the K Factor
- Weight control
- Exercise

We've seen how these are all related. So it's not surprising that the most effective way to lower your blood pressure is to combine these three factors. But the overall scientific evidence indicates that eating foods with a proper ratio of potassium to sodium, or K Factor, is usually *the* most important factor in determining whether a person with a hereditary tendency for hypertension develops high blood pressure.

Other factors, however, do have roles to play—some of them important. We have already mentioned that getting enough dietary calcium may be important; in about a third of the people with primary hypertension, it is perhaps an important factor. And dietary chloride may be almost as harmful as sodium (so table salt, which contains both sodium and chloride, is doubly bad).

We now discuss, in the most likely order of importance, these other factors.

ALCOHOL

It is very clear that heavy drinkers have much higher blood pressure than those who drink less.[1] One study of 83,947 persons with highly different occupations and ethnic backgrounds showed that this correlation is not explained by over-weight or the use of coffee or cigarettes.[2] A review of 30 studies of the effects of alcohol found that the majority reported that consumption of three or more drinks per day was associated with a small but significant increase in blood pressure.[3] But with only one or two drinks per day, the results were mixed. Forty percent of the studies actually reported that consumption of one or two alcoholic drinks per day was associated with a slight decrease in blood pressure, although this tentative conclusion is increasingly coming into doubt.

The effect of excessive amounts of alcohol on blood pressure is not surprising, since intoxicating amounts of alcohol increase the leakiness of the cell membrane to sodium.[4] Not only that, alcoholism has often been associated with decreased levels of magnesium.[5] As discussed in Chapter 4, increased leakiness can lead indirectly to an increase in the level of calcium inside the smooth muscles surrounding the small arteries, leading to narrowing of these arteries.

Fortunately, the effect of alcohol on blood pressure can be reversed. In men consuming five to seven drinks per day, either discontinuing[6] alcohol consumption or decreasing it[7] by switching to low-alcohol beer (which contains about 15% to 20% as much alcohol) results in a significant reduction of both diastolic and systolic blood pressure by 5 to 3 mm Hg, respectively.[8] Blood pressure began falling within the first two to three weeks of reduction of alcohol and was still falling after six weeks. Decrease in alcohol consumption is especially important in view of evidence that alcohol-related hypertension may contribute to the higher prevalence of strokes in drinkers.[9]

Based upon all available evidence, the Working Group of the National High Blood Pressure Education Program has concluded that consumption of three or more alcoholic drinks per day accounts for about 7% of hypertension in the United States[10] Moreover, this group (which is sponsored by the National Heart, Lung, and Blood Institute of the National Institutes of Health) has concluded that the total evidence suggests that a reduction in alcohol intake is effective in lowering blood pressure in people with hypertension *and* may help prevent hypertension. Thus, they recommend that alcohol consumption should be reduced to no more than two drinks per day.

MAGNESIUM AND CALCIUM

In the cell, the movements of calcium and of magnesium are linked to sodium and, through the sodium-potassium pump, to potassium. Adequate blood levels of calcium and magnesium are necessary to stabilize and prevent leakiness of the membrane that surrounds each body cell and are essential for normal balance of the levels of sodium and potassium across this membrane. Thus, it is not surprising that adequate amounts in the diet of calcium and magnesium are important in the prevention and treatment of some cases of hypertension.

MAGNESIUM

There are now several reasons to suspect that a dietary factor in primary hypertension is deficiency of magnesium. The incidence of hypertension is high in regions that have naturally soft water—that is, mineral-poor water—or magnesium-poor soil.[11] (Water softeners are doubly bad, since most of them add sodium in addition to removing magnesium and calcium.) Rats fed a diet deficient in magnesium develop significant hypertension within twelve weeks.[12]

Deficient dietary magnesium might be expected to result in lower levels of magnesium in the blood serum that bathes the body cells. This in turn could tend to make the cell membranes less stable and more leaky to sodium, potassium, and calcium. So an adequate level of magnesium in blood serum is probably important in stabilizing these membranes and allowing the small muscle cells that control blood pressure to remain relaxed. In fact, experiments on blood vessels in dogs have shown that increasing blood magnesium does dilate the arteries.[13] Lowering blood magnesium levels in animals and in humans is often associated with increases in peripheral resistance, with resulting increases in blood pressure.[14]

Some people with primary hypertension do indeed have low levels of magnesium in their blood serum.[15] In these people lower serum magnesium levels have been found to be associated with increased activity of a blood hormone, renin, which acts to increase blood pressure[16] (see Chapter 17). A recent study has shown that the level of free magnesium inside blood cells is about 25% lower in people with primary hypertension than in the rest of the population.[17]

Magnesium deficiency may contribute to high blood pressure in another way. Magnesium loss increases the tendency of the body to lose potassium, and administration of magnesium is sometimes required in order to enable the body to replenish its stores of potassium.[18] In fact, in patients with low blood levels of magnesium, attempts to restore blood levels of potassium to normal are ineffective until normal levels of magnesium are first restored.[19] Not only that, but administration of magnesium has been reported to increase sodium excretion by the kidneys, and magnesium deficiency decreases urinary sodium, possibly because of a decrease in a sodium-retaining hormone, aldosterone.[20] So the fact that prolonged use of the sodium-excreting thiazide diuretics results in not only a decrease in body potassium, but also a decrease in body magnesium content,[21] reinforces the desirability of using nondrug approaches—especially for people with mild hypertension.

The idea of using magnesium isn't new; it was first recommended as the treatment of severe hypertension due to kidney disease as early as 1925.[22] In one specific type of hypertension, that associated with pre-eclampsia of pregnancy, the most effective way to decrease the blood pressure has been for years, and still is, to give magnesium. And it has been reported that giving supplemental magnesium to pregnant women prevents pre-eclampsia and hypertension.[23]

In one of the few recent clinical studies testing the effects of magnesium on primary hypertension, eighteen hypertensive patients who had been taking diuretics for some time were given magnesium aspartate hydrochloride tablets each day (365 mg of magnesium per day). This resulted in an average reduction in diastolic blood pressure of 8 mm Hg.[24] Unfortunately, there were no placebo controls in this study.

Especially since magnesium deficiency can contribute to a potassium deficiency, the evidence appears strong that adequate magnesium intake is necessary to prevent or to reverse primary hypertension. Unfortunately, many of us don't get enough of this previously overlooked mineral, perhaps because of widespread areas of magnesium-deficient soil in the United States. The average daily consumption has been claimed to be as low as 200–250 mg—lower than the National Academy of Sciences Recommended Dietary Allowance (RDA) of 300 mg daily for nonpregnant women, 450 mg daily for pregnant women, and 350 mg daily for men, except 400 mg per day for 15–18-year-old men. Good food sources of magnesium include bananas, black-eyed peas, buckwheat flour, whole wheat flour, kidney beans, lima beans, avocados, and our old standby, the potato.

CALCIUM

Evidence from animal studies, from correlation of dietary nutrients with hypertension in humans, and from a consideration of the interplay between calcium, magnesium, sodium, and potassium inside the living cell all suggests that sufficient calcium in the diet is important in preventing hypertension. As far back as 1924, Addison[25] had reported that not only supplemental potassium but also calcium chloride could lower the blood pressure of hypertensive patients.

In the last few years, interest in calcium has revived. In one controlled study, half of a group of volunteers with normal blood pressure were given a daily tablet containing 1 gram of calcium and the other half received a placebo tablet (one that appeared identical but contained no calcium).[26] The group receiving the calcium showed a significant reduction in blood pressure.

In a study by Dr. Lawrence Resnick and his colleagues at Cornell University Medical College in New York City, an increase in dietary calcium decreased diastolic blood pressure, sometimes by as much as 10% to 20% in the 30% of patients with primary hypertension who had low blood levels of the hormone renin, which can affect blood pressure.[27] Increasing dietary calcium was more effective in patients with low initial levels of blood serum calcium and in hypertensives with high dietary levels of sodium.

A study in Guatemala of thirty-six pregnant women with normal blood pressure also showed that calcium supplementation can decrease blood pressure.[28] To eliminate possible psychological effects in this study, the women did not know whether they were taking placebo pills or the pills that actually contained calcium. This was a double-blind study, because both those studied *and* those doing the studying were "blind"—that is, ignorant of who got the placebo pills and who got the real thing. This information was released by the pill manufacturer only at the end of the study. Near the end of their pregnancies, the average diastolic blood pressures of the women taking placebo pills was 71.9 mm Hg; in the group taking 1 gram of calcium per day, it was 68.8 mm Hg; and in the group taking 2 grams of calcium per day, it was 64.5 mm Hg.

Still other studies have suggested the reverse: that is, the higher the dietary calcium, the higher the blood pressure. These studies were undertaken in Italy,[29] Belgium,[30] and Korea.[31] The dietary calcium was estimated by measuring calcium excretion in the urine. But this method may not always reflect the amount of calcium in the diet. Several conditions can cause loss of body calcium: certain diseases, excess sodium chloride, too little exercise. It has been suggested that too much dietary protein can also do it. Therefore, these conditions can increase calcium in the urine even when the diet is deficient in calcium.

When hypertensive rats were put on a low-calcium diet, they became even more hypertensive, whereas when they were on a high-calcium diet, the rats became much less hypertensive.[32] When normal rats are given extra sodium chloride in their diet (amounts comparable to that in the typical American diet), they begin to lose calcium from their bones into the urine. The effect of excess sodium chloride again demonstrates the counterbalance between sodium (bad for blood pressure) and potassium and calcium (good for blood pressure).

The effect of calcium on blood pressure is also consistent with our understanding of the cellular mechanisms that are involved in keeping the cell membrane "tight" so the proper balance between potassium, sodium, and calcium within the cell can be maintained, as was described in Chapter 4.

In summary, although the evidence is by no means conclusive, several clues suggest that if dietary calcium drops too low *or* is too high, this may contribute to high blood pressure.

CHLORIDE

Although the hypertensive effect of table salt (NaCl) is commonly attributed to the positive sodium ion, Na^+, there is evidence that the negative chloride ion, Cl^-, may also contribute, along with sodium, to the development of hypertension.[33] When sodium is given to people with a family history of hypertension, it raises the blood pressure only when given as NaCl. Other sodium salts, such as sodium bicarbonate,* produce relatively little elevation of blood pressure. Also, Dr. Addison had noticed that potassium citrate appeared more effective than potassium chloride in his treatment of humans with hypertension.[34] However, more recent studies have demonstrated that potassium chloride may be as effective as non-chloride potassium salts.

The fact that sodium appears to depend on chloride to do its "dirty work" may not be so surprising in light of the fact that for sodium to be reabsorbed in the kidney and thus retained by the body, most of it must be accompanied by chloride. If sodium is accompanied by another substance, such as bicarbonate or the organic ions present in natural food, then the sodium will tend to be lost in the urine. So table salt (NaCl) is double trouble.

DIETARY FAT

Beyond the small amount (probably much less than 15% of our calories) our body needs, there really is nothing good to say for dietary fat. It is true that a small amount of two unsaturated fatty acids—linoleic and linolenic acids—is necessary in the diet because our bodies cannot manufacture these essential fatty acids. As little as 5 grams per day of a liquid fat, such as corn oil or safflower oil, high in these unsaturated fatty acids is enough for good health.[35]

But saturated dietary fat (which is present only in animal products and tropical oils) is entirely unnecessary, since our bodies can make all of the saturated fats. And in excess amounts, saturated fat contributes to obesity, increases the chance of acquiring some types of cancer, and is a main factor contributing to coronary vascular disease leading to heart attacks.

Some studies have indicated that the type and amount of dietary fat also contributes to hypertension. One group of investigators reported that decreasing dietary fat to provide only 25% of energy intake *and* increasing the ratio of polyunsaturated fat to saturated fat (P/S ratio) to about 1.0—that is, eating equal amounts by weight of both—results in a significant reduction in blood pressure. This effect is independent of weight reduction and is observed in normal people as

---

*By the way, when chloride is taken in any other form, such as magnesium chloride, calcium chloride, or even ordinary food sources, once in the body the chloride becomes free and mixes with all the other ions from other food sources. Therefore, when consuming sodium bicarbonate with any kind of food, it is just like eating sodium chloride. In the experiments just described, sodium bicarbonate (and no chloride from any source) was the only thing that the people consumed during a given period of time.

well as in those with mild hypertension, although the effect appears to be greater among the latter.[36]

In these two studies, the reduction in dietary fat was accomplished by dietary substitution of vegetables and fresh fruits for fatty foods. This would be expected to increase dietary potassium. Although the amount of sodium in the low-fat, high P/S ratio diets was not changed, in the one study in which it was measured, dietary potassium was found to be increased by up to an additional 90% when the changes in dietary fat were made. Thus the decrease in blood pressure in some of these studies might have been due in part to the increase in dietary potassium.

LINOLEIC ACID

The increase in polyunsaturated fat in these diets was accompanied by an increase in dietary linoleic acid, a fatty acid "required" in the diet because the human body does not manufacture it from other foods. Since this fatty acid is required for synthesis of the hormones called prostaglandins, it has been speculated that the effect of the dietary change in these studies may be due to an increase in prostaglandin hormones, which are known to increase sodium excretion by the kidneys. This led to a study in which the effect of dietary content of linoleic acid upon blood pressure in mildly hypertensive humans was tested.

Increasing dietary linoleic acid from an average of 4.0 (plus or minus 0.3)% of total calories to 5.2 (plus or minus 0.4)% resulted in a significant reduction in diastolic blood pressure in people with mild hypertension.[37] When dietary linoleic acid was increased, excretion of potassium by the kidney was decreased by 40%. In addition, this increase of dietary linoleic acid decreased serum cholesterol by 7%, a small but significant amount. The ability of increased dietary linoleic acid (in the form of safflower oil) to lower elevated blood pressure has also been demonstrated in hypertensive rats in several studies[38] and in humans in a study done in Finland.[39]

In contrast, a summary of more recent studies[40] has led to the conclusion that it is unlikely that changes in the amount of linoleic acid affect blood pressure.

LINOLENIC ACID

Linolenic acid is another fatty acid that must be obtained exclusively from food. Based upon estimates of long-term consumption of fatty acids, a study of nonhypertensive men in New York City found evidence that increased linolenic acid consumption is associated with a lowering of the blood pressure.[41] Linolenic acid is found in linseed (flaxseed) oil, legumes, nuts (walnuts, chestnuts), and citrus fruits.

Although a role for dietary fat in hypertension is not firmly established, it is clear that a decrease of total fat intake together with some increase in linoleic and linolenic acid cannot hurt and might be of some help in reversing primary hypertension. But don't go overboard. You *can* get too much of a good thing, and it has been reported that excessive consumption of polyunsaturated fat may increase the risk for cancer.[42]

In view of the increased cholesterol levels and associated coronary artery disease that—in addition to elevated blood pressure—are part of the syndrome called hypertension, it seems especially prudent to recommend that people who have even modest elevations of blood pressure do what is good for everyone: decrease the saturated fat and cholesterol in their diet.

In view of the bad effects of dietary fat on obesity, cancer, and especially heart disease, *decreasing total dietary fat to no more than 20% of calories is a high priority for health and longevity.*

SMOKING

Remember that the 1985 British Medical Research Council study of treatment of mild hypertension found evidence that people with hypertension who do not smoke (compared to those who do) had a *much greater decrease* in rate of strokes and heart attacks than did those who received drug treatment.[43] In an editorial that accompanied the British study, that finding led to this conclusion:

> "In advising hypertensive patients we must continue to emphasise the great importance of stopping smoking, for this may turn out to be a more important therapeutic manoeuvre than the prescription of blood pressure lowering drugs."[44]

Other large-scale studies of treatment of hypertension have also demonstrated that smoking increases both strokes and coronary artery disease in people with hypertension, whether or not they are treated with drugs.

VITAMINS C AND D

The original analysis of the HANES I study indicated that people eating larger amounts of vitamin C had lower blood pressure.[45] A more recent analysis of the same data reached the same conclusion and also reported that higher levels of vitamin D in the diet were correlated with lower blood pressure. A possible explanation for these observations is that vitamin C is found in foods rich in potassium (fruits and vegetables) and vitamin D is found in milk (rich in calcium and also in potassium).

More recent evidence suggests that antioxidants such as vitamin C, vitamin E, and alpha tocopherols slow formation of cholesterol deposits in arteries.

PSYCHOLOGICAL STRESS

A commonly held view is that psychological stress can cause hypertension. In my opinion, this belief is highly speculative. As we have already discussed, it is questionable whether the people in the low-blood-pressure, non-westernized societies that have been studied are under less stress than are people in industrialized societies. Moreover, tranquilizers and sedatives are ineffective in treating hypertension. Nevertheless, there is evidence that in people with hypertension, the blood pressure is more sensitive to stress.

Stress operates through the sympathetic nervous system, which uses adrenaline to transmit signals from nerves to stimulate contraction of the smooth muscles in the walls of the arterioles. The action of the sympathetic nervous system explains how some of the drugs used to treat hypertension work. For example, the beta and alpha adrenergic blockers help lower blood pressure by blocking sympathetic nerve activity, thus allowing the small arteries to relax. So it's not surprising that in people who already have primary hypertension, there is evidence that psychological stress can make their blood pressure go still higher.

Some recent evidence indicates that some people respond to stress by losing more magnesium in their urine. This could contribute to a magnesium deficiency with consequent bad effects on blood pressure.

One thing is certain: stress often leads to behavior, such as overeating or overdrinking, that is bad not only for our blood pressure but our general health.

Even hypertension in which stress may be a contributor, however, should be helped by potassium. This is supported by the finding that humans with normal blood pressure who are given a high-potassium diet do not show as great a rise in blood pressure, when subjected to mental stress, as do people in a control group on a "normal" diet.[46]

Perhaps the main way stress contributes to hypertension is that it often leads to overeating.

MEDITATION

Although the role of psychological stress is not clear, meditation and relaxation have been reported to be effective in producing long-term reductions in blood pressure.[47] (Relaxation also produces an immediate reduction of blood pressure, so that it is very important for you to relax completely while your blood pressure is being taken, in order to avoid a falsely high reading. Just by gripping the arm of your chair firmly, you can increase your systolic and diastolic blood pressures by over 20 mm Hg.[48] Even the act of calmly talking while your blood pressure is being taken can raise your pressure readings by about 5 mm Hg.)

Although there is no doubt that regular meditation can help lower elevated blood pressure, as yet there is no evidence that it can lower elevated levels of insulin, restore cholesterol levels to normal, or rebalance the relation between potassium and sodium within the body's cells.

BIOFEEDBACK

There is little doubt that with proper training, biofeedback can lower blood pressure.[49] The power of the brain (some would say of the mind) to control basic body functions such as pulse and blood pressure has been known by yogis for centuries.

But this is just another means for regulating, or controlling, blood pressure. True, biofeedback doesn't have the side effects of drugs, but like them biofeedback is a means of treating the symptom, not of curing the primary problem. There is no evidence that biofeedback can restore the imbalance within the cell that causes hypertension in the first place.

WORKAHOLISM

It has been suggested that "workaholics" have higher than average blood pressures, but this is hard to quantify. In my opinion, good health is best maintained by a balance between work and play as well as between sodium and potassium. We need a yin and a yang. One must work in order to live and to feel a sense of accomplishment, but it is also important to laugh and enjoy life.

CLIMATE

It has been suggested that climate may have some effect on blood pressure. For example, in an extensive study of blood pressures of adults living in England, it was noted that blood pressures were significantly lower when measured in the summer than when measured in the winter.[50] Presumably this was partly due to the decreased resistance to blood flow resulting from the dilation of the blood vessels in the skin in the summertime. It may also have been partly due to the greater availability in the summer of fresh fruits and vegetables (which are rich in potassium).

To keep things in perspective, one of the low-sodium, high-potassium groups found to have consistently low blood pressures was the Greenland Eskimos, who live where the weather is cool even in the summer.

SUMMARY

There are many roads to primary hypertension. The most traveled are deficient dietary K Factor, lack of exercise, and obesity. Other commonly traveled roads are deficient dietary magnesium or calcium. Excess alcohol can also help get you there, and if you already have hypertension, smoking *greatly* increases your chance of having a stroke or heart attack.

Thus there are many things you can and should do to reduce or prevent high blood pressure. From the evidence presented here, it should be obvious that a total, or holistic, approach is required. To be really successful, you need to control your weight, get regular exercise, and—most important—eat food with a K Factor above 4!

SUMMARY: PART TWO

By now, the evidence is abundant that a lifestyle approach based upon nutrition is the *only* approach that can restore health. Let's review what we have learned:

1. Comparison of aboriginal with modern cultures demonstrates that hypertension is due to our modern lifestyle. As the Working Group of the National High Blood Pressure Education Program has pointed out, the common tendency of blood pressure to rise with age as well as the increase in the prevalence of hypertension with age is *not* a product of the aging process, but is essentially due to

   a high sodium intake many times beyond human physiologic need, overweight, physical inactivity, excess alcohol consumption, and a deficient intake of potassium.[51]

   In other words, hypertension can be prevented by avoiding obesity, sedentary lifestyle, and excess alcohol and by consuming a low potassium-high sodium (or low-K-Factor) diet.

2. The studies of different cultures, the trials of increasing dietary potassium, and our understanding of the living cell all indicate that hypertension is a consequence of an imbalance between potassium and sodium in the body. The evidence indicates that this imbalance is due in turn to a deficient K Factor in the diet. Obesity or a sedentary lifestyle produces changes in the body that can magnify the effects of a deficiency in the dietary K Factor. Alcohol and smoking can make the situation worse.

3. To keep it simple, we should remember that most vegetarians (who get their potassium in fruit and vegetables) don't get hypertension. From this it is obvious that the main aspect of lifestyle responsible for hypertension must be a lack of proper nutrition.

You have now seen five lines of evidence that all converge to indicate that a lack of proper balance between potassium and sodium in the body is an underlying factor in producing primary hypertension. This lack of balance between potassium and sodium is caused by changes in lifestyle typical of modern industrialized countries and encountered for the first time in the one hundred thousand years of human evolution: namely, a low-K-Factor diet, lack of exercise, and obesity. Those who inherit especially strong regulatory systems don't get obvious hypertension, but those who don't inherit the extra margin of error, do. In addition, the rest of us who make these mistakes in lifestyle tend to develop blood pressure above the range required for optimal health. The lines of evidence show:

1. Elevated blood pressure is not the only, perhaps not the main, problem. In addition to the elevated blood pressure, people with primary hypertension have abnormalities in their blood cholesterol, abnormalities in carbohydrate metabolism, and often elevated blood insulin levels. These effects are interrelated and are likely due in part to the presence, in people with hypertension, of an abnormal response of body cells to insulin. An abnormal response of body cells to insulin ("insulin resistance") has been shown to occur secondary to a deficiency of potassium in the body.

2. In the surface membrane of each body cell, potassium is exchanged for sodium by a mechanism, called the sodium-potassium pump, in the surface membrane of each body cell. Normal operation of this pump requires a normal amount of potassium in the body. By keeping sodium inside the cell low, this pump indirectly supplies the energy required to keep calcium out of the cell and to keep acid out of the cell.

   If the activity of the sodium-potassium pump slows down, not only will sodium inside the cells rise, but (as will be further explained in Chapter 15) potassium inside the cells *must* go down. Both effects result in a decrease in the energy of the "sodium battery." If this happens in the cells that constrict small arteries, it will result in an increase of calcium inside the cell that will lead to increased narrowing of these small arteries, thus raising blood pressure.

   The increased levels of blood insulin and of angiotensin II that often occur in hypertension probably explain the increased activity of the Na^+/H^+ exchange pump and the resulting increase in pH inside the body cells of people with hypertension. This increase in pH (or decrease in acid) can contribute to increased growth of smooth muscle cells and probably helps account for the abnormal structure that develops in the arteries of people with hypertension.

3. The fact that primary hypertension does *not* exist in some societies depends not upon the genetic inheritance of that society but upon their lifestyle. Inspection of the diets of groups who do not have hypertension reveals that all such groups consume a diet with a high K Factor.

4. Since 1904 and 1928, a few pioneering physicians have repeatedly demonstrated that increasing dietary K Factor can restore normal blood pressure—sometimes in even severe hypertension. Studies on experimental animals also demonstrate that increasing the dietary K Factor often lowers the blood pressure. But of much more importance, increasing the dietary K Factor can reduce strokes and death due to strokes *even if* blood pressure remains elevated. This has been found to be true in both humans and in experimental animals. Moreover, even people with so-called normal blood pressure, which is actually higher than optimal, are at increased risk for strokes and cardiovascular disease.

5. The evidence indicates that not only a low dietary K Factor, but also obesity and lack of exercise, by causing hormone changes, disturb normal activity of the sodium-potassium pump and thus the balance between potassium and sodium. These disturbances appear to cause changes within the small arteries that make them more prone to constrict, and to increase activity of the sympathetic (adrenaline-like) nervous system that signals these arteries to constrict.

Several factors can contribute to primary hypertension in those who have the inherited tendency. There are many ways to disturb the balance between potassium and sodium in the body: not only a deficient dietary K Factor, but obesity, lack of exercise, and other factors, such as dietary magnesium and probably calcium, also play a role. However, in view of the evidence now available, the K Factor, obesity, and lack of exercise appear to be the most important. From a practical point of view, the key point is to realize that all of these factors are under *your* control. Together with your physician, you can take charge of your life in a way that will allow your body to heal itself and reduce the dangers of high blood pressure.

No one is saying that all these ideas are completely proven (nothing in science is ever *totally* proven). But at this point, there is no longer any reasonable doubt that hypertension involves much more than elevated blood pressure. Moreover, while no one line of evidence is conclusive in and of itself, the fact that they all point to the same conclusion is impressive. There is consistency here. Everywhere you look, there is either solid evidence, or at least suggestive evidence, that potassium/sodium exchange by the sodium-potassium pump is involved in hypertension. When you see a pattern emerging time and again, it's a good sign that it reflects some approximation of the real situation.

Although much remains to be learned, we now have enough understanding of how these factors operate to realize that by changing lifestyle, we can reverse and prevent the imbalance within the body cells that leads to primary hypertension.

In the meantime, which would you rather have: diet and exercise therapy, or drug therapy? The evidence seems clear that either can reduce death due to strokes. But in the case of nutrition, there is no evidence indicating that it does harm.

Drugs affect only some of the *consequences* of this imbalance, such as retention of sodium, increased activity of the sympathetic nervous system, movement of calcium, or production of angiotensin without correcting the underlying imbalance itself. So it's not totally surprising that two studies suggest that for borderline hypertensives, aggressive drug treatment (especially with thiazide diuretics) may actually *increase* mortality. Many want to explain this evidence away. But although these studies may not be entirely conclusive, the burden of proof would seem to be on those who maintain that drugs are the preferred treatment.

Although you can't change your inheritance, if you consider the evidence presented in this section, you will realize that the changes in primary hypertension such as abnormal sodium and potassium levels, insulin levels, and blood cholesterol levels can be reversed by increasing the dietary K Factor, getting adequate exercise, and losing any excess weight. Therefore it is possible for people with primary hypertension to get their body systems back into a natural mode of operation. Moreover, by taking these same steps, it is possible for the rest of us to drastically reduce our chances of ever developing hypertension.

The next section discusses how to do this.

A Word of Caution: If you have high blood pressure for a long enough time, other secondary changes can occur (mentioned in Part Six) that can make the elevated blood pressure irreversible. This emphasizes not only the importance of early detection, diagnosis, and treatment of high blood pressure but also its *prevention*.

PART THREE

THE
PROGRAM

These lifestyle factors [that lead to hypertension] include a high sodium intake, an excessive consumption of calories, physical inactivity, excessive alcohol consumption, and a deficient intake of potassium. . . . Goals of the campaign should include promotion of foods which are lower in sodium and calorie content and higher in potassium content, and promotion of physical activity and moderation in alcohol consumption.

from the 1993 Working Group Report
for Prevention of Hypertension supported by
the National Heart, Lung, and Blood Institute[1]

In other words, the primary task in prevention—and I would add in treatment—of hypertension should be to consume foods that are high in potassium and low in sodium (have a higher K Factor), increase exercise, decrease calorie intake to prevent overweight, and promote physical activity and moderation in alcohol consumption.

The fundamental goal of the four-step program outlined in this part of the book is not *just* to get your blood pressure down, not *just* to decrease the numbers read from the blood pressure machine, but to significantly decrease and eventually eliminate the strokes, cardiovascular disease, and other damage that result from hypertension. It is intended not to treat only part of the problem—blood pressure—but, far more importantly, to allow your body to restore its normal function, which will decrease your chance of death and increase your sense of well-being. The four-step program is designed to help you be healthy, feel healthy, and live your allotted span of years.

IT'S EASY

This is not a rigid program; it does not require you to give up a lot of things you like. Moreover, you will not have to eat anything you don't like. And it is simpler and easier to stick to than other nondrug programs.

However, without understanding the program, you could make some simple oversights that would result in your not preventing or treating your hypertension successfully.

Once you do understand the simple principles we explain here, you'll be able to follow the program with relatively little effort. Soon it will become second nature to you. In particular, it wouldn't be surprising if within a few years, most Americans will be selecting and preparing their food according to these principles as well as exercising more.

BUT IT'S UP TO YOU

Although it is essential that you consult with your physician, you must realize that in the final analysis, *you* are the one responsible for your health. Neither the government, insurance companies, the medical profession, modern technology, employee programs, nor anything else can really keep you well. Only *you* can do that.

So get involved with your own health care. You're the one who is going to live (or maybe not) with the results.

THE FOUR STEPS

What follows is a brief outline of the four steps of our program. Each of these steps will be described in more detail in this part of the book. That is, Step One is described in Chapter 9, Step Two in Chapter 10, and so on.

The steps are related and work together. To take just one example: your weight will reach its proper level (Step Four) more easily if you are eating the right kinds of foods (Step Two) and exercising regularly (Step Three).

STEP ONE: SEE YOUR DOCTOR

First, see your doctor for a complete examination. In fact, you need to have your blood pressure measured on at least three separate occasions before deciding if you have high blood pressure. Even if your blood pressure is normal, you should have periodic blood pressure checks, at least once every year, especially if your parents or other close relatives have had high blood pressure.

If you have high blood pressure, you need tests for specific disease conditions that may cause high blood pressure, and you need a test for kidney function. Before you embark on our program, you need to rule out the possibility that you have some secondary condition. Such a condition, afflicting about 5% of all those with high blood pressure, often requires very special treatment and probably means that this program is not for you.

However, once you are assured that you are in the 95% group, you can begin following the other steps of our program. You will need the cooperation of your doctor. For one thing, you need professional advice about if, when, and how to change or discontinue any drug treatment you are currently on. Also, your doctor may help you determine just what kind of exercise—and how much of it—is safe for you (Step Three). Finally, the two of you together should be monitoring your progress with our program as a whole.

STEP TWO: EAT RIGHT

You need to eat food that is richer in potassium and lower in sodium—in other words, food that has a high K Factor.

To do this, you don't really have to sacrifice many things you like to eat now. The key is not so much what you eat as *how it's prepared.* You need to buy the right foods in the supermarket, and you need to avoid a couple of common mistakes in preparing your meals at home. *You can actually eat your way out of high blood pressure!* You'll see how to do this in the menu plan given in Chapter 10.

You can increase your dietary K Factor naturally by eating more of such foods as whole grains, fresh vegetables and fruits, and nonfat dairy products and eating less processed food, fast food, junk food, and—generally—food with added salt. You'll find a table to help you select high K Factor foods in Chapter 13.

You also need to cut out table salt, both on the table and in your cooking. Instead, you can use salt substitutes that contain potassium. You will find that its not difficult to eat almost anything you like and still achieve a dietary K Factor above the minimum level of about 4.

You should also include in your diet adequate amounts of calcium and magnesium, which can be found in dairy products (preferably nonfat and unsalted), nuts, whole grains, beans, and green leafy vegetables.

Finally, you need to decrease the amount of fat in your diet to no more than 20% of your total calories. And that 20% should be mostly polyunsaturated fat, such as liquid vegetable oil.

STEP THREE: EXERCISE

In some people, exercise alone is enough to restore their blood pressure to normal. A combination of eating right and adequate exercise not only can give you normal blood pressure and help you avoid heart attack but also can improve the quality of your life as well.

Exercise—aerobic exercise in particular—produces changes in blood hormones, thereby affecting the potassium and sodium balance inside the body's cells, which in turn helps reduce high blood pressure.

Also, for most people, exercise is an important or necessary part of keeping weight down to normal. Exercising even three times a week can make a noticeable difference.

STEP FOUR: HELP YOUR BODY FIND ITS PROPER WEIGHT

Quite simply, avoid being overweight. Losing excess weight is often enough to restore blood pressure to normal levels.

Obesity causes changes in the levels of the blood hormones that regulate the exchange of potassium and sodium within the body. This has been proposed as an explanation for the well-established fact that obesity increases your chances of developing high blood pressure.

One of the side advantages of Step Two, a diet with a lot of fruits, vegetables, and grains (a high-K-Factor diet), is that it is also a low-fat diet. Since fat has more than twice as many calories as the same weight of carbohydrates or protein, a diet rich in fruits, vegetables, and grains also helps you keep your weight down. Fruits, vegetables, and grains are also rich in fiber, which is necessary for a healthy diet and may help prevent some kinds of cancer.

A side benefit of an aerobic exercise program (Step Three) is that it helps you lose excess weight. In fact, 98% of weight loss programs fail *unless* regular aerobic exercise is included.

Losing excess weight and maintaining normal weight are primarily consequences of proper nutrition (Step Two) and exercise (Step Three). However, to be effective, the *balance* between nutrition and exercise must be adjusted properly. A modern concept, the setpoint, borrowed from control system theory, gives insight into this balance and is discussed in Step Four.

OTHER THINGS YOU CAN DO

Changing behavior that is bad for your general health can also help keep your blood pressure normal.

For example, avoid excessive use of alcohol. Heavy drinking clearly increases your chances of getting high blood pressure. Also, minimize or, better yet, eliminate smoking. If you already have hypertension, smoking makes such consequences as heart attacks much more likely.

Finally, minimize the effects of stress. Although stress is not a main cause of high blood pressure, it can make high blood pressure worse. Perhaps the most important aspect of stress is that it may lead to such behaviors as overeating, smoking, or alcohol abuse, which do contribute to high blood pressure.

SUMMARY

Again, we wish to emphasize that the *goal* of this program is not just to get your blood pressure down but to correct the imbalance in your body that caused the problem in the first place. This will also make you *live longer* and, equally important, *feel more healthy* during all your years.

If this program doesn't decrease your blood pressure right away, don't get discouraged. Stay with it. It will probably take weeks—and it may take months—for your blood pressure to respond to the program, especially if you've had hypertension for several years.

Remember, lowering the blood pressure with drugs does not always lead to better health or a longer life. On the other hand, evidence from studies of both experimental animals and human beings indicates that even if your blood vessels have become so damaged that your blood pressure can't come down, this program can still extend your life. So stick with the program even if your blood pressure doesn't come down. After all, what you really care about is your sense of well-being and your living a long, healthy life.

You *can* reload the dice; you can change the odds of your suffering or dying from high blood pressure.

You are the one who is ultimately responsible for your own health. To keep on top of this program, you should monitor your own progress, using the chart in Part Four.

CHAPTER 9

Step One: See Your Doctor

The very first step you should take is to see your doctor.

Please do not get involved with the other steps of this program before you do this. The results could be disastrous. Your doctor needs to examine you to verify that you do indeed have high blood pressure, and if you do, to determine just what type of high blood pressure it is.

Then, if certain types of hypertension are ruled out, your doctor should do the following:

- Advise you about any changes in whatever drugs you may currently be taking.
- Evaluate your risk of coronary artery disease to determine the type and amount of exercise that is safe or you.
- Monitor your progress with our program as a whole.

GET A COMPLETE PHYSICAL EXAM

Get a complete physical examination. Your doctor should carefully evaluate your blood pressure and test for other specific disease conditions that may cause high blood pressure. In order to get a complete picture, your doctor will have to do specific tests and will have to see you regularly.

DO YOU HAVE HIGH BLOOD PRESSURE?

On three separate visits, your doctor should measure your blood pressure while you are relaxed and not talking, at least twice on each visit and at least once on both arms. The reason for three separate visits is that both systolic and diastolic blood pressure often fall spontaneously with further visits as the patient gets used to the process. Because of this, a 1986 editorial in the journal *Hypertension*[1] recommended that if the initial diastolic pressure is above 90 mm Hg, the blood pressure should be remeasured on at least two more occasions during the next four weeks. If during this time the diastolic blood pressure falls below 90 mm Hg, the recommendation is that further measurements be made at three-month intervals for a year. The 1993 Report of the Joint National Committee makes similar recommendations.

According to the Joint National Committee's 1984, 1988, and 1993 reports, you have high blood pressure, or hypertension, if your systolic blood pressure is greater than 140 mm Hg and/or your diastolic blood pressure is greater than 90 mm Hg. But keep in mind that insurance statistics show a diastolic blood pressure over 80 is actually bad for you (see Chapter 1).

IF SO, WHAT TYPE DO YOU HAVE?

Once your doctor has verified that you do have hypertension, he or she will need to consider other specific disease conditions that may have caused it, by taking a comprehensive health history and by performing certain tests, including testing your kidneys and heart.

Although high blood pressure itself is bad, it is also a symptom, or a sign, of abnormal body function. Although the abnormality in body function is almost always caused by a nutritional imbalance such as a low K Factor or calcium deficiency in the food we eat, it is sometimes (in less than 5% of cases) an indication of other disease conditions—such as kidney disease or an adrenal gland tumor. When high blood pressure is due to another disease, it is called *secondary hypertension*. Before you embark on our program, your doctor will need to rule out the possibility that you have secondary hypertension.

Secondary Hypertension

Secondary hypertension is caused by such conditions as these:

- Kidney disease
- Narrowing of the artery to a kidney
- Primary aldosteronism
- Renin-secreting tumor
- Cushing's syndrome
- Congenital adrenal hyperplasia
- Coarctation (narrowing) of the aorta
- Pheochromocytoma
- Contraceptive, or estrogen, therapy
- Reaction to appetite suppressants
- Reaction to decongestants

- Rigidity of the arteries due to arteriosclerosis
- Leakage of the aortic heart valve
- Block of electrical signaling between the upper chambers (atria) and lower chambers (ventricles) of the heart
- Conditions involving increased blood output from the heart, including thyrotoxicosis
- Severe anemia

The last five are characterized by an increase in systolic blood pressure and so are sometimes also called systolic hypertension.

We must emphasize that the program in this book will not help those people whose high blood pressure is due to secondary hypertension. Each of the possible causes of those types of high blood pressure requires specific diagnosis and treatment—which may include surgery.

Primary Hypertension

The vast majority of people with high blood pressure, however—more than 95% of cases—have *primary hypertension* (or *essential hypertension,* which may be what your doctor calls it).

If your doctor determines that you do not have secondary hypertension, you are one of the other 95% who have primary hypertension. And it is you, your children, and your doctor for whom this book has been written. This book shows how simple—and safe—modifications in your lifestyle, especially in what you eat and in how you prepare it, can lower your blood pressure and restore your health or prevent high blood pressure from developing in the first place.

You should do something about your blood pressure, because your chances of dying are significantly increased—on the average, doubled—compared with people in your age group with normal blood pressure.

Fortunately, it is primary hypertension that can be helped by paying attention to the K Factor in your diet.

WORK WITH YOUR DOCTOR

Although it is essential that you consult with your physician, you must realize that in the final analysis, you are the one responsible for your health. When it comes to preventive medicine—and keeping you from getting a stroke or heart attack is legitimately called preventive—we in the health professions can only provide you with the information. *You* must put it into practice.

Many doctors, and many laypersons as well, realize that achieving health and maintaining it requires a transformation of the typical physician-patient relationship into a physician-partner collaboration. For this to work, the patient needs to take greater responsibility, and the physician needs to approach the patient as a co-worker.

We suggest that you take this book to your doctor and ask for his or her cooperation. If your doctor will not cooperate—that is, will not consider the K-Factor approach—seek a second, or even a third, opinion.

In the interest of facilitating this physician-partner collaboration, the rest of this chapter will provide you with this information:

- Some idea of what to expect when you visit your doctor
- Some timely warnings about discontinuing any drug therapy you may currently be following
- Some information about evaluation of exercise risk
- Suggestions for evaluating your progress with our program

WHAT TO EXPECT WHEN YOU VISIT YOUR DOCTOR

The section entitled "Do You Have High Blood Pressure?" discussed the blood pressure measurements your doctor needs to take. But your doctor needs to make several other tests as well—in particular, to rule out secondary hypertension, for example:

- Routine urinalysis
- Test for blood hemoglobin and hematocrit
- Test for serum levels of potassium, glucose, cholesterol (total and HDL), triglyceride levels, creatinine, uric acid, and serum insulin.
- Electrocardiogram

You may need to fast before the test for serum levels of glucose.

In addition, your doctor might want to do a chest X-ray and possibly a test called an *intravenous pyelogram* to look for obstruction of the urinary tract, a cause of kidney disease. Depending upon the results of these tests and the history and physical exam, other diagnostic tests may be performed.

CHANGES IN DRUG THERAPY

Stopping drugs should be done only under your doctor's supervision. The actual change can be dangerous.

NEVER WITHDRAW ANY DRUG SUDDENLY.

This should be emphasized. Any sudden change can be dangerous. For example, sudden withdrawal of Clonidine can precipitate a rebound hypertension. If you have angina, a sudden withdrawal of beta blockers can precipitate anginal attacks.

A note of caution about potassium-sparing diuretics: If you are taking a potassium-sparing diuretic, be sure to consult with your doctor about whether the K-Factor program should be used with these drugs. In any case, until further research is done, you should not take any potassium-containing pills or potassium-containing salt substitutes while you are on potassium-sparing diuretics.

GETTING A CHECK-UP BEFORE STARTING YOUR EXERCISE PROGRAM

Before you begin a new exercise program (Step Three) or make any changes in one you're already in, have your doctor measure your blood cholesterol and, if possible, blood triglycerides.

You really should get a stress test if you:

- Are over 40
- Have a blood cholesterol level greater than 200 mg/ml
- Have at least one other major coronary risk factor: (a) are (or have been) seriously overweight, (b) smoke cigarettes, (c) have diabetes mellitus, or (d) have a family history of coronary disease by age fifty
- Have a blood pressure over 145/95
- Have known cardiovascular or lung or metabolic disease

It's not a bad idea to get one even if you are under 40.

By "stress test," I am not refering to the Master Two-Step Test but to a multistage stress test that utilizes a treadmill or a stationary exercise bicycle. In the multistage test, your electrocardiogram (EKG) and blood pressure can be taken continuously while you exercise and as the level of exercise is increased.

An EKG is a tracing of electrical activity of the heart. You may have already had one taken at rest. If a resting EKG shows abnormal electrical activity, you need careful consultation with your doctor about whether and how you should begin an exercise program. If coronary artery disease has caused your heart any problems, a resting EKG may show signs of this.

However, a resting EKG often fails to show signs of coronary disease and so provides no assurance that you are not about to have a heart attack. On the other hand, abnormalities in the EKG are much more likely to show up during exercise, so a properly conducted treadmill EKG (the stress test) offers much better evidence. We discuss the value and limitations of the treadmill stress test in more detail in Chapter 11.

The treadmill stress test also gives some idea of how hard you can exercise safely. Let's say you get your heart rate up to 150 and the electrical tracing (EKG) is still normal. Although it is not a guarantee, that provides an indication that as long as your heart rate is not higher than 150 when you exercise, you are unlikely to have a heart attack.

But even the exercise EKG isn't infallible, unfortunately. Your coronary arteries could be almost two-thirds closed with cholesterol deposits and you might still pass the stress test—especially if it is not conducted according to the guidelines of the American College of Sports Medicine. However, among the simple and safe methods, it's the best we have for evaluating your cardiac health. Some of you may remember the running guru Jim Fixx, who died while running. If he had taken the advice to have a stress test, there is a good chance he would be out there today slowly jogging, or at least walking. Fixx had once been overweight and had a family history of heart trouble—both factors that increase the chance of getting a heart attack.

Especially for people new to regular aerobic exercise, the stress test is advised to help rule out coronary artery deficiency before you begin anything more than walking.

Even if you *have* been exercising regularly, you should get a physical reevaluation every year or two. And it doesn't hurt to get a stress test every few years, especially if you are going to change the amount of your exercise.

FOLLOWING YOUR PROGRESS

In order to maximize your chances of success, you will need to not only work with your physician but also follow your own progress. To do this, you need to learn to take your own blood pressure, as will be explained in Chapter 13). Using the progress chart provided in Part Four, keep a weekly record of your blood pressure, morning pulse, weight, amount of exercise, and dietary K Factor.

SUMMARY

To really take care of high blood pressure you must take charge of your lifestyle. But you can't successfully do this alone. You need information, like that in this book, and you also need a personal coach—a doctor who knows you and your health status and who will supervise you. You can't do it alone, and it can't happen without your involvement.

The first thing is to determine if you really have elevated blood pressure. Then it is *vital* that you have your doctor rule out other causes of hypertension such those listed under secondary hypertension.

You must have medical advice and supervision before any major change in diet or exercise, or in taking drugs for hypertension—or for other conditions. *Remember: Never* stop taking a drug without your physician's supervision and never stop suddenly. Before entering an exercise program, be sure to get properly evaluated, preferably with a properly conducted exercise stress test.

Finally, keep track of your progress using the forms provided.

CHAPTER 10

Step Two: Eat Right

The diet of our remote ancestors may be a reference standard for modern human nutrition and a model for defense against certain "diseases of civilization."

Eaton and Konner[1]

Cutting back on table salt, losing excess weight, decreasing alcohol consumption, and getting regular exercise—all steps recommended by the Joint National Committee in its 1984, 1988, and 1993 Special Reports—are essential steps for treating primary hypertension.

But are they enough?

The answer is no, because they do not address the need for a dietary balance we inherited from our remote ancestors: a balance between sodium and other minerals, such as chloride, magnesium, calcium, and especially potassium. Your high blood pressure is really an outer symptom of an abnormal balance in your body's cells. Establishing the proper balance of these elements—especially the ratio of potassium to sodium (the K Factor)—will usually lower your blood pressure, improve your health, and promise to increase your life span **even if your blood pressure does not return to normal levels!**

To be successful, you must eat food that is richer in potassium and lower in sodium; the K Factor should be at least 4 (four times as much potassium as sodium). This ought not to be very difficult. When food comes directly "off the vine" or "off the hoof," it has a K Factor of at least 5. The diet of our remote ancestors had a K Factor of about 16! Unsalted fruits and vegetables generally have a K Factor of at least 20 and often well over 100. But because of common mistakes we make in preparing our food, the K Factor of the average American diet is less than 1—only 0.4!

In this chapter, essentially the heart of the recommended program, you are going to see you how you can actually eat your way out of high blood pressure—or at least into improved health and longer life. As we will show, you don't have to give up many of your favorite foods; by following our simple suggestions for preparing your meals, you will be able to reap the benefits of our program with very little effort.

We will start in the supermarket, where important choices are made. Then, when you have the right foods at home, we will show you the best ways to prepare them so that your meals have a high K Factor and so that your body can regain its balance. At the end of this chapter, you will get some tips on what to avoid and what to select when you are eating out.

SELECTING YOUR FOODS: IN THE SUPERMARKET

Is this program going to impose another rigid diet, like all the other diets? Don't you have enough restrictions in your life already? Are you expected to starve, or to eat only tasteless food?

Not at all! The suggestions made here are not only good for you but are excellent-tasting as well. Mother Nature gave us foods that are fine for us. Foods with a high K Factor—that are also generally high in magnesium and low in fat—are plentiful, tasty, and healthy. In fact, you won't have to eat *anything* you don't like.

Hard to believe? A shopping list that contains foods that are tasty and healthy is included at the end of this section. But first, we want to present you with some simple nutritional principles to guide you on your way.

In most cases, it's not the food that's harmful—it's what we do to it that hurts us. That means you can eat almost whatever type of food you like, provided the K Factor hasn't been lowered in the manufacturing plant (or later in your own kitchen).

The success or failure of our program begins in the supermarket. The following are key points in selecting food that can lower your blood pressure to normal levels and make you feel better and live longer:

• Select foods with a high K Factor
• Select foods with enough calcium and magnesium
• Select low-fat foods
• Avoid commercially prepared foods with added sodium

In food shopping, these key points direct you to whole grains, fresh vegetables and fruits, and *non*fat* dairy products. Deemphasize most processed foods, fast foods, and junk foods.

In addition to this simple profile, your shopping will avoid commercially prepared foods containing added sodium, such as most canned foods and junk foods. And you will find alternatives to the use of table salt.

SELECT FOODS WITH A HIGH K FACTOR

The first point of the magic four is to buy foods that naturally have a high K Factor. These include fresh vegetables (including potatoes), fresh fruits (not just bananas), skim or low-fat milk and yogurt, grains (including rice), chicken, fish, lean meat—in fact, almost any food that has not had its naturally high K Factor diminished in commercial processing.

Potatoes—The Perfect Food

The lowly potato, as it comes out of the ground, is excellent. Why? Not only do potatoes have a potassium-to-sodium ratio of approximately 130 to 1, or a K Factor of 130, but in addition, only 1% of their calories come from fat. The potato has gotten an undeservedly bad reputation. Too many people think potatoes cause weight gain, but it's not the potatoes—it's the grease they're fried in or the gravy, sour cream, or butter they're topped with.

It's been said that milk is a perfect food, but in fact, potatoes are even better in several respects. For example, milk's K Factor is only 2.8, and 50% of the calories of whole milk come from fat, compared to potatoes with a K Factor of 130 and 1% fat.

Table 3 shows the percent of an adult woman's National Academy of Sciences Recommended Dietary Allowances (RDA) of vitamins and minerals she would get if she ate all her daily 2000 calories as milk (3 quarts of whole milk or 6 quarts of skim milk) or as 4.6 pounds of potatoes (11 medium-sized potatoes).

---

*So-called low-fat dairy products can be misleading. Two percent milk is 98% fat free only because milk is mostly water; actually, one glass of 2% milk contains as much fat as two pats of butter. One recent frozen dinner advertised itself as 98% fat free! But upon inspection of the contents, you could see that again that is because food is mostly water, and when computing the percent of fat on the basis of total calories in this particular "98% fat free" food, the fat content is 28%.

TABLE 3

PERCENT OF AN ADULT WOMAN'S RDA OF VITAMINS AND MINERALS OBTAINABLE FROM MILK OR POTATOES

VITAMIN OR MINERAL	PERCENT RDA FROM 3 QUARTS WHOLE MILK	PERCENT RDA FROM 6 QUARTS SKIM MILK	PERCENT RDA FROM 4.6 POUNDS POTATOES
Vitamin A	114	294	trace
Vitamin B$_1$	91	212	220
Vitamin B$_2$	443	667	75
Niacin	23	36	282
Vitamin C	51	78	717
Calcium	443	876	24
Phosphorus	384	725	175
Iron	trace	13	84*

*For males, it would be 151%.

A pure whole-milk diet would be deficient in vitamin B$_1$, but a skim-milk diet of the same number of calories would not, because skim milk is fortified with extra vitamin B$_1$. A milk diet (either kind) would be deficient in niacin, vitamin C, and iron. A pure potato diet would be deficient in vitamin A, vitamin B$_2$, some essential amino acids, calcium, and iron (the latter is true only for women).

Each has ample supplies of what the other lacks; in essence they are complementary. A super good combination is a baked potato with low-fat yogurt on it.

Other High-K-Factor Foods

Pasta (spaghetti, linguini, elbow macaroni, spiral and flat noodles) is excellent, since it is low in sodium and fat and high in potassium, complex carbohydrates, and fiber. Since you should get most of your calories from complex carbohydrates, you can eat pasta as often as you like—just watch what's in the sauce and remember not to add table salt to the cooking water.

All legumes have a very high K Factor. These include dried pinto, red, black, navy, garbanzo (chick-pea), and kidney beans as well as dried lentils and split peas. An added bonus is that legumes are cheap and easy to store.

Virtually all fresh fruits are excellent sources of potassium—not only the famous banana, but oranges, grapefruits, grapes, pears, peaches, apricots, pineapples, mangoes, and plums. And remember the Japanese study cited in Chapter 5 that showed that six apples a day keep both the doctor and high blood pressure away! If you like them, dried fruits, including raisins, dates, pears, apples, bananas, peaches, and apricots, are handy to have for snacks and for cooking.

Fortunately, some freezer foods do not have added sodium and offer the convenience of immediate availability. Frozen vegetables, fruits, and fruit-juice concentrates (orange juice has a very high K Factor) are good choices.

If you read about nutrition, you may worry that a plan that excludes most red meat might be deficient in iron, but many other foods are rich in iron. You can meet your iron needs by eating the dried fruits we just listed or sunflower seeds, oysters, clams, peas, or beans. Most of these also have a very high K Factor. Multivitamin supplements containing iron offer another option. Since women require more iron than men, some recommend that all premenopausal women take daily iron supplements.

Rice, especially brown rice and wild rice, is very good, as are barley, bulgur wheat, buckwheat, and bran. Flour, especially whole wheat and potato, is good and can be used in many ways.

For snacks, popcorn can't be beat if it's prepared as we describe later. Provided they aren't covered with fat or sodium-containing batter or sauces, chicken breast, turkey breast, and fish (lean fish such as bass, cod, halibut, salmon steaks, red snapper, and sole) are good for you and good to have on hand. Eating seafood is especially important. Since you will be eliminating all table salt, including iodized salt, you could develop an iodine deficiency. Seafood—from the ocean—is a good source of iodine. On top of that, seafood is rich in "omega-3" polyunsaturated fatty acids, which lower your risk of heart attack.[2]

SELECT FOODS WITH ENOUGH CALCIUM AND MAGNESIUM

Adults need at least 400 mg of magnesium and at least 1000 mg of calcium each day, according to the current U.S. RDA (Recommended Dietary Allowances set by the U.S. Food and Drug Administration, based on the 1980 National Academy of Sciences Report). The U.S. RDA for pregnant women is 1300 mg for calcium and 450 mg for magnesium. Some nutritionists recommend up to 1500 mg of calcium a day (especially for postmenopausal women), 500 mg of magnesium for all adults, and even more for pregnant or older women. There is evidence that a deficiency in either calcium[3] or magnesium[4] can contribute to the development of hypertension, especially hypertension associated with pregnancy.

Calcium is found primarily in dairy products. Skim milk or low-fat or no-fat yogurt are excellent low-calorie sources of calcium. They also have a relatively high K Factor (about 3). However, beware of cheese, which usually contains a lot of added sodium as well as a lot of fat; the payoff in calcium isn't worth it in this case. As we said before, unsalted Swiss cheese (which can be obtained at health food stores and some supermarkets), ricotta, and dry cottage cheese are acceptable. Many people who can't digest the lactose in milk do well with yogurt. You can now buy lactose-free milk in many groceries.

Getting enough magnesium is also important for preventing and alleviating high blood pressure. Fortunately, foods that have a high K Factor tend to have adequate amounts of magnesium as well. Nuts, whole grains, beans, shrimp, bananas, and green leafy vegetables are among the good sources of magnesium. Go easy on the nuts, however, for they are high in fat. Eating a few nuts is okay, since some of the fats are unsaturated, especially in walnuts. Chestnuts are low in total fat.

SELECT LOW-FAT FOODS

Whereas dietary fat may not play a large role in causing hypertension, it certainly does play a significant role in causing obesity. Chapter 7 explores the relationship of obesity itself (often the result of overindulgence in fatty foods) to hypertension.

We believe it is important to decrease your dietary fat intake to no more than 20% of the calories you take in each day. Although it is disputed, there is some evidence (discussed in Chapter 8) that a diet low in fat, and the majority of that fat polyunsaturated (that is, liquid vegetable oils), can lower high blood pressure. But the main reason for keeping fat low is to prevent heart attacks, atherosclerosis, and cancer.

A ten-year study, completed under the direction of the National Heart, Lung and Blood Institute, clearly shows that reducing blood cholesterol (by avoiding the cholesterol and saturated fats from animal fat) greatly decreases the chance of having a heart attack or other complications caused by atherosclerosis (deposits of fat in the arteries).[5] Dr. Dean Ornish[6] and his colleagues conducted studies that clearly demonstrate that changing your lifestyle, including lowering dietary fat, can actually *reverse* damage to coronary arteries. The American Heart Association (AHA) recommends that in addition to decreasing dietary cholesterol, we should keep our consumption of fat to no more than 30% of our total calories. Yet in spite of all this evidence, Americans are still obtaining, on the average, 37% of their calories from dietary fat.

If you are an American male, the chances are 1 in 2 that your blood cholesterol is elevated (above 200 mg of cholesterol per 100 ml of blood). If you are one of those with elevated blood cholesterol, the AHA recommends that you cut the fat intake down to 25%, or even 20%. The AHA also recommends that more than half of all the fat you do eat be polyunsaturated, such as that found in liquid vegetable oils. Because of all the damaging effects of fat and the fact that you don't need very much, we believe everybody should shoot for that 20% limit on fat.

Butter, sour cream, and cream are almost pure fat. On top of that, the usual salted butter also has a high sodium content. So these three items are to be avoided if at all possible. At first thought, that might seem difficult—but don't worry, there are healthy and tasty substitutes.

You do not need oil for salad dressings, as we explain later in this chapter. But for those of you who insist on dressings with some fat, use polyunsaturated oils.

For table use, safflower oil is highest in polyunsaturates and is a nice light oil for salad dressings. Buy it in small quantities and refrigerate to keep it fresh. For a butter flavor, soy oil is available with butter flavoring to use in cooking. Look for it in the popcorn section of your grocery store.

Nonstick cookware can reduce or eliminate the need for fat in your cooking. However, a small amount of oil can greatly improve some recipes without adding undue fat. For high-temperature cooking, such as deep frying and wok cooking, try corn oil; while not quite as high in polyunsaturates as safflower oil, it does have a higher smoking point. But limit the amount of deep fried foods you eat, and drain them well before eating.

In general, the longer the shelf life of a fat at room temperature, the higher it is in saturated fat and therefore the worse it is for your heart and circulatory system. Lard and hydrogenated vegetable oils (the ones that are solid at room temperature), such as palm oil and coconut oil, keep without refrigeration for many months, but unfortunately they're the ones that are bad for you. The liquid oils we recommend instead should be fresh; don't buy the giant economy size, and throw away any rancid oils.

Keep in mind that cake and muffin mixes also contain fats. They keep a long time on the grocer's shelf, a clue that the fats are saturated. These mixes are also high in sodium.

Several studies have shown that the "omega-3" polyunsaturated fatty acids found in fish oils are especially beneficial in helping to reduce blood pressure,[7] blood cholesterol level,[8] and the risk of heart attack.[9]

AVOID COMMERCIALLY PREPARED FOODS WITH ADDED SODIUM

Cut out most canned food and most junk food unless it is clearly labeled unsalted or no added salt (not just low salt). Stay away from commercial frozen dinners or prepackaged "instant" meals. Although some are now low in fat, not many are low enough in sodium. Stay away from fast foods, most of which are loaded with sodium and fat.

Commercial Food Processing

Over the past several decades, Americans have used more and more canned and otherwise processed foods. Before canning, the food companies may put some vegetables into a salt solution to separate the ripe ones, which float, from the overripe ones, which sink. Canned whole tomatoes and some canned or frozen fruits may be bathed in a solution of sodium hydroxide to remove their peel. The canning process usually involves boiling the food, which leaches out the potassium. The tasteless result is then flavored with sodium chloride. All this tends to replace the potassium with sodium. So with too little potassium and all the added sodium, most processed food has a very low K Factor.

Processed Vegetables and Fruits

Whereas fresh peas contain almost no sodium and have a K Factor of 160, most canned peas contain very large amounts of sodium and have a K Factor of only 0.4. So canned peas have a K Factor that is three hundred times lower than fresh peas. The same large decrease in the K Factor is usually found in canned corn and beans as well. Pass up most canned food. To take just one example: Campbell's cream of mushroom soup contains 400 mg of sodium per *half* can. But Campbell's *also* makes some low-sodium soups with only about 100 mg of sodium per can.

Much frozen food should also be avoided. Plain frozen peas may not have sodium added, but those frozen with prepared sauce usually do. Your job is to learn to pick and choose. For example, the amount of sodium in frozen apples ranges from 2 to 200 mg per 100 grams. Watch out for frozen green beans in butter sauce; not only do they have a lot of fat, some have as much as 255 mg of sodium per half-cup serving. Some frozen lasagna has as much as 855 mg of sodium per package. One half of a small frozen pizza may have 1000 mg of sodium.[10] That's 11 times your minimum daily requirement and half of your *maximum* daily allowance!

Processed Meats

Sodium salts are added to processed meats. Although most fresh meats have a reasonably high K Factor, processed meats, including hot dogs, pork sausage, bacon, smoked ham, and cold cuts such as bologna and salami, not only have unacceptably low K Factors but are also high in fat. Spam has 840 mg of sodium per 3-ounce serving. Ordinary fresh beef may be 30% fat, even with the visible fat trimmed off. Compare this to the wild animals our ancestors ate, which were less than 5% fat.[11] Fish, skinned chicken, and turkey have less fat than beef and pork. Thus, unsalted turkey or chicken breast, or unsalted water-packed tuna, makes good sandwich meat. An occasional thin slice of roast beef is okay.

Breads

Unless they are marked low salt, beware of most commercially baked breads. As you can see from the table in Chapter 13, most commercially prepared English muffins have an unacceptably low K Factor of about 0.1. Some bakeries are making unsalted bread, or you can bake your own without table salt. Yeast does not need added salt. You can get away with a couple of slices of commercial whole grain bread if you're sensible about the other foods you eat.

Desserts

Unfortunately for those of you with a sweet tooth, most commercially prepared desserts have a low K Factor. Besides, sugar is bad for your teeth and may overstimulate the secretion of insulin, a hormone that stimulates both appetite and the conversion of calories to fat. So most commercially prepared desserts should be avoided.

Fortunately, there are some exceptions. Packaged gelatin dessert mixes have only moderate amounts of sodium. At home, with some flavorful fruit juice and plain gelatin, you can make no-sodium ones. For added interest, whip the gelatin when it has just begun to gel and add some fruit. You can even add a dollop of "whipped cream" made by beating together equal parts of powdered milk and water, and adding a few drops of lemon juice, vanilla, and perhaps some artificial sweetener.

Rice or tapioca puddings and cornstarch-based puddings can be made without table salt. Since angel-food cake and meringues are made with egg whites and not yolks or shortening and can be made without table salt, they are also good. If you hanker for cheesecake, try avoiding the fat this way: Dissolve a package of lemon gelatin dessert in 1½ cups of hot water, cool until slightly firm, then whip. Put a pint of cottage cheese through a sieve or puree it in the blender, then add to the whipped gelatin, sweeten to taste, add a few drops of vanilla, and pour into a cake pan and leave in the refrigerator until firm.

Except for the sugar, sherbets or fruit ices are healthy low-salt, low-fat desserts. If you like fresh fruits, which have a high K Factor, these are excellent for dessert.

Surprise—we saved the best for the last: you can make a *hot fudge banana split* (with nuts no less) that has only 29% of the calories from fat and a K Factor of about 8! Split one banana, use one cup of ice milk (*not* ice cream), top with 1 tbs. cocoa powder dissolved in about 2 oz. boiling water (no sugar and you don't need sweetener), and sprinkle with ¼ oz. walnuts. Don't eat this *too* often though, because it does have 365 calories and there's a good deal of sugar in the ice milk.

Junk Foods

The term "junk food" is no misnomer. Junk food contains not only too much sodium but also too much fat. Avoid all salted nuts, potato chips, and most crackers (Ritz crackers, for example, have 240 mg of sodium per 1-ounce serving). Some low-salt whole-grain crackers are available.

Caution: "Low-sodium" is not sodium-free. If you like, eat the low-sodium food—but keep the sodium very low in the other things you eat that day. Some newer canned foods are really low in sodium.

Other Foods to Avoid

Most people would recognize the following foods as salty: olives, anchovies, canned sardines, commercially prepared dill pickles, soy sauce, and bacon. Other high-salt foods include most breads, cheeses, most peanut butters, canned tomato juice (unless it's unsalted), V-8 juice (unless it's the low-salt variety), creamed cottage cheese, instant pudding, and most instant hot cereals. Most of the regular hot cereals are fine if you don't add table salt. Most cold cereals should be avoided as well; for example, Wheaties has 200 mg of sodium per 1-ounce serving. But several low-salt brands, such as Nabisco Shredded Wheat, are very good. Club soda has 93 mg of sodium per 12-ounce serving, and low-sodium sparkling water has almost none.

Avoid Softened Water

Most water softeners work by replacing calcium, magnesium, and other minerals that make water "hard" with sodium; thus, softened water is loaded with sodium. Not only that, the magnesium and calcium that are removed would have been good for you. If you have a water softener, make sure it is hooked up only to the hot water side of your plumbing, and avoid using hot water for cooking or drinking. You might also want to check to see if your local water supply has a significant amount of natural sodium. Check with the local water treatment companies; some of them have water treatment systems that replace sodium with potassium.

Over-the-Counter Drugs

Finally, watch out for nonprescription drugs. According to *Consumer Reports*, Vicks' Formula 44 has 105 mg of sodium per 2-teaspoon dose. Rolaids antacid has 70 mg per 2-tablet dose. Alka-Seltzer has 935 mg per 2-tablet dose—this is one half the maximum daily allowance of sodium in our recommendations! So if you're getting an over-the-counter medicine, first read the label or ask your pharmacist.

THE GOOD NEWS

Fortunately, not all food processing lowers the K Factor. Bulk packaged oatmeal, creamed wheat cereal, and other hot cereals cooked without added sodium chloride have a high K Factor. Beware, though: while individual serving packets of instant hot cereal are convenient, they are likely to be presalted. Several types of dry breakfast cereals, including puffed wheat, puffed rice, shredded wheat, and some of the granolas, are unsalted and have a high K Factor. Unfortunately, many of the granolas contain saturated fats such as palm or coconut oils.

Gradually, food companies are responding to the demand for low-sodium, healthy foods. Campbell's, Hunt's, Del Monte, several of the supermarket chain brands, and others have come out with various unsalted canned foods. Herb-Ox makes very good salt-free chicken and beef instant broths, which can be used in soups and also as a seasoning in a wide variety of dishes. More unsalted food products are appearing on the market every day.

Most cheeses have added sodium salt, but unsalted cheese can be obtained at health food stores and some supermarkets. Unsalted Swiss cheese tastes just as good as the regular Swiss: A single thin slice is flavorful and won't add too much fat to your diet. Ricotta and dry curd cottage cheese (not creamed) have less sodium than creamed cottage cheese and are low in fat as well.

Nonfat dry milk, cornstarch, low-sodium baking powder, gelatin, and quick-cooking tapioca are good items to have on hand. Several old standby products never did have added sodium. Tomato paste is good and, when diluted, will do many of the things a salted tomato sauce will do. In recipes calling for tomato sauce, you can still add the herbs, wine, mushrooms, green pepper, onion, garlic—everything tasty but sodium chloride (table salt).

Remember your goal: good health. It's worth the effort to look for unsalted prepared foods. Ask the store manager to order them if you can't find them.

Study the table in Part Four and avoid the items in italics except on rare occasions, go for the boldfaced items, and use your judgment on the others (they are okay in moderation). If you shop around, it is possible to buy unsalted mustard, catsup, potato chips, crackers, low-fat cheeses, and so on.

How Can You Tell?

How can you determine the K Factor in processed foods? Only if the label lists both the potassium and the sodium content. If it does, divide the milligrams of potassium by the milligrams of sodium to get the K Factor. It's as simple as that. A glance will tell you if the K Factor is over 1 (there is more potassium than sodium). Until the amount of potassium is listed on all labels, your best bet is to *avoid foods with more than about 100 mg of sodium per serving.*

The U.S. Food and Drug Administration (FDA) now requires the sodium content to be stated. Unfortunately, potassium content labeling is left entirely up to the manufacturer.

Use Substitutes for Table Salt

As you should recognize by now (and see Chapter 16), you just do not need table salt (sodium chloride). It doesn't belong on your table or in your cooking. Food in its natural state has plenty of sodium—all you need. So don't buy table salt, and get rid of the supply you already have at home.

Potassium-Containing Salt Substitutes

At the table and in your cooking, potassium-containing salt substitutes can be used instead of table salt.

It's best that the increase in potassium intake be achieved primarily through a return to a more natural diet. The natural potassium in food is generally safe because it is absorbed slowly and because it occurs as organic salts rather than as just potassium chloride. But moderate use of commercially available potassium-containing salt substitutes helps increase the K Factor in your diet, both by replacing salt (sodium chloride) and by increasing potassium.

These salt substitutes are commonly available on grocery shelves. Be aware that some contain sodium: read the label.

Do read the precautions on the label, and also consult with your doctor before using a salt substitute, as too much potassium could cause problems if you are taking a potassium-sparing diuretic or if you have kidney or heart disease.

Other Ways to Season Without Salt

There are other ways around salt besides just salt substitutes. Vegit is a versatile seasoning, Lawry's Seasoned Salt-Free adds more familiar flavor to many saltless dishes, and Mrs. Dash adds a peppery note where appropriate. Mrs. Dash steak sauce is a tangy blend of herbs and spices that is good on many things other than steak, for example, spaghetti, rice, Chinese cabbage, and vegetables. Bitters is a neglected but very useful addition to many salt-free dishes. Bell's poultry seasoning can be used for more than stuffing a turkey; many meats profit from the touch of sage it provides. Lemon and its juice are very useful for many foods besides fish. Lemon juice dresses salads, with or without a little oil.

Curry is certainly an authoritative flavor, as are chili and Tabasco. Dry mustard enlivens many foods, especially salad dressings and sauces for vegetables. Horseradish can be found fresh in some markets (Caution: the jars of prepared horseradish usually contain salt).

It's amazing how much savory flavoring onion or garlic, sauteed in a little unsaturated oil, can provide a dish. Without salt, in any recipe, the flavors of onion and garlic—and most other spices as well—will be more pronounced.

Avoid Baking Soda and Baking Powder

Actually, salt (sodium chloride) is not the only sodium compound you should avoid. Common baking soda is sodium bicarbonate, which is also one of the ingredients of baking powder. Remember, you're cutting sodium, so don't use ordinary baking powder in foods you bake. Low-sodium baking powder, such as Golden Harvest, is available at health food stores. (This brand contains potassium bicarbonate and thus actually helps boost your K Factor.)

SHOPPING LISTS

The following shopping lists provide a quick look at the foods that are healthy and unhealthy if you are working toward lowering your daily sodium intake and boosting the K Factor in your diet. With lists like these, you will be selecting foods that prolong your life—and keep your palate happy.

HEALTHY SHOPPING LIST

FRESH MEATS

chicken or turkey breast
fresh fish (or frozen without
  sodium)
clams or oysters

VEGETABLES AND FRUITS

potatoes
fresh peas, beans, corn
romaine, escarole, and other
  lettuces
fresh spinach
fresh green or red peppers
fresh mushrooms
onions, garlic
fresh horseradish
lemons, oranges, and apples
bananas
frozen orange juice concentrate
dried dates and apricots
raisins

GRAINS AND CEREALS

pasta (spaghetti, noodles, etc.)
brown rice
dried beans, lentils, peas
flour
bulgur wheat
shredded wheat (unsalted)
puffed rice or puffed wheat
  (unsalted)
cooked oats (when cooking hot
  cereals, do not add salt as per
  instructions on the package)
creamed wheat cereal
any other "unsalted" brands
low-sodium breads
matzo crackers (no sodium, egg,
  or fat)
"no salt added" crackers

DAIRY

skim milk
lowfat yogurt
ricotta cheese
unsalted Swiss cheese

CONDIMENTS, PACKAGED FOODS, OTHERS

orange sherbet
low-sodium baking powder
unsalted mustard
sunflower seeds
curry powder, chili powder
fresh-ground peanut butter
  (unsalted)
safflower oil (small bottle)
"no salt added" catsup, tomato
  paste, and spaghetti sauce
wine vinegar (or other brands)
low-sodium creamy garlic salad
  dressing
cranberry sauce or cranberry-
  orange relish
Angostura bitters
low-sodium tuna in water
"no salt added" pink salmon
"no salt added" soups
water chestnuts (not canned)
vegetarian chili (unsalted)
some brands of dry ("instant")
  potatoes (but check label and
  do not add sodium as per
  instructions)
any brand of canned or bottled
  fruit or fruit juices (apple sauce
  or juice, pineapple, etc.)
any brand of canned vegetables *if
  labeled "no salt added"*

For those of you who already have hypertension, it is *vital* that you avoid foods on the following list. (For the one out of three or four people who have a genetic potential to develop hypertension, the following food shopping list is a sure way to produce hypertension and its consequences.)

AN UNHEALTHY SHOPPING LIST

MEATS

smoked ham
hot dogs
pork sausage
bacon
bologna
frozen chicken (breaded and
    seasoned)
canned meats

VEGETABLES AND FRUIT JUICE

canned peas, canned corn (unless
    unsalted)
canned tomatoes (unless un-
    salted)
tomato juice (unless unsalted)
frozen french fries (salted)

DAIRY

butter
creamed cottage cheese
cream
sour cream
ice cream
most cheeses

OTHER FOODS

soy sauce
table salt (NaCl)
potato chips (unless unsalted)
English muffins
dill pickles
olives
the vast majority of frozen
    dinners (look at the label)
most frozen pizza

Using the Shopping Lists for Decreasing Blood Pressure

Feel free to eat anything on the healthy shopping list. On a day that you might get stuck with a meal with a low K Factor, eat only items on the healthy list or boldfaced items from the table in Chapter 13 for the rest of the day.

Again, the key to our approach is what you eat *and* how it's prepared. We want to emphasize that not only is this program good for your blood pressure, but it should decrease your chance of having a heart attack as well, since it automatically cuts the fat you eat to levels at or below those recently recommended by the American Heart Association in order to prevent heart attacks. Not only that, but it turns out that low fat, high-fiber eating programs such as this one probably decrease your chances of getting some kinds of cancer.

This program is good for your blood pressure and good for your heart, and helps prevent some types of cancer. So it's your choice. You will live with the consequences. You can either adopt this eating program, or go ahead eating your way into not only hypertension but heart attacks, strokes, and perhaps cancer. You can eat to live and be healthy, or you can eat so you will ruin your health, live poorly, and maybe die before your time. If you want to live longer and not only enjoy good health but enjoy your food, read on.

PREPARING YOUR MEALS: IN THE KITCHEN

Now that you've selected your foods in the grocery store, it's time to use them in preparing healthy—and appetizing—meals. Once you understand the simple principles we described here, it's easy. Because this eating program is based upon natural principles, it will allow you to eat almost any food you want—provided it is prepared correctly. So once you've made the change, you'll forget you ever ate food prepared the wrong way—the way that leads to high blood pressure.

This section will show you how to plan your meals to obtain the highest possible K Factor, thereby reducing (or avoiding) high blood pressure, and it also offers you some tips in food preparation to ensure that foods with a naturally high K Factor do not lose potassium in the cooking.

At the end of this chapter two weeks' worth of specific menus are given to get you started, as well as some general suggestions for planning your menus.

Before looking at the specific suggestions for meals, consider the following general guidelines for breakfasts, lunches, dinners, and snacks:

BREAKFAST

Nutritionists say that breakfast is the most important meal of the day, since you have been the longest without food. A recent study done in Minnesota indicates that this is especially true if you are overweight. A large number of overweight women who volunteered for this study were randomly divided into two groups. Both groups ate exactly the same foods, totaling 2000 calories, every day. One group ate all of their food in the morning; the other group ate all of their food in the evening. Almost all of the women in the first group lost weight, whereas the women in the second group either gained weight or maintained the same weight they started with. This is because activity gears your metabolism to burn calories, whereas rest gears your body to store calories as fat. So don't skip breakfast!

For breakfast, always have fruit and/or fruit juice. Fresh whole fruits are best. If you use canned tomato or V-8 juice, use a brand that doesn't have added sodium. In the menus that follow, we often list orange juice because it's easily available year-round, but substitute fresh fruit when possible. Low-fat yogurt with fruit or preserves stirred into it makes an excellent breakfast.

If you have toast, use unsalted bread. (If you can't find it in a health food store or in the supermarket, you can make it at home.)

If you make hot cereal, don't add table salt. Use cinnamon or a salt substitute if it tastes too flat to you. Because of the saturated fat problem, we recommend 1% fat, ½% fat, or—best of all—skim milk on your cereal. Almost any fruits are good on cereal—bananas, strawberries, blueberries, peaches, apricots, dates, raisins. For more sweetening, add a sugar substitute or a small amount of brown sugar, molasses, or maple syrup. The last three have more flavor than white sugar, and provide some minerals as well, but nevertheless are primarily sugar (sucrose) and should be used sparingly.

One good idea is the breakfast potato, which is rich in potassium and low in fat. Having a potato for breakfast is actually an old American practice first used by farmers and cowboys, and it is still popular in the South and parts of the West. An interesting breakfast variation is our modern version of the potato pancake. Simply shred one or two potatoes, without peeling, add some minced onion, and fry in a pan coated with a thin layer of unsaturated cooking oil. Serve with applesauce or yogurt. Potatoes and milk complement each other's nutritional deficiencies.

LUNCH

Include fresh fruit in your lunch. Raisins, dates, dried apricots, or other dried fruits make a nice addition. Since unsalted nuts are loaded with potassium, they make a good choice, but take it easy, because they do contain a lot of fat.

Whenever possible, use unsalted bread for sandwiches. Between the slices use lettuce or sprouts, unsalted mustard, and unsalted tuna (from the health food store), or chicken, or turkey. As we mentioned earlier, a thin slice of unsalted Swiss cheese or a moderate layer of unsalted peanut butter is okay. Salads are excellent for lunch. If you brown-bag it, try carrot sticks, florets of broccoli or cauliflower, radishes, or slices of zucchini; they're all refreshing and rich in potassium. If you don't carry your lunch, head for the salad bar for lots of almost any raw vegetables and fruits. But do watch out for pickled vegetables, which have an alarming amount of sodium, and for dressings, which are usually salty and loaded with fat. Be a purist and use vinegar or lemon juice with a small amount of unsaturated oil such as safflower oil, sunflower seed oil, or olive oil (or even better, skip the oil).

Soups that do not contain cream or whole milk or added table salt are excellent. They tend to be low in calories yet filling as well as tasty and nutritious.

DINNER

What if your hectic schedule leads you to arrive home late, too bushed to cook? Are high-K-Factor meals out of the question? By no means! It takes just a bit more time than using a frozen dinner. Broil lean meat, or broil or steam fish. Microwave potatoes in 5 to 10 minutes. Pasta cooks quickly; add herbs instead of table salt to the cooking water. Combination meals can be thrown together in minutes with leftovers and previously cooked rice. You'll have a meal in short order.

Keep fresh fruits and vegetables in your refrigerator for quick salads. Some unsalted canned vegetables, including beets, corn, beans, and sweet potato, are still tasty. However, beans are not very tasty when unsalted, so add spices and a little salt substitute. Frozen vegetables (without prepared sauces, which are invariably salty) can be heated in very little time, especially in a microwave oven.

Many traditional recipes work out very well with the simple omission of table salt. With any recipe, this is worth a try.

Onion can be the cook's best friend. When in doubt about how to prepare a good sodium-free meal, fry a few slices of onion in a little unsaturated oil in a pan and the aroma will give you confidence that the rest of the meal will materialize. This is also a boost for the spouse who arrives home first, so the one who arrives home second, starving, will find olfactory comfort wafting from the kitchen to the hall, driveway, or sidewalk. Garlic is as useful as ever, and the whole array of fresh and dried herbs and spices can provide new sodium-free excitement.

Remember, potatoes aren't fattening as long as you don't use fatty toppings like butter or sour cream. You can make a topping that tastes almost the same as sour cream by using low-fat yogurt with a touch of lemon blended in.

Use more fish and poultry, which are also excellent sources of complete protein, as you cut down on the sodium and fat in meats, eggs and cheese. Vegetables and whole grains also provide protein. For example, legumes (beans, peas, and lentils) have almost as much protein as an egg.

In order for your body's cells to make proteins, all of the essential amino acids must be present in the body's cells at the same time. Because plant proteins are sometimes low on one or more of the essential amino acids, the building blocks of proteins, it is good practice to combine two or more types of vegetables or grains in a meal to make a more complete mixture of amino acids. Rice and beans are the classic example. The essential amino acids that are low in the rice are plentiful in beans, and vice versa. Other good protein pairs include corn tacos with beans, chili with corn bread, or skim milk on rice pudding.

It's not necessary to worry about this with each meal because no plant protein is totally deficient and some amino acids are present in your intestine and blood to help tide you over until the next meal. However, if you were to eat only one thing, such as rice, routinely, you would have to eat huge quantities to get enough of each essential amino acid.

For a complete explanation, see *Diet for a Small Planet*, by Frances Moore Lappé (Tenth Anniversary Edition, Ballantine Books). In this book, Lappé points out that provided you don't eat one single food or a diet that is almost completely fruits, or sweet potatoes, or junk food, it is almost impossible not to get enough complete protein if you eat enough calories to maintain your ideal weight. For example, per calorie, spinach is 49% protein—more than a cooked hamburger patty, which on a calorie basis is only 39% protein (and 58% fat). Spinach is also rich in magnesium; perhaps Popeye knew what he was doing after all!

One word of caution: Spinach contains oxalic acid, which ties up calcium so that you can't absorb it. You can neutralize the oxalic acid by adding calcium when you cook spinach (milk, for example). Also, since spinach is low in calories, you won't get much protein from a normal portion.

SNACKS

The bad snacks are the ones that are high in fat, sodium, and/or sugar, such as commercial doughnuts, ice cream, fatty cheeses, candy bars, and salted potato chips. Good snacks should not have added sodium or sugar and should be low in fat.

Don't despair—popcorn can be great for you! If possible, use a hot air popper or use a very small quantity of oil. Flavor with brewer's yeast or no-salt seasoning, or use a potassium-containing salt substitute instead of table salt. Prepared this way, popcorn is not only tasty but low in fat while high in fiber and complex carbohydrate.

Because of their high K Factor, fruits or raw vegetables make excellent snacks. Nuts have a very high K Factor, but go lightly because of their high fat content. Unsalted pretzels, low-fat crackers, and corn or flour tortillas (buy them fresh and toast them) all make healthy snacks (unsalted or salted with salt substitutes, of course). To make a dip for your crackers, chips, or tortillas, mix some unsalted hot pepper sauce and/or some unsalted fresh horseradish into some low-fat yogurt.

Eat snacks early in the day, so that you will burn off the calories. *Just before bed is probably the worst time to eat,* because most of the calories may end up as fat.

SELECTING YOUR MEALS: IN THE RESTAURANT

Obviously, you will need to select foods high in the K Factor when you are dining out just as much as when you are shopping in the supermarket. Since you cannot control how the food has been selected or prepared in a restaurant, you need to be especially wary. While you are somewhat at the mercy of our habits of food preparation, there are some things you can do.

First we'll give you a few specific examples of good things to order. For breakfast: fresh fruit (orange, grapefruit, melon, banana, etc.) and pancakes (no butter, light on syrup), oatmeal, poached egg white on whole wheat toast, or shredded wheat. For lunch: turkey breast sandwich on whole wheat bread with no table salt, no pickle, but lots of tomato and lettuce, or salad in a pita bread pocket (preferably whole wheat). For dinner: fish, other seafood, white meat of chicken or turkey, or go vegetarian. For a beverage: skim milk, low-salt sparkling water (e.g., Perrier) with lemon or lime, or fruit juice. For dessert: fresh fruit (apple, berries, peach, pineapple, mixed fruit cup, melon, etc.).

If your physician has okayed your use of a salt substitute, take it with you when you eat out, and use it instead of table salt.

A number of restaurants are now specializing in the preparation of "heart-healthy" meals, which are low in sodium and fat. The American Heart Association is encouraging restaurants to do this through their Creative Cuisine program; call your local affiliate to see what's available in your area.

Other than fast foods, all cuisines offer some choices with a high K Factor. Be selective and give some thought to the foods as well as the method of preparation. Don't despair if nothing you can order is low in sodium. You can ask the chef not to add table salt and to go light on fat. Be creative about balancing the meal: If the filet of sole has a delicious sauce that contains sodium, balance it with a high-potassium salad and a baked potato topped with a grind of pepper and yogurt or cottage cheese (if the restaurant has it; you'll have to ask). When you order, consider how the food is prepared. Boiling causes the potassium to leach out of foods, whereas steaming, baking, and stir-frying produce no significant drop in the K Factor.

Beware of fast foods: almost all are high in sodium chloride and in fat. But don't just give up if trapped at a fast food restaurant—you can ask the chef not to add table salt! Even McDonald's will make unsalted fries on request. Salad bars are now available at many fast-food franchises (if you order chicken, though, don't eat the skin: you'll be able to eliminate most of the sodium and fat). A few pizza parlors now offer low-salt pizza with whole-wheat crust and healthy toppings such as tuna, mussels, chicken, or vegetables.

On the other hand, don't overcerebrate. Enjoy!

GETTING THE FAMILY TO GO ALONG

If you are starting the high-K-Factor diet because you have high blood pressure, it is a good idea for you to encourage your children to adopt the same diet. Since the tendency for high blood pressure is inherited, your children are likely to develop high blood pressure when they reach your age if they continue eating the usual American diet. Not only that, there is some evidence that even in people who have inherited the tendency, eating excess table salt in childhood may reset their system to make them even more sensitive to sodium in adulthood. You can prevent this by starting them on the proper diet now.

If your children live at home, they probably eat the same food you do. My co-author for *The K Factor,* Dr. George Webb, has found that his teenagers have gotten accustomed to high-K-Factor, low-fat foods, and they like most of them. Healthy snacks are on hand, so they can get their caloric needs with foods like unsalted whole wheat bread, sliced turkey, locally ground unsalted peanut butter, low-fat yogurt, a variety of fruits, oatmeal-raisin cookies, 0.5%-fat milk, cider, orange juice, cranapple juice, and the like. If your spouse doesn't have high blood pressure, he or she will probably want to eat the same food you do just to share the experience. The diet we are recommending has added appeal, since it is not only good for keeping your blood pressure down but also helps prevent coronary artery disease as well as some types of cancer.

COOKING TIPS

Keep in mind three principles:

- All cooking should be done without table salt.
- All vegetables should be steamed, baked, stir-fried, or microwaved rather than boiled.
- All meats should have as much fat removed as possible.

As we have said, many familiar recipes taste just as good without added table salt. Salt-free bread is just one example. Just omit the table salt from a standard recipe. We have made some delicious bread without table salt. Many of the quick breads (coffee cakes, muffins, cornbread) can be made with a low-sodium baking powder, such as the one made by Golden Harvest. Follow directions on the label: one and a half times the usual quantity of baking powder may be required.

If you must add salt during food preparation, use a recommended salt substitute to avoid the sodium.

And if you *must* use canned food for a favorite recipe, rinse and then wash the food first. One study found that draining water from canned food and then rinsing the food under tap water for 1 minute reduced the sodium content of canned green beans by 41% and that of canned tuna by 79%.[12] This probably removes some potassium also, but canned food often is deficient in this mineral to begin with; you'll have to get the extra potassium from other foods.

In the few cases where leaving out table salt makes the recipe unpalatable, some modifications are in order. The list of salt-free cookbooks increases almost daily. *Craig Claiborne's Gourmet Diet,* by Craig Claiborne with Pierre Franey (Ballantine Books, 1985), is good. An excellent guide for changing sodium-potassium balance is *How to Up Your Potassium,* by Corinne Azen Krause (William G. Johnston Company, 1979). If you can't find the latter in your book store, write to Potassium Cook Book, 7 Darlington Ct., Pittsburgh, PA 15217. The American Heart Association has published a good cookbook entitled *Cooking Without Your Salt Shaker.*

Boiling is out—but broiling, steaming, stir-frying, baking, or using a microwave oven are in. Boiling not only causes food to lose vitamins, but really lowers the K Factor. For example, raw potatoes have a K Factor of about 130. If the potatoes are boiled in even slightly salted water, the K Factor drops from about 130 down to between 1 and 3.[13] The same holds true for carrots, beans, and peas. Vegetables cooked in the microwave oven are crisply appealing, as well as rich in vitamins and minerals. Since some nutrients and flavors escape when you steam vegetables, save the small quantity of water remaining for a soup stock.

Since many traditional protein sources are high in saturated fats, we emphasize proteins from plant sources. When you do use meats, trim or skin off as much fat as possible.

MAKING THE TRANSITION

No matter how desirable, any change can be dangerous if it is made too quickly. If you turn the wheel of your car too fast, if you lose weight too fast, if you increase the amount of exercise you do too fast—all these sudden changes can get you in trouble. This is also true when increasing your K Factor. **It is very important that you** *do not* **change your eating style suddenly—this could be** *dangerous*. Remember, if you're like the typical American, your dietary K Factor is only about 10% of the minimum it should be. Paradoxically, when your body is deficient in potassium, it cannot tolerate as much as it would normally.[14] So it's necessary to build up slowly for about a week.

Therefore, we recommended in the beginning that you take at least a week to eliminate the salt you add at the table. The next two weeks can be spent changing your diet, using a 14-day menu plan like the one we provide in this section. Our intention in spelling out menus in detail is to offer you security and peace of mind by showing you exactly how to change your eating habits. Then for the first week of this plan, you should stop adding salt in your cooking as well as at the table.

The menus for the second week—Day 1 to Day 7 of the menu plan—are scientifically designed to provide a progressive increase in the K Factor of the average American diet. We gradually increase your K Factor from just under 1 to almost 4. **It is essential that this first seven days of menus be taken** *in order* **and** *not repeated*. If you have already been on a low-sodium diet, you should start at Day 3 or later. Otherwise you'll be taking a step backward.

The suggested meals represent standard American fare. If you have a healthy diet already—one high in fruits and vegetables, complex carbohydrates, and monounsaturated fatty acids—you may not suffer from hypertension. In any case, you should view these menus as suggestions and should not eat something you don't like. Comparable substitutions for many foods can be found in the table in Chapter 13. With growing awareness about healthy food choices, it is becoming easier all the time to eat a healthy diet.

This menu plan provides about 2000 calories per day, approximately the amount required for maintaining constant weight for an average middle-aged woman. Larger women and men and more active people will generally need to eat more. Smaller women, less active or older people, those who are reducing, or those whose metabolism is geared for storing fat will need to eat less. You can adjust for your particular caloric requirements by increasing or decreasing the portion sizes. Obviously, the sensible serving sizes for a petite great-grandmother and for a high school athlete are very different.

The menus for the third week—Day 8 to Day 14 of the menu plan—begin the maintenance period. They contain adequate vitamins, minerals, and amino acids.* These menus also contain sufficient iron for men, but several days are short of meeting the U.S. RDA for women (18 mg, as opposed to 10 mg for men). *Therefore, women should take daily iron supplements.*

Each day's plan is summarized in terms of total calories, percent of calories from fat sources, total potassium, total sodium, and, finally, the potassium-to-sodium ratio (the K Factor). The nutritional summaries given at the end of each day's plan allow for typical commercial bakery bread (except where specified otherwise), but you can probably find low-sodium bread instead, or bake your own, and thus lower your total sodium intake for the day.

Most of the fat you see listed is from plant sources and is high in polyunsaturates.

If you want recipes that emphasize reducing the fat in your diet and increasing unsaturated fats, a good one is *The American Heart Association Cookbook*, published by Ballantine Books. We also recommend the new booklet *Eating for a Healthy Heart*, which is available from your local affiliate of the AHA.

The snacks as listed can be shifted to the time of day you need them most; just remember, you're likely to store calories as fat at the end of the day. They can also be eliminated if you need a much lower caloric intake. Conversely, if you need more calories, enlarge the portions.

POINTS TO KEEP IN MIND

Remember the first seven days of menus should be taken *in order,* since they are planned to increase your K Factor at a rate designed to allow your body's cells sufficient time to adapt.[15] Do not return to the menus of Days 1–7 after you have completed them. For Days 8–14 you may shift days around, since all the menus have healthy K Factors. When an alternative choice is listed, nutritional data apply to the first choice. Eating the alternative food will make little, if any, significant change in the day's nutritional totals.

---

*These were checked using food tables and the Nutritionist III computer program by N-Squared Computing Co., Silverton, Oregon. The U.S. RDAs for all major vitamins, essential amino acids, iron, magnesium, and calcium were exceeded for the total recipes of the last week (see text regarding iron for women). An occasional day was short on one vitamin, which was more than compensated for on the next day.

Remember, once you get the hang of it, you can personally create substitute meals using the master chart given in Chapter 13.

As an example of getting used to this program, a registered nurse who read *The K Factor* wrote:

> I had been on blood pressure medication for about ten years when I decided that I wanted to find a way to live without medication. It was just then that I happened on your book, which I read avidly, and immediately set about implementing the formula . . . It was only three months until [with the advice of her doctor] I was able to stop medication. It has now been over a year and I'm still doing very well. I must admit that it took a long time before I could eat without calculating with pen and paper the milligrams of sodium and potassium—I would say the whole adjustment took about a year to be comfortable with and that's nothing compared to the 10 years on medication. . . . My internist is very pleased with the results. I gave him a copy of your book. . . . [Before starting the K Factor program] my blood pressure had been running about 145/95 with symptoms of dizziness whenever it was 140/90 or above. It now reads 110/70 most of the time. . . .
>
> Incidentally, keeping sodium that low is no problem anymore. My diet consists of fresh fruit, raw or steamed vegetables (in abundance), Baker's Bread (a brand made locally with low sodium and high multigrain taste), other simple whole grain cereals (such as oat bran, brown rice, buckwheat), skim milk, low sodium cheese, small amounts of chicken and fish cooked plain, occasional nuts. Everything is so simple and plain that I don't need to calculate anymore. Once in a blue moon I have some junk food, like fruit cobbler, and rationalize that at least it has fruit.

So once you get the hang of it, it's simple. But before you start, remember: No table salt should be added in the kitchen or at the table for any of these meals (and for the rest of your life).

THE PLAN

THE TRANSITION PERIOD

First Week

Eliminate table salt at the table and in cooking.

Second Week

Start the transition week of menus on Day 1—**do not repeat these menus**—and keep Days 1 through 7 in order. If you've been on a low-sodium diet, start with Day 3.

THE MAINTENANCE PERIOD

Third Week and Beyond

Starting with Day 8, your food has a K Factor of at least 4. By the end of the third week, you should be able to plan your own menus so that your daily K Factor is above 4.

Note: Calories are rounded to the nearest 50; sodium and potassium are rounded to the nearest 100 mg, except to the nearest 50 if under 1000.

DAY 1

BREAKFAST
8 oz Orange juice (from frozen concentrate)
1½ oz Cold cereal
8 oz Whole milk
1 Corn muffin

LUNCH
Lean hamburger on roll (catsup, 2 slices pickle)
1¼ oz Pretzels (adieu to these after today)

SNACK
1 Slice coconut custard pie

DINNER
10 oz Fish and chips dinner
½ cup Broccoli with cheese sauce
½ cup Instant butterscotch pudding

Calories (total for the day): 2000; **Fat (total for the day):** 74 g; **Calories from fat:** 37%; **Potassium (total for the day):** 2800 mg; **Sodium (total for the day):** 4200 mg*; **K Factor for the day:** 0.7 (potassium to sodium ratio = 0.7 to 1)

This day's total was calculated using values for a frozen fish and chips dinner, which definitely has too much sodium in it for later in the program. DO NOT REPEAT THIS DAY.

---

*If you are a heavy user of table salt, we are tapering your sodium down gradually. If you are already on a low salt diet, you should enter the menu program at day 3.

DAY 2

BREAKFAST
8 oz Orange juice
1½ oz Shredded wheat with 1 tsp sugar
½ cup Whole milk
English muffin (or buttermilk biscuits from packaged refrigerated dough would have about the same K Factor, but the fat content would be higher)
1 tbsp Jam

LUNCH
1 Bagel (or hard roll)
1 oz Lox (smoked salmon, or use other lean meat)
1 tbsp Cream cheese
4 oz Apple juice

SNACK
1 Oatmeal cookie and 1 apple

DINNER
11 oz Zucchini lasagna
½ cup "Boil in bag" green beans, onions & bacon bits, frozen vegetables
2 Hard rolls (bakery type)
4 oz Whole milk
1 cup Cherries (frozen, sweetened)

Calories: 2000; Fat: 34 g; Calories from fat: 15%; Potassium: 3100 mg; Sodium: 3500 mg; K Factor: 0.9

On this day, you have eaten slightly less potassium than sodium; if the amounts were equal, the K Factor would be 1. The ratio, or K Factor, of 0.9 is slightly higher than yesterday's. Each day during this first week, you will see a gradual increase. This small daily increase gives your system a chance to readjust. Remember, this slow increase is very important. DO NOT REPEAT THIS DAY.

DAY 3

BREAKFAST
8 oz Orange juice
1 Egg, scrambled (no table salt, no butter; oil the pan sparingly)
1 Breakfast patty (sausage substitute)
2 Slices whole wheat toast, no butter
1 tbsp Jelly

LUNCH
Turkey or pastrami sandwich (1 oz of turkey or other lunch meat, lean as possible), unsalted mustard, extra lettuce
1 Medium-size kosher dill pickle (make this your last pickle)
8 oz Skim milk

SNACK
Strawberry shake

DINNER
3½ oz Chicken, fried, without skin
⅔ cup Frozen spinach, rice and mushrooms, no sauce
Medium baked potato
1 roll
Lime ice served on a split banana

Calories: 1950; **Fat:** 39 g; **Calories from fat:** 16%; **Potassium:** 3300 mg; **Sodium:** 2700 mg; **K Factor:** 1.2

Today your foods have slightly more potassium than sodium, giving you a K Factor greater than 1. By the end of this week, your system will have had a chance to adjust to the higher K Factor and you will be eating menus with a healthy K Factor of 4 or above. DO NOT REPEAT THIS DAY.

DAY 4

BREAKFAST
8 oz Orange juice
¾ cup Oatmeal, cooked without table salt
10 Dates cooked with the oatmeal
8 oz Skim milk

LUNCH
Very large fruit salad with lots of greens, dressed with lemon juice or orange juice
Iced tea

DINNER
16 oz. Mexican combination platter (frozen dinner or at restaurant)
2 Glasses of beer (or soft drinks)
1 cup Lime ice

Calories: 1950; **Fat:** 39 g; **Calories from fat:** 18%; **Potassium:** 3200 mg; **Sodium:** 2100 mg; **K Factor:** 1.5

This is an example of a day on which you might be stuck with eating a Mexican (or other) dinner that is high in sodium. By keeping the sodium low at breakfast and lunch, you can eat the Mexican dinner without ruining your progress. DO NOT REPEAT THIS DAY.

DAY 5

BREAKFAST
8 oz Orange juice
½ cup Stewed prunes (cook without sugar and mix with:) ¾ cup Creamed wheat, cooked without table salt
8 oz Skim milk

LUNCH
Tuna salad, made from 3¼ oz water-packed unsalted canned tuna, plenty of lettuce, small amount of mayonnaise, preferably unsalted
1 Apple
2 Slices low-sodium whole wheat bread
8 oz Skim milk

SNACK
Freeze-type citrus drink, made with fruit ice, not ice cream

DINNER
11¼ oz Frozen pork loin dinner or Swiss steak
Large salad of greens and tomato, dressed with wine vinegar and a sprinkle of sugar if you like
8 oz Skim milk
1 cup Sliced peaches

Calories: 2100; **Fat:** 38 g; **Calories from fat:** 16%; **Potassium:** 4100 mg; **Sodium:** 1900 mg; **K Factor:** 2.2
DO NOT REPEAT THIS DAY.

DAY 6

BREAKFAST
9 oz Grapefruit juice
¾ cup Oatmeal cooked without table salt, 10 dates added for flavor
8 oz Skim milk

LUNCH
Large fruit salad with 1 cup cottage cheese and lemon/honey dressing

SNACK
1 Slice sweet potato pie

DINNER
3½ oz Curried fish and ⅘ cup of rice, cooked without table salt, ⅔ cup of raisins added
⅔ cup Green beans, steamed, no butter
8 oz Skim milk

Calories: 2000; **Fat:** 27 g; **Calories from fat:** 12%; **Potassium:** 4300 mg; **Sodium:** 1600 mg; **K Factor:** 2.7

Here is an example of a day with steady progress in spite of a piece of sweet potato (or similar) pie. DO NOT REPEAT THIS DAY.

DAY 7

BREAKFAST
8 oz Orange juice
¾ cup Oatmeal, cooked without table salt
Banana or melon in season
8 oz Skim milk

LUNCH
Chef's salad: all types of raw vegetables, greens, sprouts, strips of Swiss cheese (1 oz), and slices of hard-boiled egg; oil and vinegar dressing
8 oz Skim milk
1 cup Grapes (or other fruit)

SNACK
Mixed dried fruit

DINNER
Noodles Romanoff from mix (¼ package) or spaghetti with meatless tomato sauce
Baked acorn squash, brown sugar, no butter
⅔ cup Asparagus with lemon
8 oz Skim milk

Calories: 1900; **Fat:** 45 g; **Calories from fat:** 21%; **Potassium:** 5000 mg; **Sodium:** 1300 mg; **K Factor:** 3.8

You have now completed the week of "break-in" menus to gear your body up for food with a naturally high K Factor of 4 or more. DO NOT REPEAT THESE DAYS.

From now on (Days 8 through 14) you can change the order or repeat days as you choose.

DAY 8

BREAKFAST
8 oz Orange juice

3 Pancakes, made with no table salt and using low-sodium baking powder (just whisk together 1 egg, 1 cup of water, and 2 tbsp oil; then add ¼ cup nonfat dry milk, 1 rounded tbsp of low-sodium baking powder, and about 1½ cups flour)

2 tbsp Maple or other syrup

8 oz Skim milk

LUNCH
2 cups Bean soup made from dry or unsalted canned beans, using low-sodium bouillon

2 Pieces cornbread

8 oz Skim milk

SNACK
10 halves Dried apricots

DINNER
3½ oz Veal, cooked without butter

⅔ cup Peas and carrots, steamed, unsalted, no butter

Green salad, Italian dressing used sparingly

8 oz Skim milk

⅔ cup Strawberry ice milk

Calories: 2000; **Fat**: 52 g; **Calories from fat**: 23%; **Potassium**: 4800 mg; **Sodium**: 1200 mg; **K Factor**: 4.0

DAY 9

BREAKFAST
½ Grapefruit

2 oz Shredded wheat

1 Banana

8 oz Skim milk

LUNCH
Super hamburger (e.g., McDonald's Big Mac)

French fries without table salt (ask for them that way—you may have to wait a few extra minutes for a special order, but it's worth it)

8 oz Orange juice

DINNER
1½ cups Beans (cooked from dry beans, no table salt, add molasses and dry mustard for flavor, tomato paste, unsalted flavorings)

2 Corn muffins, made with low-sodium baking powder (whisk together 1 egg, 1 cup water, 3 tbsp oil, then add ¼ cup each of sugar and nonfat dry milk, then 1 cup each of flour and cornmeal, and 2 tbsp low-sodium baking powder; stir and bake in preheated oven at 425° F for about 15 min)

⅔ cup Frozen broccoli, steamed cauliflower and red pepper, no sauce

Calories: 2050; **Fat:** 60 g; **Calories from fat:** 26%; **Potassium:** 6600 mg; **Sodium:** 1400 mg; **K Factor:** 4.7

Today you'll be able to accommodate a commercial super hamburger with all the fixings and still achieve a K Factor of over 4. For instance, you might be going on an outing with the grandchildren.

DAY 10

BREAKFAST
8 oz Orange juice
1 cup Whole-wheat hot cereal cooked without table salt
1 Banana (on cereal)
8 oz Skim milk

LUNCH
Sandwich of sliced turkey (2 oz) on low-sodium bread, lettuce and cranberry, with a little mayonnaise
8 oz Skim milk

DINNER
4 oz Steamed fish
1 cup Brown rice
½ cup Chopped spinach
Salad of ½ avocado with grapefruit sections
2 Whole-wheat muffins
1 cup Mixed frozen fruit, sweetened

Calories: 1900; **Fat:** 36 g; **Calories from fat:** 17%; **Potassium:** 4900 mg; **Sodium:** 1200 mg; **K Factor:** 4.1

DAY 11

BREAKFAST
½ Grapefruit
¾ cup Creamed wheat, no table salt, with ⅔ cup raisins
8 oz Skim milk

LUNCH
Sandwich of tuna salad using low-sodium, water-packed tuna
8 oz Skim milk
1 Apple

SNACK
3½ oz Mixed dried fruit

DINNER
6 oz. Lean club steak
Medium-sized sweet potato, baked
½ cup Succotash, no table salt or butter
8 oz Skim milk
1 cup Strawberries, sweetened

Calories: 1950; **Fat:** 21 g; **Calories from fat:** 9%; **Potassium:** 5100 mg; **Sodium:** 800 mg; **K Factor:** 6.4

DAY 12

BREAKFAST
8 oz Orange juice
½ oz Puffed rice
1 Banana
8 oz Skim milk

LUNCH
1⅓ oz Lentil soup, made with dry
    lentils, chopped carrot, low-sodium
    broth*
1 slice Boston brown bread (or
    French-, Vienna-, or Italian-style
    bread)
1 oz Swiss cheese
1 cup Red cabbage and apple salad
8 oz Skim milk

SNACK
1 Soft ice cream cone

DINNER
16 oz Eggplant and rice casserole,†
    using unsalted canned tomatoes
2 Whole-wheat rolls, no table salt
⅗ cup Brussels sprouts
8 oz Skim milk
1 cup Frozen cherries, sweetened

Calories: 2050; **Fat:** 26 g; **Calories from fat:** 11%; **Potassium:** 4600 mg;
Sodium: 1000 mg; **K Factor:** 4.6

*Unlike other legumes, lentils don't require long soaking; simmer the soup that day to use,
or simmer it one day and reheat it when you need it.
† Sauté diced eggplant in a light oil with garlic and onion; add eggplant and unsalted
canned tomatoes to cooked rice in a casserole dish. Cover and bake for 45 minutes at 350°
or until eggplant is tender.

DAY 13

BREAKFAST
8 oz Grapefruit juice
1 cup Shredded wheat
1 cup Strawberrries
8 oz Skim milk
1 Slice whole wheat toast, low
    sodium
1 tsp Jelly

LUNCH
Low-sodium canned soup
1 oz Swiss cheese
2 Zwieback crackers
8 oz Skim milk

SNACK
1 cup Fruit-flavored low-fat yogurt
5 Dried peach halves

DINNER
½ Chicken breast, without skin, rolled
    in chopped walnuts (2 tbsp) and
    baked
1 medium-sized baked potato, no
    table salt or butter
⅔ cup Turnip
Salad of fresh spinach and mush-
    rooms, oil/vinegar dressing
8 oz Skim milk

Calories: 2050; **Fat:** 37 g; **Calories from fat:** 16%; **Potassium:** 4900 mg; **Sodium:** 950 mg; **K Factor:** 5.2

DAY 14

BREAKFAST
½ Grapefruit
1 cup Creamed wheat, cooked without table salt, ⅔ cup raisins added
8 oz Skim milk

LUNCH
2 Blueberry muffins, made with low-sodium baking powder (or 4 graham crackers)
1 cup Low-fat yogurt
3 Medium-sized fresh apricots or 1 large peach

DINNER
Noodles (2 oz dry) and goulash, made with 3½ oz chicken previously simmered and chilled, with fat and skin removed, then simmered again with paprika, carrots, cabbage, a little yogurt at serving time
Beet salad, using ⅗ cup canned unsalted beets, lettuce, and onions
8 oz Skim milk

SNACK
1 slice Rhubarb pie*

Calories: 2000; **Fat:** 38 g; **Calories from fat:** 17%; **Potassium:** 4300 mg; **Sodium:** 850 mg; **K Factor:** 5.0

*Some days it may seem a social necessity to eat a friend's masterpiece dessert, such as a rhubarb pie, but with judicious choices made earlier in the day, you can avoid disaster and maintain a K Factor of 5.

All the data for calculating the nutritional summaries for each day were obtained from J. A. T. Pennington and H. Nichols Church, *Food Values,* Harper & Row, New York, 1985; or the *Agriculture Handbook No. 8 Series,* U.S. Dept. of Agriculture, U. S. Government Printing Office, Washington D.C.; or by using a personally edited version of the Nutritionist III computer software program by N-Squared Computing Co., Silverton, Oregon.

CHAPTER 11

Step Three: Exercise

The finding that exercise lowers blood pressure significantly in a group of sedentary hypertensive patients suggests that "essential" (or primary) hypertension is a result primarily of lifestyle and can be prevented or treated effectively by reasonable physical activity.

Robert Cade, M.D., et al[1]

The theme of this book is that high blood pressure is due to an imbalance of lifestyle, particularly nutrition and exercise. Therefore, the proper prevention and reversal of high blood pressure is to be found in lifestyle changes, not only in the K-Factor approach to nutrition but, as Dr. Robert Cade says, "in reasonable physical activity."

Unfortunately, not many of us are engaging in "reasonable physical activity." According to the Surgeon General and the American College of Sports Medicine, fewer than 10% of Americans are exercising at the level they recommend. Worse yet, as many as 20% to 25% are totally sedentary and unfit. So there is a lot of room for improvement for many of us here.

This chapter discusses additional benefits of exercise, from helping you keep your weight down to maintaining a proper hormone balance in your body to enhancing your mood, and answers the typical arguments against exercise. It then provides some principles and guidelines for a comprehensive aerobic exercise program that you and your physician can tailor to your own personal situation.

BENEFITS OF REGULAR EXERCISE

Regular aerobic exercise is beneficial because it

- Returns blood pressure toward "normal"
- Decreases body fat
- Restores hormone balance

- Decreases blood lipids (fats), which cause heart attacks
- Increases blood levels of the "good" cholesterol (high-density lipoprotein cholesterol, or HDL-C)
- Increases stability of electrical activity of the heart
- Increases resistance to fatigue
- Decreases craving for smoking
- Adds life to your years
- Probably adds years to your life

RETURN OF BLOOD PRESSURE TOWARD "NORMAL"

It is probably no surprise to you that exercise helps you lose weight (and thereby helps bring down your blood pressure). But several scientific studies (discussed in Chapter 7) have shown that regular exercise programs are effective in lowering blood pressure even if you're not overweight and even if you don't lose excess weight. In fact, the drop in blood pressure during physical training correlates not with weight loss but with decrease in plasma insulin levels.[2] That chapter discussed the study of Dr. Cade and his co-workers, which demonstrated that aerobic exercise can be a remarkably effective way to enable your body to better regulate its blood pressure and can even produce a fall in blood pressure in patients with severe hypertension.

Several studies have shown that keeping fit by regular exercise also helps prevent the development of high blood pressure.[3] A study of 6,000 women and men showed that people whose blood pressure was in the "high normal" range (130–139/85–89) and who had a low level of physical fitness were ten times more likely to develop hypertension than those with blood pressure in the normal range (120–129/81–84) and who were physically fit. Even when the blood pressure was less than 120/80, lack of physical fitness resulted in a 50% increased probability of getting hypertension.[4]

DECREASE OF BODY FAT

As discussed in the next chapter, losing excess weight may be essential for reducing your blood pressure. And exercise (at least three times a week) plays a very important—in many people a necessary—role in maintaining normal weight. In fact, any effective weight (and blood pressure) reduction program requires at least some aerobic exercise, especially in the long run (pun intended).

RESTORATION OF HORMONE BALANCE

Exercise makes muscles more responsive to insulin and decreases the blood level of this hormone.[5] As you'll remember from Chapters 4 and 7, lowering an elevated blood insulin level should help correct some of the imbalance in your body cells, thus improving cholesterol levels and lowering your blood pressure. Lower levels of insulin also decrease any tendency of your body to convert calories into fat, and some studies suggest that lower insulin levels suppress feelings of hunger. The resulting weight loss also helps your body rebalance itself and lowers your blood pressure.

DECREASE OF BLOOD LIPIDS

Blood cholesterol occurs primarily in two forms: low-density lipoprotein cholesterol (LDL-C), and high-density lipoprotein cholesterol (HDL-C).

It is the LDL, which contains a large amount of cholesterol and other fat, that is "bad," because it contributes to the formation of fat deposits in your arteries. Another type, very-low-density lipoprotein (VLDL), is also bad. VLDL contains more fat (mostly triglycerides) than protein and explains why high levels of blood triglycerides should be avoided.

As you'll remember from Chapter 7, exercise helps reduce elevated insulin levels. In view of the fact that insulin stimulates production of triglycerides, it is then not surprising that exercise can lower the level of blood triglycerides, VLDL cholesterol, and LDL.[6]

INCREASING BLOOD LEVELS OF THE "GOOD" CHOLESTEROL

On the other hand, HDL (specifically HDL-2) carries the bad cholesterol to your liver, where it can be converted into bile and excreted.

In view of the fact that elevated levels of insulin lower HDL, again it's not surprising that several studies have shown that exercise can raise the amount of HDL in your blood while lowering the level of LDL. The ratio of total cholesterol to HDL should be less than 5.0 for men and less than 4.5 for women. There is some dispute as to what the total cholesterol level should be. Although it is generally considered normal if below 220 or 240 mg per 100 ml of blood (220 or 240 mg/dL), there is good reason to be more conservative and say that the total blood cholesterol should be no more than 200 mg per 100 ml of blood. In fact, life insurance statistics show that your chances of death rise once your total cholesterol level rises above 170 mg per 100 ml. On the other hand, in the 40 years of the scientific study of the people living in Framingham, Massachusetts, there evidently has not been even one death due to heart attack in a person whose blood cholesterol is below 150 mg per 100 ml.

INCREASED STABILITY OF ELECTRICAL ACTIVITY OF THE HEART

Of course, the all-important muscle that can benefit from exercise is your heart. Evidence suggests that regular exercise increases your chances of surviving a heart attack. This may be because the electrical activity of your heart muscle is more stable if you exercise regularly.

In a study of animals, the chances of heart fibrillation (abnormal electrical activity that makes the heart stop pumping blood) was decreased in those animals that had experienced exercise training.[7]

INCREASED RESISTANCE TO FATIGUE

Regular aerobic exercise increases the number of mitochondria, or "powerhouses of the cell" (tiny membrane "sacks" within the cell that contain special proteins that combine oxygen with food products to provide energy to the cell), which allows your body to increase the percent of energy you can get aerobically (aerobic means "using oxygen"). Therefore, your body places less reliance on the more inefficient anaerobic (without oxygen) metabolism and so is more resistant to fatigue.

Initially, as you get in shape, you may well need a bit more sleep than usual. But joggers who regularly cover at least 20 miles (or expend about 2000 calories) a week frequently report that they require less sleep than before they took up regular exercise. In fact, you may find that once you've made it a habit, regular exercise may not decrease the number of hours you have for other activities. Regular aerobic exercise also increases your stamina for everyday work.

DECREASED SMOKING

A frequent observation is that many people who take up regular aerobic exercise either decrease the amount they smoke or stop altogether. Remember that the British study of antihypertensive drug effectiveness found evidence that indicates that not smoking (versus smoking) is associated with a much greater decrease in rate of strokes and heart attacks in people with hypertension than is drug treatment.[8]

ADDING LIFE TO YOUR YEARS

People who exercise regularly also know that it makes them feel better and even changes their mood. Exercise stimulates the brain's production of opiate-like substances called beta-endorphins, which may explain why exercise is often beneficial for mild depression. "Runner's high" describes a common experience in which euphoria or elation is felt during or immediately after a good aerobic workout.

THE BOTTOM LINE: ADDING YEARS TO YOUR LIFE

Although the medical profession is still debating this, the life insurance companies are already betting their money that exercise will make you live longer. Allstate

Life Insurance Company has given up to a 35% discount for those who exercise regularly. Most of the companies giving discounts on premiums for life insurance require a minimum of 30 minutes of aerobic exercise (such as running) at least three times each week.

Recently there has been controversy about the safety of exercise, and about whether or not exercise can extend your years. The discussion that follows should help demonstrate that, with proper precautions, exercise can be safe and that it almost certainly can extend your life span.

THE CONTROVERSY ABOUT EXERCISE

During the 1970s, exercise, especially jogging, became almost a national obsession. The popular opinion has been that exercise makes us more healthy, and many joggers believe it will make them live longer.

IS AEROBIC EXERCISE SAFE, OR IS IT DANGEROUS?

For several years, the view circulated that enough exercise could "immunize" you against a heart attack. For a while it was claimed that no one who finished a marathon had ever died of a heart attack. But then it was found that marathoners like U.S. Congressman Goodloe Byron, age 49, who had run six Boston marathons; New Zealander Dennis Stephenson, who held records for 100-mile runs; and 48-year-old Frenchman Jacques Bussereau, who died of a heart attack during the 1984 New York City marathon, had died because of their cholesterol-filled coronary arteries. And then in 1984 Jim Fixx, the well-known author of *The Complete Book of Running* and a finisher in 20 marathons, collapsed and died of a heart attack at the end of a jog on a Vermont road.

WHAT ABOUT JIM FIXX?

When one of the main running gurus, a man who regularly put in about 60 miles per week, dropped dead at the end of a four-mile jog, the antiexercise group sallied forth claiming that exercise not only doesn't make you live longer but can kill you. So many uncertainties were triggered by Jim Fixx's death that some thought the exercise boom would begin to die. Certainly Fixx died while, or immediately after, exercising. But did exercise kill him? Or was it something else?

The autopsy of Jim Fixx revealed that of the three coronary arteries in his heart, one was almost completely plugged by fat deposits, one was 70% closed, and the third was 80% closed. Not only that, scar tissue was present on three regions of his heart, each a record of a previous myocardial infarction, or heart attack. One of these heart attacks had occurred about two weeks and another about four weeks before he died.[9]

These heart attacks had not felled him but probably had been associated with classic symptoms that were, unfortunately, not recognized. For example, during that last month, Jim Fixx had mentioned to friends that at times he felt a tightness in his throat when he was at rest. In Kenneth Cooper's newsletter *Aerobics,* Jim's son John was quoted as saying, "It turns out that when he was running all that summer he would have to stop because of the tightness in his chest about five minutes into a run. He would walk a little and then he would be fine and go on and do his miles."

It's not unusual for people with coronary artery disease to experience chest or throat tightness or pain about 6 minutes after starting to run, only to have it get better if they continue for a while at a slower pace. This happens because it takes about 6 to 10 minutes for the body to get "warmed up," and for blood vessels in the muscles to open, decreasing blood pressure and thus decreasing the load on the heart.

The two heart attacks before the fatal one were probably associated with symptoms. On one occasion, Fixx complained of pain in his jaw. The other nonfatal attack probably occurred when he was running with his son John just two weeks before he died. Very early in the run, Jim remarked that he had to go to the bathroom. The two then walked to a nearby airplane hangar, where they stopped to talk with someone for about 10 minutes, before resuming their run. When the son questioned Jim's bathroom remark, Jim said he was all right now and did not have to go. It's possible that he was having a mild heart attack and the brief rest, plus the warm-up effect, decreased the load on his heart enough to diminish any symptoms.

Not only had he had at least three previous heart attacks, not only were his coronary arteries almost completely plugged, but the autopsy showed that Jim Fixx had an enlarged heart—probably since birth. This type of enlarged heart, known as biventricular hypertrophy, is fairly rare and has been associated with sudden death in athletes, usually at a much younger age. Running didn't kill Jim Fixx, but heart disease and a congenital heart condition probably did.

But could this sudden death have been prevented? Or does this mean that you shouldn't exercise because you might have heart disease? Let's take a look at the coronary artery disease—and the three heart attacks that resulted. Jim Fixx had had several risk factors for heart attack. He had a family history of heart trouble (his father died at age 43 of a second heart attack), and before Jim took up running at the age of 36, he had smoked, worked in a high-stress environment, eaten a high-fat diet, been obese, and lived a sedentary life. In addition to these risk factors, or warning signs, Jim's blood cholesterol had been found to be elevated: his cholesterol level was 253 mg per 100 ml in 1980 and was 254 at autopsy. Although his ratio of total cholesterol to HDL was in the normal range—2.91 in 1980 and 3.48 at autopsy—his total cholesterol level was abnormally high.[10]

So before Jim Fixx died, there were plenty of indications that there might be something seriously wrong with his heart. These included

- Recent unexplained fatigue
- Recent chest pain while running
- Family history of heart disease
- Previous high-fat diet
- History of being overweight
- Formerly led a high-stress lifestyle
- History of smoking
- Elevated blood cholesterol

PUTTING EXERCISE-ASSOCIATED DEATH IN PERSPECTIVE

The examples of Jim Fixx, Goodloe Byron, Dennis Stephenson, Jacques Bussereau, and others clearly show that exercise doesn't immunize you against heart attacks. Dr. L. E. Lamb, of the U.S. Air Force School of Aerospace Medicine, has emphasized that most American men over age 40 have "silent" coronary artery disease—a condition that does not produce symptoms, may not show up in a stress test (treadmill electrocardiogram, or EKG), and may not even prevent completion of a marathon. Nonetheless, according to Lamb, a fatty-cholesterol deposit in the coronary arteries of these men may eventually trigger a blood clot that clogs an artery, causing a heart attack, especially during or just after exercise. Dr. Lamb does not claim that exercise actually causes a heart attack, just that it can trigger one.

Frequency of Sudden Death During Exercise

In a six-year study of joggers in Rhode Island, only one death during jogging occurred per year for every 7,620 joggers.[11] Similarly, in King County, Washington, with a population of 1.25 million, only nine cardiac arrests occurred during vigorous exercise during one fourteen-month period.[12] To put things in perspective, another Rhode Island study found that of 81 people who died during recreational exercise, the largest number of deaths (23% of the total) occurred during golf! Jogging was second (20%) and swimming third (11%).[13] In almost 90% of these deaths, the underlying cause was hardening of the arteries, or atherosclerosis, and 93% of those who died either had a medical history of heart disease or had recognized risk factors. Another way to keep this in perspective is to realize that of all sudden deaths that occur, very few occur during exercise. In a study of 2,606 sudden deaths studies in Finland, only 22 were associated with exercise.[14]

The statistical evidence suggests that overall, among people most of whom have not had a stress test, the chance of sudden death during exercise is about seven times that of death during sedentary activity.

If you exercise 2 hours per week, you do accept a slightly higher incidence of sudden death during those 2 hours. But as will be discussed, during the other 166 hours, you may be decreasing your chance of death. In any case, the overall chance, if we judge by Rhode Island, as we noted, is only about one jogger out of every 7,620 during a whole year.

Not only that, but with today's medical knowledge, it's possible to improve the odds a good deal more. As an example of the value of proper medical evaluation, as of 1985 at Dr. Kenneth Cooper's Aerobics Center in Dallas, over five thousand participants have been followed who have collectively run more than six million miles (an average of over 1000 miles per person), with only two cardiac-related events and no fatalities. These people had all been screened with an exercise tolerance stress test as well as a complete physical and history.[15]

Can anything be done to identify whether exercise is dangerous for you? If anything, the running death of Jim Fixx demonstrates that sudden death during exercise rarely if ever happens unless there is underlying disease, usually heart disease. And usually there are previous symptoms and/or risk factors that can provide warning signals that heart disease is present. As cardiologist-runner George Sheehan has said, "Nobody with a normal heart is going to drop over while exercising."[16]

Most important, an adequate medical examination by your physician can catch many of these cardiac problems in time, especially if a proper stress test is done. Even as far back as 1973, a physical exam of Jim Fixx had picked up some signs of problems with his heart. That exam revealed abnormalities in his resting EKG (heart tracing) as well as an enlarged heart on X-ray and a heart murmur. Today we have not only better techniques, such as echo cardiography, lithium angiography, and advanced types of EKG stress tests, but also more knowledge and more insight with which to detect and evaluate the existence of heart disease. Had physicians known then what is known today, or had Jim Fixx been tested with a modern treadmill stress test, the likelihood is high that his underlying heart disease would have been revealed before it was too late.

Shortly we will go over the main things you and your doctor should check to decrease the odds of sudden death during exercise. Along with Nathan Pritikin,[17] Dr. L. E. Lamb[18] has pointed to several studies showing that major diet changes can reverse the effects of coronary artery disease.

On the other hand, because of the high fat content typical of the Western diet that most of us have been eating, there is some risk of having a heart attack while exercising, especially if you haven't had a medical workup before you start. But you can exercise without worry if you meet the following conditions:

- Your blood cholesterol is "normal" (see Chapter 9).
- Your doctor evaluates you for certain other risk factors (see Chapter 9 and page 190).
- You can pass a properly conducted treadmill stress test (see Chapter 9), even if you're over 40, have risk factors, or have a diastolic pressure above 95 mm Hg.
- You have been eating a low-fat diet (see Chapters 10 and 12).
- You follow the recommendations in the section "Aerobic Exercise Guidelines" on page 196.
- You to get a complete medical evaluation, and you start the exercise program *slowly* as described.

Keep in mind that because high blood pressure is a major risk factor for heart attack and because some drugs interfere with exercise, the last item on the foregoing list is especially important.

DOES EXERCISE LENGTHEN YOUR LIFE?

But how about the other 166 hours in your week when you're not exercising. Does exercise influence your chance of death during the hours you are not exercising?

Although the interpretation has been disputed, in 1978 the first study of 16,936 graduates of Harvard University—the Paffenbarger Study[19]—appeared and indicated that regular aerobic exercise every week may significantly lower the risk of heart attacks.

In 1984, Dr. Paffenbarger published an updated report of his study of those 16,936 Harvard alumni.[20] This recent report shows that men who expended over 2,000 kilocalories (kcal) per week on physical activity had about half the death rate from heart disease as did men who were sedentary (expending less than 500 kcal per week), even though both groups of men were living similar lifestyles in other respects. Expending 2,000 kcal per week on exercise is roughly equivalent to jogging twenty miles per week.

Incidentally, this same report shows that having hypertension puts a man (the alumni were men) at greater risk for having a heart attack than do a sedentary lifestyle, cigarette smoking, obesity, or a family history of coronary artery disease.

The Paffenbarger report contained another unexpected, but pleasant, finding. The death rate *due to cancer* of those men expending more than 500 kcal per week on physical activity was 25% lower than the cancer death rate of men expending less than 500 kcal each week. This means that men who jogged even five miles each week apparently had less chance of dying of cancer. While this is not "proof," it certainly is a strong clue.

Other evidence supports the view that regular aerobic exercise can help extend life. In a study published in late 1984, Dr. David Siscovick and co-workers compared the exercise history of 133 men who had cardiac arrest without prior known heart disease to that in a random sample of healthy men of the same age, marital status, and similar lifestyle. The overall risk of heart attack—during vigorous exercise as well as the rest of the time—was 60% lower in the men who exercised regularly than in those who didn't.[21]

One of the most complete studies, published in 1989, followed 10,244 men and 3,120 women for an average period of almost eight years. Thanks to this study, we now know that you can gain health-related benefits from modest levels of exercise that do not lead to improvement in cardiorespiratory fitness. The results showed that the rate of overall mortality progressively decreases as the degree of physical activity is increased. Moreover, although the protective effect of exercise increases with each increase in activity level, the biggest drop in mortality occurs when activity is increased from the lowest level to a moderate level of exercise.[22] So low-level fitness activities that don't necessarily make one much more fit can nevertheless increase health benefits

As might be expected, much of the decrease in overall mortality in this study was due to reduced rates of cardiovascular disease in the more fit men and women. But surprisingly—at least to some of us—part of the reduction in mortality was due to a decrease in cancer deaths. At least one other study has reported that a reduced rate of cancer may be associated with increased exercise.[23] It is possible that exercise has a beneficial effect on the immune system. All this raises the possibility that we may be able to decrease the rates of some cancers if people become more physically active.

In summary, it is clear that exercise has several desirable effects, each of which reduces your chance of death:

• Exercise helps decrease body fat.
• Exercise helps reduce blood pressure.
• Exercise helps reduce the "bad" (LDL) blood lipids.
• Exercise helps increase the "good" (HDL) blood lipids.
• Exercise helps stabilize electrical activity of the heart.
• Exercise helps normalize hormones that affect the body's ability to balance sodium and potassium.

So if you look at the whole picture, it's a pretty safe bet that, with the proper precautions, exercise is on your side. As Dr. David Siscovick and his co-workers conclude, "even though intense physical activity may be one of the factors that can precipitate primary cardiac arrest, habitual participation in such activity is associated with an overall reduction in the risk of primary cardiac arrest."[24]

DANGERS OF EXERCISE

SUDDEN DEATH

The chance of sudden death during exercise is quite small, only 1 in 7,600, but it is there. The problem for older people with unrecognized coronary artery disease is that strenuous exercise can precipitate a heart attack. Because of this, it is wise for everyone over 30 to obtain a serum cholesterol level before embarking on an exercise program. If the serum cholesterol is above 200, a properly conducted exercise stress test EKG should also be done. With this information, your doctor can advise you as to your risk of having a heart attack and any special precautions you should take.

INJURIES

Of course, exercise can cause such minor problems as "runner's heel" (achilles tendinitis), strained muscles, and sore feet. But as will be mentioned in the next section, there are ways you can prevent this.

How about joints? Won't running for years wear out your knees? Some people, apparently considering bones and joints as just another machine, have maintained this, but the evidence doesn't bear it out—provided you don't have arthritis or other joint disease, are not greatly overweight, and take proper precautions.

Actually, there is no evidence whatsoever that regular exercise increases risk for joint damage such as osteoarthritis. In fact, there are a number of reasons that exercise should reduce the risk of osteoarthritis. When you run, your joints develop more synovial fluid, stronger ligaments, and thicker cartilage. The argument that properly conducted exercise is not bad for normal joints is supported by a study of several thousand men and women that could find no relation to risk of developing osteoarthritis. Indeed, women who ran were actually slightly less likely to get osteoarthritis than those who were sedentary.[25]

The argument that exercise must be bad for joints was an intuitive one based upon the assumption that the body acts like a machine. But the body is *not* a machine. True, over a very short period (seconds or minutes), the body acts like a machine: after all we can break a bone or wreck a knee. That mechanistic view is part of an old scientific paradigm that is outdated. But in the new paradigm, we realize that over time—periods of days or weeks—the body is a dynamic self-renewing living organism with remarkable potential for self-repair. Recent basic research has shown that, to an extent far greater than previously thought, your body can actually rebuild itself.

The Tarahumara Indians in northern Mexico virtually make running a way of life. For fun, they play kickball games in which they run as far as 200 miles, they have been known to run 500 miles in five days, and they run well into their sixties and seventies. No joints made out of a nonrenewing substance could hold up to a lifetime of that sort of activity. And it's not just this group, or anything special about their inheritance. Early American Indians used running as a means of communication, and it was part of their ritual of relating to nature. In the last century, one Hopi Indian was asked by the local Indian agent to deliver a message 78 miles away. He set out at three in the morning, reached his destination at about noon, rested half an hour and got rubbed down, and resuming his gait, ran back home, covering the round-trip of 156 miles in less than 24 hours. He was almost a hundred years old when he died.[26]

Regular exercise helps strengthen your bones as well as your muscles. Thus, regular exercise can help prevent osteoporosis (weakening of the bones), which is especially frequent in older women.[27] Conversely, if you have been sedentary, your bones may be weak, and this emphasizes, once again, the recommendation that sedentary people begin their exercise program gradually, preferably with walking. Otherwise you're more likely to develop "stress" fractures or joint damage. But, since the body is a self-renewing organism, if you don't overstress it, and if you give it a chance to respond, moderate exercise will stimulate your body to renew itself, strengthening your bones, muscles, and, some evidence suggests, even the ligaments that stabilize your joints.

I have a trick knee that was uncomfortable and would occasionally "lock." When I began jogging, I really had to take it easy and slow down every time the knee bothered me. Now, after several months of jogging four to six times a week, I tend to forget that the knee ever bothered me.

In 1985, the then head of the ski patrol at Sugarbush, in Vermont, had badly damaged his knee with several severe sprains during bike racing, basketball, and tennis. The damage was so bad that he experienced pain walking and his knee would dislocate and buckle under him when he played tennis. Then he began gradually to jog, slowly increasing his workouts. Two years later, he was skiing and running foot races of over five miles without any pain in his knees.

Don't jump to the conclusion that we're saying exercise is good for all bone, ligament, and joint ailments. Some orthopedic conditions could be made worse by exercise, especially if it's too strenuous or the changes are too sudden. Remember, with *sudden* stress, the bones do act like a machine—and break. There's still a lot we don't understand about how the body maintains itself, but provided you take proper precautions, the evidence is that running not only won't hurt your joints but may even be good for them.

Remember also that the effect of exercise upon elevated blood pressure is not limited by age.[28] Even in 70- to 79-year-old men and women with moderate hypertension, endurance training results in modest (4 to 8 mm Hg) reductions in blood pressure.[29]

AEROBIC EXERCISE GUIDELINES

The key to increased physical endurance—and an aid to loss of weight and to achieving normal blood pressure—is aerobic exercise. Aerobic exercise refers to repetitive movements involving the large muscles of the legs or arms. These movements require more oxygen (hence, aerobics) and thus make us breathe more heavily.

Because only one fifth of all the energy released actually moves your muscles, the remaining four fifths appears as heat, causing you to get warm and sweat a lot. In aerobic exercise, motion is the name of the game, but not motion so strenuous that it prevents you from exercising continuously for many minutes.

In contrast to aerobic exercise, power weight lifting (pumping iron), or progressive resistance exercise, may require comparatively little continuous motion of the large muscle groups and so may use relatively few calories. It therefore may not increase your breathing or heart rate very much. In addition, during power weight lifting the blood pressure may rise to extreme levels. In five young body builders, even a one-arm curl raised the blood pressure to an average of about 255/190 mm Hg, and during maximum exercises, such as the double-leg press, the pressure rose to an average of 320/250 mm Hg![30] Even in those who aren't body builders, lifting as little as 50% of their maximum weight can raise blood pressure from normal resting values to about 170/108 mm Hg.[31] If you recall Chapters 4 and 6, there is pretty good reason to believe that the blood vessels in people with hypertension are "muscle-bound" and weakened. Therefore, since power weight lifting is not aerobic and since at present there isn't sufficient information about its dangers in people with hypertension, it seems the wiser for people with hypertension to refrain from this activity until further information becomes available.

However, if you do repetitive resistance exercises involving high numbers of repetitions with small weights with little rest in between, you can raise your heart rate sufficiently and for a long enough time to obtain the benefits of aerobic exercise.[32] Also, as will be mentioned under "Preventing Injuries," for some sports, such as jogging or running, you may need to do some work with very small weights in order to maintain balance between opposing groups of muscles.

Outdoor forms of aerobic exercise include bicycling, jogging, running, cross-country skiing, swimming, rowing, active skating or singles tennis, and fast walking. The exercise that burns the most calories per hour is cross-country skiing, followed by rowing, and then by running.[33] Indoor aerobic exercises include aerobic dancing, riding a stationary bicycle, using a rowing machine, a cross country ski simulator (NordicTrack®), or an exercise treadmill. Tennis or racquetball may qualify if performed vigorously enough over a sufficient period of time. Jumping rope is another option.

There is now evidence[34] that aerobic dance can cause as large an increase in the capacity for aerobic exercise and endurance as jogging. A note of caution: Be sure to wear proper shoes and to exercise on a resilient surface rather than on something hard like concrete. Also remember that in any exercise, you should progress slowly under the supervision of a well-trained instructor who will be sure not to place you in a class with "young turks" ahead of your fitness level. You can do aerobic dancing at home, either to your own music or to videotapes. Videotapes can be a good motivator, providing discipline and some instruction. But since they can't be tailored to your particular degree of fitness, be careful to not let yourself be overworked by them especially if you're just starting. Also be certain to avoid those videotapes that have a lot of stretches that involve bobbing. Slow, constant stretching is not only much more effective for flexibility but much safer.

Those who are significantly overweight (20 pounds) or who have orthopedic problems should probably start by riding a bike, swimming, or walking leisurely followed by faster walking. These are good ways to get aerobic exercise without overstraining joints and ligaments.

Remember that we now know you can gain health-related benefits from modest levels of exercise that do not lead to improvement in cardiorespiratory fitness.[35] So low-level fitness activities that don't necessarily make one much more fit can nevertheless increase health benefits.

If you are interested in starting to jog, take a look at any of several good introductory books for advice on how to prevent injuries. Still hard to beat are *The Complete Book of Running* by James Fixx, (Random House, New York, 1977) (don't do what he did—skip an exercise EKG—do what he said and take one) and *Dr. Sheehan on Running* (World Publications, Mountain View, California, 1975.)

Here are seven basic points to keep in mind as you begin your exercise program:

- Begin with a proper medical examination.
- Start your program slowly.
- Pay attention to the intensity and duration of your workout. Never overexert yourself.
- Listen to your body
- Exercise frequently.
- Warm up and cool down.
- Take steps to prevent injuries.

BEGIN WITH A PROPER MEDICAL EXAMINATION

The very first thing is to check with your doctor, who will want to do a physical examination as well as perform some blood tests, including a blood cholesterol. This is Step One of the program. (See Chapter 9 for details.)

SEE YOUR DOCTOR *before beginning your exercise program!* This step is extremely important!

START SLOWLY

As with most activities dealing with your health and body, it's important not to make sudden changes. Begin your exercise program only after you have had a medical evaluation, and begin it slowly.

To emphasize the importance of increasing the intensity of exercise gradually, consider the following: In a study of 2606 sudden deaths, Vuori and co-workers found that the chance of death being triggered by strenuous physical exercise was highest if the exercise had been intensified without a gradual increase in training.[36] If you have high blood pressure, the importance of *gradually* increasing the level of training is even greater. So don't start off by taking an all-out fitness test. Begin gradually.

Especially if you have severe hypertension (diastolic pressure of 100 mm Hg or above) or are taking antihypertensive drugs, begin very slowly, walking at a pace that allows you to carry on a conversation at the same time. If you can carry on a conversation, that means your metabolism is still aerobic; that is, your body is getting enough oxygen to use more fat and less carbohydrate for energy.

Your doctor may need to consider the drugs you take before you begin your exercise program. For example, if you are taking a beta blocker, this drug will prevent your heart rate from rising as much as normal and so would be expected to limit your exercise capacity. This is borne out in the studies done so far that conclude that taking a beta blocker for hypertension will probably decrease your ability to exercise easily, especially if it's endurance exercise lasting more than 30 minutes.[37] It is essential to discuss this with your doctor: he or she may want to replace your present drug with one that has less effect on your exercise capacity. If you do exercise while taking a beta blocker, keep in mind that it may make you tire more easily, so be very careful to not overdo it, and keep the sessions under 30 minutes but at least 5 times per week. Finally, a slow warm-up may help reduce the effect of the beta blocker, and a longer, slower cool-down will prevent you from feeling lightheaded, a symptom often experienced by exercisers who take beta blockers.

In summary, it is recommended that you be very careful not to overexert if you are taking a beta blocker. If you stick to the K-Factor program, your physician may be able to take you off of these drugs eventually. But never stop any drugs, especially beta blockers, except under your physician's supervision. Suddenly stopping these drugs can cause rebound hypertension and can be *lethal*.

If you have an elevated blood cholesterol level, I believe you should be in a supervised program and should have an exercise stress test before you start the program. However, so that you can reach your maximum heart rate during the test (which some consider important in order to perform the stress test properly), some exercise physiologists point out that it may be necessary for you to do a few weeks of very gentle exercise first. This is important not only to improve muscle tone but to get you used to detecting the symptoms of normal fatigue.

The exercise stress test has been underrated, in my opinion, and it is not a bad idea for anyone who is out of shape to take one before beginning an exercise program. This is especially recommended for those with hypertension, certainly if the diastolic pressure is 95 mm Hg or above, and if coronary risk factors are present. According to the American College of Sports Medicine, if you wish to perform low- to moderate-intensity exercise, you do not need an exercise stress test unless you have symptoms of disease or other known cardiopulmonary or metabolic disease. On the other hand, if you wish to participate in high-intensity exercise, then you should undergo exercise stress testing if you are male and over age 40, female and over age 50, or irrespective of age if you have two or more coronary heart disease risk factors, or symptoms of disease or known cardiopulmonary or metabolic disease.

Dr. Lamb recommends that until the blood cholesterol has been down to normal levels for at least three months, the only unsupervised exercise that you should do is walking at a conversational pace and light calisthenics.

If you haven't been exercising regularly or are overweight, start out by taking walks—even if your diastolic pressure is less than 100 mm Hg. This will help strengthen your bones and muscles before you start fast walking or jogging. Your muscles, joints, ligaments, and cardiovascular system need time to toughen up a bit before you take on anything more vigorous. This is especially important if you're overweight. It's surprising how a few extra pounds put extra strain on your joints and can increase the chance of injuries to the knees or ankles.

The American College of Sports Medicine points out that beginning joggers tend to have "increased foot, leg, and knee injuries when training was performed more than 3 days per week and longer than 30 minutes duration per exercise session."[38] Also, keep in mind that elderly people apparently need longer to get the benefits of training.[39]

Dr. Rachel Yeater, of West Virginia University, recommends walking at a leisurely pace for 10 minutes each day if you are out of shape. Increase your daily walk by 5 minutes each week. Keep increasing the duration until you walk 30 to 60 minutes each day. Don't be in a hurry; this will take at least 6 weeks.

Don't start jogging until you can cover two miles in your half hour walk. Then, if your blood cholesterol level is normal and your resting diastolic blood pressure is not above 90 mm Hg, you can begin jogging a few paces every couple of minutes during your walk. Slowly increase the amount of the distance covered by your short jogging periods. Play it by ear. As you proceed, you'll automatically jog more and walk less, until you can do the whole two miles at a slow jog. It should now take you about 20 to 25 minutes—not much faster than a brisk walk. During these early stages you may need a little more sleep; listen to your body. Later on, you'll probably actually need less sleep!

For older persons, walking may be enough exercise. If you are jogging, just keep up an easy pace, and over a period of time, as your conditioning improves, you will find you gradually speed up automatically, thereby covering more miles in the same time. Take it easy; don't rush; be patient. Don't force it. It may seem slow at first, but progress is inevitable with this approach. You'll be surprised how much progress you've made after three or four months. It must be emphasized that you must not overdo it initially or you will risk becoming discouraged from unnecessary soreness or injuries and not continue your regular exercise program long enough to see those satisfying results.

INTENSITY AND DURATION

Intensity

Never overexert yourself. Overexertion is dangerous—and completely unnecessary. In fact, during overexertion, the systolic blood pressure can rise to levels that might present a danger to a person with hypertension. And too great an intensity of exercise can make hypertension worse.[40] Fortunately, you need never strain or work to exhaustion to get in shape and lower your blood pressure.

Patience is the name of the game. If you are a beginner, during the first few months you should never push yourself. Even when you get into better shape, I don't think you should push yourself until you have been evaluated with a properly conducted treadmill stress test. If you feel muscle pain, or if afterward your muscles are more than slightly sore or your resting pulse upon awakening is elevated, you are pushing yourself. Don't push yourself into injuries.

Don't ignore any unusual sensations during or after exercise. Pain caused by a heart attack isn't felt in the heart; it's carried by nerves, or "referred" to other parts of the chest, arm, throat, neck, jaw, or stomach. And it may not cause pain at all, just a feeling of tightness, discomfort, nausea, severe dizziness, extreme breathlessness, or fatigue. Therefore, if you have pain in either the front or the back of the chest, a choking sensation, or a tightness in your chest or throat—as Jim Fixx did about a week before he died—don't ignore the warning: *Stop exercising and see your doctor.*

If you have orthopedic or other health problems, your physician may advise you to limit your exercise to brisk walking, which is still very beneficial but much less stressful on the joints.

How do you determine the intensity of your exercise? There are three indicators:

1. How you feel.
2. Whether you can carry on a conversation.
3. Your heart rate.

How you feel, whether you are relaxed or straining—in other words, "listening to your body" is a constant indicator to you about your level of exercise.

An excellent indicator is whether you can carry on a conversation. If you can, you are going at a pace that will help burn off fat but not unduly strain your heart.

Your heart rate is an objective measure of your pace, and this will be discussed further.

Use all three of these signs. Work out at a pace that allows you to feel comfortable, carry on a conversation, and keep your pulse at about 50% to 60% of its maximum value.

If you are just beginning to get in shape, most exercise experts would say that your intermediate goal should be maintaining a heart rate of 60% to 70% of its maximum for about 20 minutes. But if you keep your heart rate to between 50% and 60% of its maximum predicted rate, it will help you lose weight just as well. If you really want to get in shape, aim for 70% of the maximum rate for over 20 (preferably over 30) minutes—once you have your weight at a good level (percent of body fat preferably below 15%).

There are two methods of estimating your predicted maximum heart rate (PMHR). According to Dr. Kenneth Cooper,[41] who started the aerobics movement in the 1960s, if you are a male and have been exercising regularly, simply subtract one-half your age from 205. For a 52-year-old, that gives 179 beats per minute. Sixty percent of that is about 107. So the target range for that person would be a pulse of 107 while exercising.

If you are a woman, your predicted maximum heart rate is determined by subtracting your age from 205. This formula also applies if you're an out-of-shape male. If our 52-year-old were a woman or a man who was out of shape, that would give a predicted maximum pulse rate of 153. So, if that person were just beginning to get in shape, her or his pulse should be raised to between 76 and 92 while exercising (50% to 60% of the maximum). After a few weeks, he or she could move into the higher range.

Many exercise physiologists prefer a different formula for calculating your maximum heart rate: 220 minus your age for males and 215 minus your age for females.[42] For a 50-year-old male, this gives a predicted maximum pulse of 170, as compared to 180 which is arrived at using Cooper's formula. This difference emphasizes that the predicted maximum pulse is an estimate only.

If you have been steadily active in athletics, your actual maximum pulse may be higher. For example, cardiologist-runner Dr. George Sheehan is 66 years old and his actual (not predicted) maximum heart rate determined during a treadmill stress test is 179. One of the exercise physiologists who critiqued this chapter, a former member of the Canadian Olympic Team, Dr. Robert Kochan, at age 36 had a treadmill-determined actual maximum pulse of 209.

On the other hand, keep in mind that if you are taking a beta blocker, your actual maximum heart rate will be much lower than the predicted maximum.

For a quick and easy way to measure your heart rate while exercising, count the pulse on the inside of your wrist for 6 seconds, then multiply by 10 (just add a zero). Checking your pulse while exercising will help keep you from overdoing it. If you overdo, you will fall back and risk quitting because of discouragement. Haste makes waste when you are getting your body back in the condition it was meant to be in.

And even if you do feel comfortable with longer workouts, don't go to 85% of your maximum heart rate, especially if you are over 40 or have been obese, *unless* you have been told that your EKG is normal during at least that heart rate while doing a stress test, your resting diastolic blood pressure is below 90 mm Hg, and you do not have other coronary risk factors such as these:

- A blood cholesterol level above 200 mg/100 ml blood (200 mg/dl)
- A history of cigarette smoking
- Family history of heart attacks
- High-stress lifestyle
- Diabetes
- High-fat diet
- Obesity

Don't *ever* go above 85% of your maximum heart rate without a coach and special medical evaluation. World-class athletes can do it, but most of us would be playing Russian roulette.

This cannot be overemphasized enough: *Don't force it!* Sudden changes in intensity could trigger silent heart disease into becoming a heart attack. So—**make no sudden changes in intensity, and never change intensity and duration at the same time.**

Duration

Time is the important thing. At least initially, don't set goals of distance in your exercising—particularly if you're jogging, swimming, or cycling. It is more important to increase the time you spend exercising than it is to achieve a distance goal. By emphasizing time spent exercising rather than competitive goals, you reduce the chance of overdoing it and injuring yourself. You don't need to be competitive to get into really good shape.

Apparently there are two important time thresholds for aerobic exercise. The minimum amount of time you should spend exercising depends on the intensity of the exercise. To get a good training effect if you're walking, 30 minutes is the minimum and 45 to 60 minutes is better. If you're jogging or running, 20 minutes is the minimum and 30 to 45 minutes is better.

If you find you can't spare at least 20 minutes a day, even a 5- or 10-minute walk, especially when you're starting your program, is better than nothing. But try for the 20-minute minimum if you're jogging, or the 30 minutes if you're walking.

If you feel lazy and don't want to go for a 20-minute jog, remember that the real trick is to get out the door and take those first steps. Once you have gone 10 minutes, it's easy to say, "Well, let's do another 5," and at 15, "Well this feels good," so 5 more minutes isn't much time out of the day. And there you are—you did your 20 minutes even though you hadn't felt in the mood.

Whatever the form of exercise, the same guidelines apply: Start off slowly, and gradually work up to 30 or more minutes of walking or 20 or more minutes of jogging, running, or other more active forms of aerobic activity.

Exercising at your target heart rate for 20 to 30 minutes (enough to expend 300 kcal of energy) at least three times per week (1.5 total hours per week) is the minimum to help reduce body fat.[43] This is also enough to produce a significant increase in your body's ability to use oxygen (maximum oxygen uptake, or Vo_2 max). However, depending upon the fat "setpoint" of your own body (see Chapter 12), you may well need to spend more than 1.5 hours per week to get a significant weight reduction effect. Some people need to do aerobic exercise for at least 3 hours per week to maintain a normal weight, and some people (who have a lot of fat cells) are going to have to do 3 or 4 hours per week and also cut down on calories. You will just have to find out for yourself by doing it.

To get the optimum effect on your blood pressure, you also may need to exercise more than 1.5 hours (90 minutes) per week, although the total amount required is well within reason. It is documented that three 55-minute sessions of aerobic exercise (including jogging, dancing, and light gymnastics) per week (a total of 165 minutes per week) can produce a significant lowering of blood pressure.[44] The study by Dr. Cade and co-workers showed that once people had been jogging two miles per day, seven days per week (a total of about 140 minutes per week) for three months, half of those being treated with drugs for *primary* hypertension achieved normal blood pressure and were able to stop taking their medicine without changing any other factor such as diet.[45] And 96% of the 105 patients in the exercise program achieved a significant reduction in blood pressure. More recently, Dr. John Holloszy and co-workers at Washington University School of Medicine in St. Louis have reported that in men who previously had insulin resistance, running fifteen to twenty-two miles each week is enough to normalize the insulin response to glucose.[46]

Thus, the evidence so far is that to get your blood pressure down, you need to spend a total of about 2¼ to 2¾ hours per week doing aerobic exercise. This should be divided into at least three, and preferably five or six, sessions a week. This probably is enough to help you maintain both normal weight and normal blood pressure.

I agree with the American College of Sports Medicine that because of the greater chance of discouragement or of injuries associated with high intensity activities, "lower to moderate intensity activity *of longer duration* is recommended for the non-athletic adult," especially older people.[47]

If you want to go beyond this level for other reasons, for example, to help lose weight, do it gradually. After a few weeks or so, start increasing your daily jog by about 5 minutes each week until you can comfortably jog for 45 minutes. After several months, as you really begin to get in shape, you may have a few 45-minute and eventually 60-minute workouts.

But remember, as was discussed in Chapter 7, Dr. Cade and his co-workers showed that more than 70% of their younger patients achieved blood pressure in the "normal range" within three months of when they were able to run only two miles every day.

LISTEN TO YOUR BODY

To get the most benefit while not overdoing exercise, you'll need to keep track of your heart rate—your pulse. This is one of the best ways of monitoring whether you are overdoing it, underdoing it, or doing it right.

Your heart rate at rest is important, too. One of the best indicators of progress is your resting heart rate upon waking in the morning. As you achieve better cardiovascular fitness, the resting morning pulse will decrease. As you really get fit, it should come down to about 60 and may approach 50. If one morning you notice your resting pulse is higher than usual, especially if you feel tired, you probably have been overdoing it and need to take it easy for a couple of days or even skip a day to give your body some extra rest.

Other signs of overdoing it include lack of energy for other activities, trouble with sleeping, and the development of aches and pains that don't go away. As time goes by, you will become better tuned in to your body and find it easier to notice small aches or signs of tiredness before they become serious. You will develop the ability to judge your exercise level by "listening to your body."

FREQUENCY

The importance of regular exercise has already been stressed. This is the main point: At least three or four times a week, do some active, or aerobic, exercise such as jogging or swimming. If you're only walking, try to make it more often than that; there's nothing wrong with a walk every day.

Remember:

* The most dangerous exercise is infrequent sporadic exercise.
* Never increase intensity, frequency, or duration at the same time or too quickly.

WARM UP AND COOL DOWN

Warm up slowly during the first 10 minutes of exercise session. Even world-class Olympic athletes start their warm-ups jogging at a pace not much faster than walking. It's the amateurs who want to get off to a flying start.

The warm-up is especially important for those who have high blood pressure or heart disease. When you first start exercising, both your systolic and your diastolic blood pressure increase. However, later, as your body begins to warm up, the tiny blood vessels, or arterioles, in your muscles open, or dilate, allowing easier flow of blood. As a result of this vasodilation, your diastolic blood pressure then begins to drop, placing less strain on your heart. It is very important that you go slowly until this decrease in peripheral resistance occurs. That way you will be placing a smaller load on your heart while you exercise.

The cool-down (or "warm-down") period is also important. It allows the blood in the muscles you've been using to get back into your main circulation. (This point can be underscored by the experience of a man who ran in a park and then drove home without a cool-down and fainted at the wheel.) So at the end of your exercise, slow down for the last 3 to 5 minutes.

Dr. George Sheehan, cardiologist and noted runner, doesn't think cooling down is so important.[48] He says at the end of a run he just sits—and watches the others cool down. Dr. Kenneth Cooper, the aerobics expert, disagrees.[49] He believes that a warm-down is *very* important. Cooper points out that at the end of a run, blood tends to pool in your legs, slowing its return to the heart. This can decrease the amount of blood delivered to your coronary arteries and, if they are narrowed with cholesterol plaques, could trigger a heart attack. Cooper points out that the first marathon runner, who brought Athens the news of the Greek victory on the Plain of Marathon, didn't die until after he stopped. He died during the cool-down, not the run. Cooper points out that we still don't fully understand the importance of the cool-down period and suggests that this may be what happened when Jim Fixx died right at the end of his run. So Cooper recommends that you continue brisk movement for a few minutes, slowing to a walk before stopping.

Dr. Sheehan does point out that lying down right after a run allows blood from your legs to return to your heart faster than normal and so can place an extra load on your heart. In addition, the increased output of the heart, plus the fact that it doesn't have to push the blood against gravity to your head, would increase the blood pressure within your head. If you already have high blood pressure, this could be very dangerous. So don't lie down right after a run. Wait five or ten minutes for your system to readjust.

A Comment

Slowing down during the last 3 to 5 minutes of your exercise can't hurt. Look at it this way: Even though you're slowing to a walk, that last 3 to 5 minutes of cooldown is still exercise. It counts. So it seems wise to make sure that the last few minutes of your exercise are done at a progressively slower pace. If you want to put out some hard effort, do it before the last 5 minutes of the workout.

PREVENTING INJURIES

Perhaps one of the most common reasons that people stop exercising is that they get hurt. So take steps to prevent injuries. If you're jogging, proper running shoes are essential. Tennis shoes or sneakers won't provide adequate support or cushioning for your foot, and if you jog or run in these shoes, you'll likely end up with painful foot problems. Running on dirt roads or on grass (beware of hidden stones and holes) is better than running on harder surfaces, such as asphalt and concrete. This is especially important when you are beginning. If you do aerobic exercise, stay off floors without resilience, such as concrete. If you jog or run, try to stay off concrete.

Jogging and running tend to result in an imbalance between major muscle groups. For example, the gastrocnemius, or calf muscle, becomes much stronger than the small muscles in the front of your shin. This muscle imbalance can cause a continuous pull on your achilles tendon (the strong tendon you can feel at the back of your ankle), which can result in achilles tendinitis. Since this tendon attaches to bone on the bottom of your heel, achilles tendinitis causes pain on the bottom of the rear of your foot, so you may confuse it with a bruise and not recognize the cause.

Of course, the best medicine is to prevent injury. Fortunately, you can take simple steps to prevent the bad effects of muscle imbalance. Light weight training and stretching are necessary to prevent this type of muscle imbalance. For example, stretching will increase blood flow to the shin muscles and help prevent shinsplints. Perhaps the most important stretching is to prepare the calf muscle by slowly leaning into a wall for 1 minute, as illustrated in Figure 17.

Do this stretching exercise both before *and* after your walk, jog, or aerobic dancing. Stretching not only helps preserve muscle balance and prevent injuries but helps your workouts. Stretching is especially effective when done at the end of your exercise period. Not only does it help prevent muscle cramps, but because your muscles are warm, you can stretch them further and help keep them from shortening. So after cooling down, do some stretching exercises for at least 2 to 5 minutes.

Light weight training to strengthen arm, shoulder, and back muscles and the muscles in the front of your thighs also helps maintain a proper balance among your muscles. See *Running and Being* (Simon and Schuster, New York, 1978) by

Dr. George Sheehan for his "magic six" stretching and weight exercises. Dr. Sheehan has since modified the "magic six" by changing the "backover" (or yoga plow) to the "knee clasp" and has added two extension exercises for the low back. As Dr. Sheehan emphasizes, stretch slowly and only to the point of tension, not pain.

FIGURE 17

STRETCHING THE ACHILLES TENDON

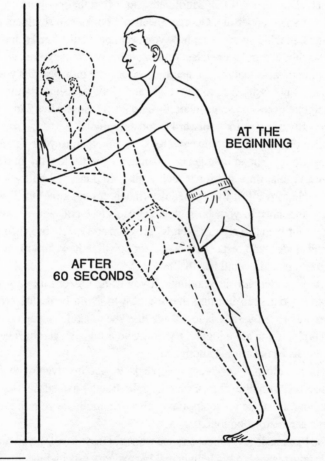

AT THE
BEGINNING

AFTER
60 SECONDS

Fig. 17. This exercise is the one that can prevent, or reverse, "runner's heel," a painful condition that occurs when the achilles tendon pulls on the back of your heel. Simply stand a distance equal to about one-half to two-thirds of your height from a wall, leaning forward with your arms outstretched, and then over a 60-second period slowly pull in your arms so your head approaches the wall. Keep your body straight and your feet flat on the ground. This slowly pulls on the achilles tendon, lengthening the gastrocnemius to counter the shortening effect of running. Take it easy; stretching exercises should never cause pain, just a sense of tension in the muscles being stretched.

An excellent book on stretching exercises for any sport is Bob Anderson's *Stretching* (Shelter Publications, Bolinas, California, 1980). Yoga is another way you can increase body flexibility.

Learn to listen to your body. If you feel tired and if your resting heart rate is higher than usual, take it easy for a day or two. (On the other hand, be sure to do something, such as walk.)

MOTIVATION

I hope this chapter itself helps motivate you. I find that periodically reviewing it helps light a fire under me. George Sheehan's books and seminars are excellent motivators, making you wonder how you ever could have lived (maybe you really haven't) without regular exercise; running is his particular game.

Keeping in mind that regular aerobic exercise not only benefits your health, but is virtually a necessity for proper weight and blood pressure, should help you use the discipline necessary to get started—and keep going. After 2 to 4 months, you will probably begin to look forward to most sessions.

Realize that regular aerobic exercise is as important to your health as sleeping or eating. So it is not an indulgence or something to try to work in when you can. Reserve a regular time slot for it each week, and don't feel guilty if this requires some people to readjust their schedules (lunch, for example) to fit yours. To the contrary, announce to your boss, your spouse, close colleagues, and friends that you are committed to a regular exercise program and it *must* be scheduled. Most of them will understand, especially when they realize how important it is to your blood pressure and overall health.

Try to pick pleasant surroundings. If you walk, jog, or run, vary your route to give variety, but keep in mind that it's best to avoid hard surfaces if you can. Another way to get variety is to change the type of exercise you do occasionally. For example, if you are a jogger, try riding your bike, an aerobics dance class, or swimming as an occasional alternative.

Another motivator for many people is to get involved with a group—an exercise class, a running club, a friend. An Irish setter named Charley got me back into running. Exercise videotapes may also help motivate you, but remember the precautions already mentioned.

If you like music (ever meet anyone who said they didn't?), you may find that a portable tape player is a big help in making exercise especially enjoyable. Just one word of warning: Don't listen to songs such as Laura Branigan's "Gloria" while you run unless you're in almost competitive shape. If music gets to you, songs like that can put you into overdrive and you may wind up really overdoing it without realizing it—until the aches and pains set in afterward.

If you stay with it during those first slow weeks, you will feel encouraged as your body begins to remember what it is to feel young.

Finally, following your progress will help as you see your resting heart rate drop and the distance you cover in a given time go up (see Chapter 13). Seeing that progress charted out will help encourage you. But be patient—you can't reverse the effects of a lifetime of sedentary living in a couple of weeks or months.

SUMMARY

Several points appear well established:

- Exercise decreases your blood pressure.
- Exercise helps restore normal insulin function.
- Exercise helps decrease obesity
- Exercise can be safe if proper precautions are taken.
- Exercise increases the quality of life and helps keep you out of hospitals.

The total evidence strongly suggests that exercise also increases your chance of having a longer life. Beside the fact that some statistical studies indicate this, it's hard to see how something that helps normalize both your blood pressure and your weight, helps balance your body's hormones, and helps relieve psychological stress can do anything other than lengthen your life.

To the point of this book, regular aerobic exercise certainly can help lower your blood pressure toward the normal range *and* normalize your blood insulin and blood cholesterol levels.

CHAPTER 12

Step Four: Help Your Body Find Its Proper Weight

In overweight patients with Stage 1 hypertension [diastolic pressure between 90 and 99 and systolic between 140 and 159 mm Hg], an attempt to control blood pressure with weight loss and other lifestyle modifications should be tried for at least 3 to 6 months prior to initiating pharmacologic therapy.
                    The Report of the Fifth Joint National Committee, 1993[1]

The fourth step in the program for lowering your blood pressure and increasing your well-being is to shed excess body fat.

Of course, observing Step Two (eating right) and Step Three (exercise) overlap considerably with this step. Nonetheless, since overweight people have particular problems not shared by people with normal weight, losing excess weight deserves a discrete focus.

We hardly need to tell you that losing weight is not easy, and keeping it off is even more difficult. But hypertension occurs twice as often among obese people as it does among people with normal weight. In its 1993 recommendations for dealing with hypertension, the Joint National Committee warns obese people with high blood pressure to shed some of those excess pounds.

In an obese person, some of the blood hormones do not work properly; they do not maintain a correct balance between sodium and potassium in the cells, thus contributing to hypertension. Getting rid of excess fat helps return the blood hormones to normal levels, allowing the body to maintain a more normal balance between sodium and potassium. For example, shedding extra pounds lowers blood insulin, and in many people this helps the kidneys excrete more sodium, thereby lowering blood pressure.[2]

Losing excess weight alone, without doing anything else, can sometimes bring blood pressure back to normal. In clinical studies, loss of one third to one half of excess body weight has led to significant blood pressure reduction.[3] On the other hand, if you *don't* get rid of the extra fat, your abnormal blood hormone levels may prevent the K Factor or even drugs from reducing your blood pressure. So if you have hypertension and are overweight, it is *very* important that you reduce your weight.

Getting your weight toward normal has other benefits, too. There is a good deal of evidence that maintaining normal weight decreases your chances of having a heart attack, and it is a major factor in preventing you from developing adult onset (NIDDM) diabetes. Normal weight, along with good physical fitness, increases your energy. You just plain feel better.

ARE YOU OVERWEIGHT?

How do you know if you are "obese" or have "normal" weight? Actually it's not weight but the amount of *fat* in your body that counts. You can have normal weight and be too fat! If you haven't put on any weight since high school, when you weighed in at 195 and were "all muscle," don't brag too much. Unless you work out a lot, there is a good chance that a lot of that muscle has wasted away, or atrophied, from lack of use. You may have gained several pounds of fat even though your weight is the same.

The most accurate way to tell if you're obese is to determine, with the underwater immersion test, the percent of your body weight that is fat. This involves some special equipment that measures your naked weight when you are completely submerged in a water tank. This weight is compared with your naked weight in air. Since the fat part of your body is lighter than water and the rest of your body is heavier, the percent of your body that is fat can be calculated from the difference between your weight in air and your weight in water.

There is also a more advanced way to determine your body fat, based upon an electrical property (called conductivity) of your body,[4] but this method is not yet widely used.

Once you know the percentage of your weight that is fat, you can compare that with the "average" to determine whether you are overweight. For men, the national average is about 15% to 20%; about 22% to 23% is considered healthy for a woman. Some people who exercise a lot have only about 9% body fat. The lowest value is found in some world-class male athletes: about 5% body fat. For women, the figures are somewhat higher.

Tables for ideal body weight are of limited help for many people because they cannot take into account the wide variations in the amounts of bone and muscle. As an example, I had my body fat measured scientifically in the water tank. After subtracting body fat from total weight, the resulting lean weight was still 3 pounds over "ideal" total body weight as listed in one table! Even if all fat were removed from my body (which is impossible), I would still be 3 pounds "overweight."

Of course, there is a much easier guide: skin fold thickness, which you can estimate right in your own home. Pinch the skin of your abdomen. If while sitting, you can pinch more than one inch, your body has too much fat. By using calipers, you can estimate your percent of body fat more accurately. This requires determining the skin fold thickness in several body locations and then using a table to estimate the percent of fat in your body. Some of the fancy calipers have a built in microchip that contains the information of the table and does the calculation for you. You need to determine the thickness in several locations because body fat tends to go to different places on different people. In fact, you probably have abnormal insulin function, and recent studies indicate that if your body fat tends to accumulate in the abdomen, your chances of having a heart attack are increased.

Finally, just looking at yourself nude is not only one of the simplest but one of the best ways to determine if you are overfat. If you can see folds of fat sagging, you are too heavy. If you look trim, you probably aren't.

WHAT DETERMINES YOUR BODY FAT?

We used to be convinced that if you were overweight, you ate too much—period. That's all there was to it. I remember a physician friend of mine examining a very obese teenager whose mother insisted, "Doctor, she eats just like a bird," to which my young physician friend wryly replied, "Yeah, like a giant condor." Neither he nor I could believe anyone could be that overweight without overeating. Why? Because the First Law of thermodynamics, or the Conservation of Energy Law, says that energy can neither be created nor destroyed. This law, which was discovered in the 1840s, is well established and has appropriately influenced not only physics and medical thinking but the thinking of society at large. The obvious solution for losing weight was simple: Don't eat so much. But decreasing your calorie intake does not necessarily decrease your weight. It's just not that simple. Some obese people really do eat like birds, yet they stay fat. In fact, many overweight people actually eat fewer calories than thin people.

How could this be? Well, the energy law does hold true; none of us, the obese included, can create energy out of nothing. But the situation is a bit more complicated. We need to follow a newer scientific approach and look at the whole picture.

Perhaps we can most easily see the true situation by looking at the way energy enters and leaves the human body.

Figure 18 shows what happens to the calories you eat:

• As much as 80% are "burned off": they are turned into heat (#1) (that's what keeps your body warm).

- Some are burned off in doing work (#2).
- Some are turned into proteins and other structural components of your body (this is less than 1% in an adult).
- Some are lost in the stool.
- The rest are stored as fat (#3).

You want to eliminate the last possibility; you want to avoid having "the rest" left over for fat. In fact, if you don't take in enough calories to provide for the other possibilities adequately, the fat you already have will be burned off and you will lose weight.

FIGURE 18

WHAT HAPPENS TO THE CALORIES YOU EAT

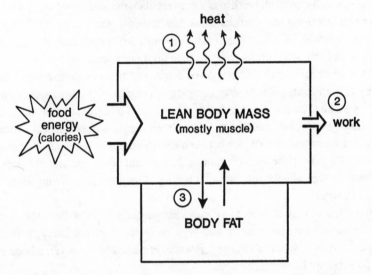

Fig. 18. A simplified diagram of the energy input and output of the body. (Not shown is the normally small amount of calories lost through feces and urine, although in people in diseased states, such as diabetics losing sugar through the urine, or in people with diarrhea, this amount can become great.)

Let's look at this in more detail.

Almost all your energy comes into your body in the form of food. The two main ways we lose energy are by the body giving off heat and by the body performing work on the environment (exercise). Any energy left over must, according to the energy law, be used to increase body protein (such as muscle) *or* be stored as fat (#3).

So far, so good. Eating more should make you gain weight, and vice versa, right? Not necessarily; if we look closer, we see that there are other possibilities.

Inside your body are several mechanisms that determine the balance between the energy stored as fat (#3) and that given off as heat (#1) or work (#2) (see Figure 18). To oversimplify a bit, these mechanisms can be divided into those that primarily regulate the amount of energy that goes into fat, and those that primarily regulate the amount of energy given off as heat:

- **Factors that increase energy going into fat:** insulin, white fat cells.
- **Factors that increase energy lost as heat:** thyroid hormone, brown fat cells, sodium-potassium pumps.

Insulin prevents fat from being used up; thyroid hormone increases heat production; sodium-potassium pumps also produce heat both directly and indirectly. Brown fat cells tend to burn fat more than store it. On the other hand, white fat cells tend to store fat.

These mechanisms all work together to regulate the amount of fat in your body. The balance among these mechanisms determines if you will be "fat" or not. No one can "control" your amount of fat; your body itself does that. But we will see that within fairly wide limits, you can help your body reset the fat level.

To look at this, scientists borrowed a concept from modern control systems theory (which deals with the way complex systems, such as airplanes or computers—or human beings—are regulated) called the set point. Just as the thermostat in your home establishes a set point, or target temperature, mechanisms inside your body that determine the balance between energy stored as fat versus that given off as heat tend to keep the amount of body fat constant at a target amount *even if you cut back on the calories you eat.* That is why in the long run, dieting alone won't and can't work!

Since the extent to which we can change the set point depends upon our genetics and upon the number and type of fat cells in our body, part of this regulation is beyond our ability to influence. Fortunately, however, a large part of this fat set point *can* be influenced.

All this means we've got some good news and some bad news. The good news is that you *can* change the amount of fat in each of your white fat cells: you can change your body's set point for body fat. If you have a lot of white fat cells you'll just have to change the set point further. But you *can* do it—naturally. How?

It should be obvious from Figure 17 that doing more work—exercising—is one way to get rid of excess calories. Some people used to downplay this, saying that the amount of energy lost through exercise isn't enough to make a difference. But for each mile you walk or jog, you lose at least a hundred calories—and each pound of fat contains 3500 calories. So walking or jogging just nine miles each week would be enough to burn off about a pound of fat a month. Maybe that doesn't sound dramatic, but that's 12 pounds in a year.

But exercise also changes the set point that determines the balance between energy going into heat or into fat. Not only do we lose more heat during exercise than we do during rest (the body temperature actually increases a degree or two—and we sweat), but regular exercise produces changes in blood hormones, involving insulin, adrenaline, and thyroid hormones, which cause the body to lose more heat *even between exercise sessions.* So the effect of exercise actually reflects more than just the amount of energy it takes for each mile, or hour, of aerobic exercise.

Merely decreasing caloric intake changes the levels of some of your blood hormones, such as thyroid hormone and insulin, which signals your body to waste fewer calories in heat and hold onto its fat. The purpose of this is to prevent your body from using up spare fuel (fat) and thus to help you survive longer if you are faced with starvation. Of course, this is a great advantage if the possibility of actual starvation is imminent, but for most of us, surrounded by plenty of food, it's a Catch-22. To make matters worse, the fatter you are, the fewer calories you need to eat just to maintain the same weight. And as you become older, the problem gets more acute. Fat cells of obese people have a defect that makes them give off less heat than the fat cells of thin people.

A major part of the calories you eat, perhaps a quarter to a third, goes into running the pumps that move sodium out of your cells and potassium into them.[5] Most of the energy used by these pumps eventually winds up as heat. Some overweight people apparently have fewer of these sodium-potassium pumps in their cells than do people with normal weight.[6] This means that obese people expend fewer calories as heat than do thin people; their calorie needs are therefore a few hundred less per day. The altered sodium-potassium balance might also help explain the fact that obese people are twice as likely to have high blood pressure as people with normal weight.

Interestingly, a potassium deficiency has been shown to decrease the number of sodium-potassium pumps in skeletal muscle (which makes up most of your lean body mass).[7] So it's possible that restoring the proper K Factor in your diet may provide some assistance in resetting your body fat set point.

Another problem is that being overweight tends to increase your blood levels of insulin, a hormone that works to promote the storage of fat (and may also make you feel hungry).

Unfortunately, you can't decrease the *number* of your fat cells.[8] Worse, you can *increase* the number of fat cells by gaining and losing weight—which is common in obese people who try one diet after another. Most of the diets work temporarily, few work permanently. Also, white fat cells just store fat, but brown fat cells actually help turn energy into heat—they can actually help keep body weight down. Recently there has been a lot of talk about brown fat cells. But only a few lucky people have enough brown fat cells to waste enough energy to lessen their tendency to gain weight. The rest of us have mostly white fat cells—so we have a harder time losing weight than those who have more brown fat cells. Well, you win some and lose some.

Fortunately, by changing the set point you change the *amount* of fat in each fat cell. A person who has more fat cells will have more body fat at a given set point than one who has fewer fat cells. Thus to lose weight, a person with more fat cells will have to change his or her set point more than a person with fewer fat cells will have to do.

THE VICIOUS CIRCLE

So the more overweight you are, the tougher it can be. Being obese is a vicious circle: The more obese you are, the more your body hormones and metabolism change to make you even more obese from the calories you eat. Not only that, but since the fat surrounding your body is a good insulator, just having more body fat tends to decrease the energy you lose as heat. And being obese makes it more difficult to work off calories during exercise.

In addition, some people have so many fat cells or predisposing genetic factors that it's extremely difficult to achieve healthy weight even using the principles outlined here. Those people especially need the help of a physician-nutritionist in order to handle their problem.

Fortunately, the new paradigm, with the systems approach and its set point concept, shows that by working *with* nature, most of us can influence our body's fat storage—we can break out of the vicious circle.

HOW TO LOSE WEIGHT

In order to lose weight, you must

- Pay attention to your diet and restrict calories.
- Increase the number of calories you use up doing work.
- Change your body's fat set point to increase the amount of calories you burn off.

PAY ATTENTION TO YOUR DIET

So what else is new? Am I just telling you to eat less—as though you hadn't heard that already countless times? Not exactly. It's important not just to eat less but also to manage the kinds of foods you do eat. If you are following our recommendations from Chapter 10 you're probably doing the right thing. However, it is important to make a significant, and simple, distinction between kinds of foods: high-energy-density foods, which have a high ratio of calories to bulk, and low-energy-density foods, which have a low ratio of calories to bulk. It helps to avoid the first kind (in spite of its nice-sounding name) and concentrate on the second kind. The high-energy-density foods tend to make you obese.

Some nutritionists say simple carbohydrates are absorbed rapidly into the bloodstream. This raises your blood levels of insulin, a hormone that, among its many actions, causes storage of fat. Alcohol is also absorbed fast; it is readily metabolized by the body for quick use, or its energy can be converted into fat. Fat is absorbed more slowly than either simple carbohydrates or alcohol but has about twice as many calories as the same weight of carbohydrate or protein. Simply put, fat is fattening. In contrast, the low-energy-density foods release their energy slowly and gradually, over a sustained period and in a form your body can use.

TABLE 4
CLASSIFICATION OF FOODS BY ENERGY DENSITY

HIGH-ENERGY-DENSITY FOODS	LOW-ENERGY-DENSITY FOODS
FAT FOODS	**LOW- OR NONFAT FOODS**
butter, margarine, nuts, gravies, marbled beef, etc.	low-fat yogurt, skim milk, non-fat dry milk, etc.
SIMPLE CARBOHYDRATES*	**COMPLEX CARBOHYDRATES† AND FOODS CONTAINING FIBER**
refined sugars, foods with added sugar white bread, etc.	fresh vegetables (potatoes are great), fruits, whole grains (including rice), pasta
ALCOHOL	**PROTEIN FOODS**
	skinned chicken, fish

*Simple carbohydrates include table sugar (sucrose), milk sugar (lactose), and dextrose (glucose). Honey contains sucrose predigested by the bee into a mixture of glucose and fructose. Sucrose is composed of one molecule of glucose joined with one of fructose. Lactose is composed of one molecule of glucose joined with another sugar called galactose. Some people don't have the enzyme to break lactose into these two sugars. Lactose-free milk is available for these people.

†Complex carbohydrates include starch and cellulose, both of which are made of hundreds or thousands of glucose molecules bonded together. In starch, these glucose molecules are bonded in a single chain, which our digestive system breaks down into glucose molecules; but in cellulose, the glucose molecules are bonded in a way that can't be digested by people. So cellulose, which is one type of fiber, doesn't give us calories even though it helps satisfy hunger.

There is evidence that high-energy-density foods increase your hunger. One study showed that people who ate high-energy-density foods, containing lots of fat and refined sugar, required almost twice as many calories to satisfy their hunger as did a group who ate low-energy-density foods. The high-energy-density foods tend to stimulate your appetite, whereas the fiber in low-energy-density foods produces bulk to help satisfy your hunger.

When you eat high-energy-density foods, the level of insulin in your blood increases far more than it does when you eat low-energy-density foods. This insulin stimulates your hunger, according to some researchers. And the extra insulin raises your blood pressure by causing the kidneys to retain sodium and by stimulating activity of the sympathetic nerves.

In contrast, low-energy-density foods are high in K Factor and fiber and low in fat. Eating them will not only help you avoid overeating but will provide you with the nutrition you need to keep your blood pressure down and also decrease your chance of getting coronary artery disease or cancer.

EAT LOW-FAT FOODS

Avoid butter, cream, margarine, sour cream, nuts, gravies, and other fats.

Since fat contains about twice as many calories per gram as does dietary protein or carbohydrate, cutting dietary fat intake is the most effective way to cut calories. Besides, eating fat stimulates your appetite and thus encourages you to overeat.

Fat may be even more "fattening" than previously thought. A study published in 1984 reported that laboratory animals eating a diet containing 42% to 60% of the calories as fat became obese (51% body fat), whereas the control group, which ate a low-fat diet containing *the same number of calories,* ended up with "normal" (30%) body fat.[9] This thought-provoking study indicates that it is not only fat's extra calories and ability to stimulate hunger but the way the body processes fat that makes it especially fattening. From what we know of basic biochemistry, this isn't too surprising. When food is turned into body fat, some of the energy is wasted in the conversion process. When protein is converted to fat, 25% of the calories are lost as heat, with carbohydrate the figure is 20%, but when dietary fat is converted to fat, only 4% of the calories are lost as heat—the rest go into fat.[10]

So the next time you're tempted to pour on the butter, yogurt, sour cream, or add whole cream to your coffee, go ahead if you must—it's your choice. But in your mind's eye, visualize almost all of that pat of butter going straight into those unsightly bulges on your abdomen or legs.

In 1984 Americans derived, on the average, 44% of their calories from fat. This may help explain why Americans today are more obese than in 1910, when they obtained only 27% of their calories from fat.[11] And the evidence indicates that we need even less than that.

But can we get too little fat in our diet? Your body manufactures most of the fat it needs: several fatty acids (both saturated and unsaturated), cholesterol, and other steroids. (There is one fat though, that the body cannot manufacture: an unsaturated fat called linoleic acid, which, incidentally, helps to keep your blood pressure normal. Linoleic acid is contained in most vegetable oils (e.g. safflower oil, corn oil). If you are an active adult, you need about 30 to 60 calories—7 grams, or about one-half a tablespoon—of linoleic acid every day. In addition, you need some fat in order to absorb vitamins A, D, E, and K, which are all fat soluble. If you were to cut your dietary fat to below 10%, you might not get enough of these essential vitamins.)

The 1984 American Heart Association recommendation was a step in the right direction. They suggested that you cut your fat consumption down to 30% of your caloric intake—and if you have a cardiac risk factor, to 20% of your total caloric intake. But there is no reason *everyone* shouldn't strive to cut it to 20%.

To put things in perspective, keep in mind that you couldn't eat a totally fat-free diet even if you wanted to. Everything we eat, whether animal or vegetable, is made of cells, and all cells have membranes that contain fat. Therefore, even crisp iceberg lettuce has 7% fat (by calories), and looseleaf lettuce has almost 15% of its calories in fat! Hardly anything—except such starchy foods as potatoes, rice, and beans—has less fat than lettuce.

The menu plan in Chapter 10 helps you do just that: cut your fat intake to 20% or less.

EAT FOODS CONTAINING COMPLEX CARBOHYDRATES

If you avoid simple sugars and processed carbohydrates (candy, sugar cookies, white bread, cakes, etc.), you can eat a fair amount of complex carbohydrates (carrots, cucumbers, broccoli, green beans, fresh fruits, cornstarch, brown rice, potatoes, beans, whole-grain breads and cereals, etc.) and still lose weight.

Remember, carbohydrate doesn't make as much body fat as does dietary fat.

RESTRICT THE TOTAL CALORIES YOU EAT

Exercise and changing your set point can do a lot, but if you want to lose excess fat, keep a cap on your calories—don't *over*eat.

Listen to your body—not to the situation or the environment. Avoid temptation. Don't keep fattening foods in the house. If everyone else is going to indulge at dessert, explain that you must leave the table—and then do it! Use vegetables such as celery or carrots as a substitute for fattening desserts or snacks. If you find it helpful, join a weight-reduction group or class.

INCREASE THE AMOUNT OF CALORIES YOU USE UP DOING WORK

Decreasing the amount of calories you take in is not enough. Remember, when you diet without exercise, your body actually wastes *fewer* calories as heat. This slows the loss of body fat. Worse than that, some of the weight you lose may be muscle.

In order to lose weight, you also need to increase the amount of calories your body burns. Unfortunately, as we've already pointed out, even at rest, overweight people tend to give off less heat than do people of normal weight. And studies have shown that obese people automatically learn to do tasks with the smallest amount of body movement. For example, they actually expend *less* work making a bed than thin people do. Therefore, it's down to work: You must burn off calories by doing work—that is, by exercising.

The previous chapter discussed exercise in detail. Here I want to present some ideas specifically for those of you who are overweight. Obesity and lack of exercise are closely related. Obesity makes it more difficult to exercise, and without exercise, many of us have difficulty keeping our weight down. This can become another vicious circle, as illustrated in Figure 19.

FIGURE 19

A VICIOUS CIRCLE

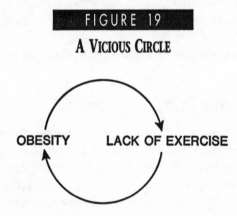

By the same token, exercise does help you lose weight, and losing weight makes it easier to exercise, especially if you jog or run. In a slow jog for 1 hour, a 110-pound woman would burn up about 500 calories. For a 150-pound man, the figure would be 650 calories, and a 200-pounder would burn about 800 calories. Aerobic exercises, such as cross-country skiing or swimming, can burn off as many calories per hour as jogging.

If you are very overweight, instead of jogging, you can walk, ride a bike, or swim. If the 110-pound woman were to walk briskly for 1-hour, she would burn off 230 calories; the 150-pound man would burn off 300 calories, and the 200-

pounder would burn off 360 calories. For a 1-hour leisurely walk, the figures are 150, 180, and 220.

As an example of the value of walking, one group of women who had a sedentary lifestyle and had repeatedly failed to lose weight were instructed to walk for a half hour each day. After a year, they had all lost at least 10 pounds. Those who walked more lost still more weight.

Try to get in the habit of taking advantage of everyday opportunities. For example, use the stairs instead of the elevator; if you have to take things to the basement, make two or three trips instead of one; if you are walking, do it at a brisk pace and don't take the shortcut. Use your imagination.

The bottom line is: You must have patience. Regular exercise may take fat off slowly, but it will *stay* off as long as you continue exercising.

CHANGE YOUR BODY'S FAT SET POINT TO INCREASE THE AMOUNT OF CALORIES YOU BURN OFF

Exercise not only uses more calories while you are working out but also helps reset your set point to cause your body to "waste" more energy, in the form of heat, during the rest of the day—even when you sleep. Exercise builds up your muscles and at the same time actually increases the activity of the fat-burning enzymes in your body.

Even moderate regular physical activity helps elevate the level of hormones such as adrenaline that *promote* fat breakdown and decrease the blood level of the hormone insulin, which *inhibits* fat breakdown.[12] Thus exercise tends to prevent the calories you eat from being turned into fat (since, again, a high level of insulin tends to shift calories into making more fat) and allows fat to be released from the fat cells so the muscles can burn it up. The lower levels of blood insulin may also be the reason exercise helps match your appetite to your body's needs.

CUT BACK ON FOODS CONTAINING SIMPLE CARBOHYDRATES (SUGAR)

Besides exercise, *how* and *what* you eat can influence your body's setpoint. For example, carbohydrates in the form of sugar cause your blood insulin level to rapidly increase, or "spike," more than complex carbohydrates do. The increased level of blood insulin promotes the production of fat and the retention of sodium by the kidneys, and the combination of elevated blood sugar and elevated blood insulin tends to stimulate the sympathetic nervous system, thus raising your blood pressure[13] (remember Chapter 7?). One study showed that in people on low-calorie ("reducing") diets with lots of simple sugar, blood pressure did not drop, whereas people whose diets had the same number of calories but very little sugar did obtain a reduction in blood pressure.[14]

TIMING

Timing is important: It helps if you coordinate your eating with your physical activity. As you recall, a high blood level of insulin tends to shift calories into making more fat. From this, you can correctly conclude that eating just before going to sleep will spike your blood insulin and maximize the storage of the calories in fat at a time when you are going to do *no* exercise to burn calories or to lower the insulin. So midnight snacking may be one of the worst things you can do. Taking in more of your food in the early part of the day can decrease the number of calories used to make fat. A few minutes of *mild* exercise, such as a leisurely walk or a bike ride after a meal, will help keep the blood insulin level from rising and will thus decrease the number of calories in the meal that are converted into body fat. Taking a 15-minute walk after supper, for example, can burn off about 50 calories. That amounts to about 5 pounds of fat per year! Walking after meals seems to be especially effective for those who have trouble losing weight.

Finally, remember that if you not only want to lose weight but want to keep the weight off, you will need to do regular aerobic exercise.

STRESS

Stress can contribute to obesity in at least two ways. From your own experience, you may already know that stress tends to promote overeating and binge eating. But stress also causes the release of certain hormones, such as adrenaline, that stimulate insulin release, thus decreasing fat breakdown. In this way, stress tends to increase the fat setpoint.

If you know stress is a problem, make an effort to learn what you can do about it; there is a lot of literature on the subject. For starters, though, you might try listening to music or taking a short walk as a substitute for binge eating when you feel stress driving you to the icebox. You might also consider various relaxation techniques, including yoga and meditation, to counter the effect of chronic stress on your fat set point. A swim, or a long walk, or a jog outdoors is also good for relieving stress.

PRECAUTIONS

Do not begin a new exercise regimen, or substantially change the one you are currently on, without first consulting your doctor. If you are dieting (decreasing your caloric intake), do not exercise as strenuously as you would if you were not dieting; balance the two activities. Never exercise strenuously after a meal, because more blood is flowing to the stomach and intestines then, and less to the muscles.

GROUP AND PROFESSIONAL SUPPORT

Many people can adjust their life on their own so that their body finds its healthy weight. But many others, especially those with too many fat cells, will have difficulty achieving a healthy weight. Most overweight people have already tried to lose weight and are now discouraged.

In that case, you really have to consider getting into an organized program. It helps to realize that for most obese people, there *is* a way to lose weight. Many of us can't do it on our own but must participate with others. If you insist on doing it on your own, you will probably get very discouraged. A program can give you structure, support, and guidance, such as do *this* this week and *that* next week. Although you can monitor your progress, a program can help monitor you and provide reinforcement.

Finally, a few people are going to have a very difficult time achieving a healthy weight. They should not feel guilty but should realize that they *especially* can't do it on their own and need to participate with others and receive professional help.

SUMMARY

Actually this is a simple illustration of the change in the way scientists think about things, an illustration of the paradigm shift (the framework of the working scientific philosophy or viewpoint) that is currently under way. The Energy Law (from the earlier paradigm) is not only still true but necessary for us to understand fat regulation. But it's not enough. Alone, it is misleading. Thinking in terms of the earlier paradigm, which emphasized only the Conservation of Energy Law, led us to "blame overeating as the major cause of obesity and has stimulated the development of hundreds of diets and other techniques [including pills] to 'control' how much we eat."[15]

We need more than the Energy Law; we need to look at the whole system and focus on the *relationships* (or feedback loops, as they are called) inside the system.

You can participate with your physician—and with nature—to achieve a more healthy weight in the following ways:

1. Change your set point by (a) exercising more, (b) watching *what* you eat, especially your sugar intake, and (c) relieving stress.
2. Restrict calories by (a) decreasing the percentage of calories in your food obtained from fat, (b) cutting back on alcohol, (c) eating fiber-containing foods, such as fruits and vegetables (which fill you up more quickly and also have a high K Factor), and (d) regulating the amount you eat (some may need to restrict calories).

PART FOUR

THE
WORKBOOK

CHAPTER 13

The Workbook

The next breakthrough in medicine is the patient taking responsibility for his own health.

John Knoll, M.D. 1950

In the early months of adopting our program, it is important that you keep records of your progress. Otherwise it will be too easy for you to slack off on some days or make a major mistake (such as eating commercial pickles or several olives for lunch) and thus sabotage your possibility for success.

At the end of this part, we will provide you with a sample chart on which you can record your progress.

Earlier in the book we emphasized that lowering your blood pressure is not enough. You must give your body the care it needs to restore the normal balance between potassium and sodium in your body's cells. So in contrast to the past, when only a symptom (actually a sign)—blood pressure—was treated, we want you to record other signals that reflect the actual condition of your body.

The most important things for you to do for your blood pressure are the following:

• Keep track of your K Factor.
• Keep track of your exercise.
• Keep track of your weight.
• Keep track of your blood pressure.

There is a small section in this part devoted to each of these. In addition, for your general health, you should

• Keep track of your dietary fat intake.

Again, you need to record your progress on the chart provided at the end of this part.

226

KEEP TRACK OF YOUR K FACTOR

It's important that you monitor your progress on our program by keeping track of the K factor in your body. You can do this by monitoring your diet, your urine, and your blood.

MONITORING YOUR DIET

While you follow our sample fourteen-day menu plan, you can look up your daily K Factor, which is given at the end of each day's menus. Then, when planning your own menus, you can determine your K Factor by using the table provided in this chapter.

After a while, you'll become familiar with the potassium and sodium contents of various foods, and you won't have to do any calculations. But in the beginning, you may find it reassuring to double-check the sodium and potassium content of your foods by looking over the table.

POTASSIUM AND SODIUM CONTENT OF FOODS

The items printed in boldface in the table are very good in terms of sodium (Na) and potassium (K) balance and were selected because their sodium content is less than 65 mg and their potassium-to-sodium ratio (K Factor) is greater than 5, or their sodium content is less than 40 mg and their potassium-to-sodium ratio is greater than 3. The italicized foods should be avoided because their sodium content is greater than 200 mg and their potassium-to-sodium ratio is less than 1.0, or their sodium content is greater than 20 mg and their potassium-to-sodium ratio is less than 0.5, or their sodium content is greater than 400 mg. Even though beer and wine are in boldface, they are not recommended (except in moderation), because long-term alcohol consumption has been shown to cause hypertension. Although nuts have a high K Factor, they are not recommended in large quantities because their fat content is high.

The usual portion size for some foods is close to 100 grams (g). Many of the portion sizes were rounded to exactly 100 g to simplify comparisons. For your computations it helps to know that 100 g weighs 3.5 ounces, 100 g of water has a volume of 3.4 fluid ounces, and 1 ounce weighs 28 g. Beverage ounces are given in fluid ounces; all other ounces are avoirdupois weights. Remember that a K/Na ratio of less than 1 means that the food has more sodium than potassium, whereas when it's greater than 1 there's more potassium than sodium. The K Factor of some of the food brands in the following list may have changed since these tables were compiled, so by all means check the labels. New and healthier products are appearing all the time.

Go for the **boldface items** and avoid the *items in italics*. The normal print items are O.K.

Food	Portion Size	Calories Per Portion	K Content (mg)	Na Content (mg)	K/Na Ratio (K Factor)
BEVERAGES					
Apple juice	6 oz (182 g)	86	184	1	180.00
Beer (Pabst)	12 oz (351 g)	147	128	6	22.00
Beer (Natural Lite)	12 oz (353 g)	96	105	7	15.00
Club soda (Seagram)	12 oz (358 g)	0	1.4	93	0.02
Coffee	3.4 oz (100 g)	1	36	1	36.00
Coke	12 oz (373 g)	146	2.5	1	0.16
Cranberry juice*	8 oz (253 g)	147	61	6	10.00
Dr. Pepper	12 oz (370 g)	144	1.4	31	0.05
Ginger ale (Schweppe's)	12 oz (370 g)	115	0.7	26	0.03
Grapefruit juice	6 oz (184 g)	72	298	2	140.00
Milk, skim	12 oz (368 g)	132	532	190	2.80
Mineral water	12 fl oz (360 g)	0	1	1	1.00
Orange juice	8 oz (250 g)	112	500	2	250.00
Orange pop (Sunkist)	12 oz (370 g)	170	1.8	38	0.05
Perrier water (although it has 26 mg calcium)	6.5 fl oz (192 g)	0	0	3	∞
Root beer (Hires)	12 oz (370 g)	152	1.8	66	0.03
7-Up	12 oz (370 g)	160	1.4	39	0.04
Tap water (Burlington, Vermont)	12 oz (355 g)	0	0.7	2.8	0.25
Tomato juice:					
canned	6 oz (182 g)	35	413	364	1.10
canned, unsalted	6 oz (182 g)	35	413	5	83.00
V-8 juice*	8 oz (242 g)	47	493	653	0.74
unsalted*	8 oz (242 g)	53	527	47	11.00
Wine, red	3.5 oz (102 g)	87	94	5	19.00
Wine, sherry	2 oz (59 g)	81	44	2	22.00
Wine, white	12 oz (345 g)	293	248	3.9	64.00
BREADS/CEREALS					
Bagel	1 (55 g)	163	41	198	0.21
Barley, dry	½ cup (100 g)	349	160	3	53.00
Biscuit	1 (35 g)	92	29	156	0.19

Food	Portion Size	Calories Per Portion	K Content (mg)	Na Content (mg)	K/Na Ratio (K Factor)
Blueberry muffin	1 (40 g)	112	46	253	0.18
Bread, corn	1 piece (78 g)	161	122	490	0.25
Bread, cracked wheat	1 slice (25 g)	66	34	132	0.26
Bread, Italian	1 slice (30 g)	83	22	490	0.12
Bread, raisin	1 slice (30 g)	79	70	110	0.64
Bread, rye	1 slice (25 g)	61	36	139	0.26
Bread, white	1 slice (27 g)	74	33	134	0.25
Bread, whole wheat	1 slice (25 g)	61	68	132	0.52
English muffin*	1 (57 g)	135	319	364	0.88
Flour, enriched white	1 cup	400	129	2	64.5
Flour, whole wheat	1 cup	400	444	4	111.0
Grapenuts flakes*	1 oz (28 g)	102	99	218	0.45
Noodles, egg, cooked, no salt	1 cup (160 g)	200	70	3	23.00
Oatmeal	1 oz (28 g)	109	98	0.7	140.00
Puffed wheat	1 cup (14 g)	50	35	1	35.00
Quaker 100% Natural	¼ cup (28 g)	130	120	15	8.00
Raisin Bran (Post)*	2 oz (57 g)	171	370	285	1.3
Rice, brown, dry	¼ cup (46 g)	166	99	4	23.00
Rice, white, dry	¼ cup (46 g)	168	42	2	19.00
Roll, white, hard	1 (50 g)	156	49	313	0.16
Spaghetti, dry	2 oz (57 g)	209	112	1	110.00
Sugar pops*	1 oz (28 g)	109	20	63	0.32
Wheat germ	¼ cup (28 gm)	108	268	1	268
CRACKERS					
Cheese Nips	100 g	479	109	1039	0.10
Graham	100 g	384	384	670	0.57
Ritz	100 g	438	113	750	0.15
Ry-Krisp	100 g	344	600	882	0.68
Saltines	100 g	433	120	1100	0.11
DESSERTS					
Angel food cake	100 g	269	88	283	0.31
Animal crackers	100 g	429	95	303	0.31

Food	Portion Size	Calories Per Portion	K Content (mg)	Na Content (mg)	K/Na Ratio (K Factor)
Apple pie	100 g	256	80	301	0.27
Applesauce (unsweetened)	100g	41	78	2	39.00
Apricots (canned)	100 g	66	239	1	240.00
Banana custard pie	100 g	221	203	194	1.00
Brownies	100 g	485	190	251	0.76
Cherry pie	100 g	261	105	304	0.34
Chocolate cake	100 g	369	154	235	0.66
Coffee cake	100 g	322	109	431	0.25
Custard, chocolate*	½ cup (112 g)	142	186	153	1.22
Doughnut, plain	3 (100 g)	391	90	501	0.18
Fig newtons	5½ (100 g)	358	198	252	0.79
Fruitcake, dark	100 g	379	496	158	3.10
Fruitcake, light	100 g	389	233	193	1.20
Lemon meringue pie	100 g	255	50	282	0.18
Orange sherbet	100 g	134	22	10	2.20
Peach pie	100 g	255	149	268	0.56
Pecan pie	100 g	418	123	221	0.56
Pumpkin pie	100 g	211	160	214	0.75
Raisin pie	100 g	270	192	285	0.67
Vanilla pudding (instant)*	½ cup (148 g)	147	207	422	0.49
Vanilla tapioca	100 g	134	135	156	0.86
Vanilla wafers	100 g	462	72	252	0.29
FATS/OILS					
Butter, salted	1 tbsp (14.2 g)	102	3	140	0.02
All cooking oils	1 tbsp (13.6 g)	120	0	0	—
French dressing	1 tbsp (16 g)	66	13	219	0.06
Margarine	1 tbsp (14.2 g)	102	8	140	0.06
Mayonnaise	1 tbsp (14 g)	101	5	84	0.06
FISH/SEAFOOD					
Catfish	100 g	103	330	60	5.50
Clams, cherrystone	6–7 (100 g)	80	311	205	1.50
Clams, soft	100 g	82	235	36	6.50

Food	Portion Size	Calories Per Portion	K Content (mg)	Na Content (mg)	K/Na Ratio (K Factor)
Cod, fillet	100 g	170	407	110	3.70
Flounder, or sole	100 g	202	587	237	2.50
Haddock	100 g	165	348	177	2.00
Halibut, steak	100 g	171	525	134	3.90
Lobster, cooked	100 g	95	180	210	0.86
Oysters, fried	100 g	239	203	206	0.98
Oysters, raw	100 g	66	121	73	1.70
Pike, walleye, raw	100 g	93	319	51	6.30
Salmon, canned	100 g	141	361	387	0.93
Salmon, steak	100 g	182	443	116	3.80
Sardines, Atlantic, canned in oil	100 g	311	560	510	1.10
Scallops	100 g	81	396	255	1.60
Shrimp	100 g	91	220	140	1.60
Tuna, white	½ can (100 g)	288	301	800	0.38
canned in oil	¾ can (184 g)	381	506	1159	0.44
in water	¾ can (184 g)	237	487	865	0.56
in water, low salt	¾ can 184 g)	230	487	72	6.8
Whitefish	100 g	155	299	52	5.80
FRUITS					
Apple	1 medium (150 g)	80	152	1	150.00
Apricots	3 (114 g)	55	301	1	300.00
Avocado	100 g	167	604	4	150.00
Banana	1 medium (175 g)	101	440	1	440.00
Blueberries	1 cup (145 g)	90	117	1	120.00
Cantaloupe	½ (477 g)	82	682	33	21.00
Cherries	100 g	70	191	2	96.00
Coconut	100 g	346	256	23	11.00
Cranberries	100 g	46	82	2	41.00
Dates	10 (80 g)	219	518	1	520.00
Grapefruit	1 medium (400 g)	80	265	2	130.00
Grapes	10 (40 g)	18	42	1	42.00
Olives, green	100 g	116	55	2400	0.02
Orange	1 medium (180 g)	64	263	1	260.00

Food	Portion Size	Calories Per Portion	K Content (mg)	Na Content (mg)	K/Na Ratio (K Factor)
Peach	1 (175 g)	58	308	2	150.00
Pear	1(180g)	100	213	3	71.00
Pineapple	1 slice (84 g)	44	123	1	120.00
Plantain	1 medium (365 g)	313	1012	13	77.00
Plums	10 medium (110 g)	66	299	2	150.00
Raisins	1 tbsp (9 g)	26	69	2	34.00
Strawberries	1 cup (149 g)	55	244	1	240.00
Watermelon	100 g	26	100	1	100.00
MEATS/POULTRY					
Bacon	1 slice (15 g)	86	35	153	0.23
Beef, ground	3.5 oz (100 g)	287	270	60	4.50
Beef, rib roast	1 piece (85 g)	374	189	41	4.60
*Bologna (beef)**	1 slice (23 g)	72	36	230	0.16
Chicken, baked	2 pieces (50 g)	83	206	32	6.40
Egg	1 medium (50 g)	72	57	54	1.10
Ham	2 pieces (85 g)	318	220	48	4.60
Hot dog	1 (45 g)	139	99	495	0.20
Lamb chop	3.4 oz (95 g)	341	234	51	4.60
Liver, beef, cooked	100 g	229	380	184	2.10
Liver, chicken, cooked	100 g	165	151	61	2.50
Pork chop	3 oz (85 g)	308	233	51	4.60
Pork sausage	1 patty (27 g)	129	73	259	0.28
Steak, sirloin	8 oz (226 g)	876	583	127	4.60
Veal cutlet	3 oz (85 g)	184	258	56	4.60
Veal breast	8 oz (226 g)	684	471	103	4.60
MILK PRODUCTS					
Cheese, American	1 slice (14 g)	52	11	159	0.07
Cheese, cheddar	1 slice (24 g)	96	20	168	0.12
Cheese, cottage	1 ounce (28 g)	30	24	65	0.37
Cheese, cream	1 tbsp (14 g)	52	10	35	0.29
Cheese, Swiss	1 slice (14 g)	52	15	99	0.15
unsalted	1 slice (14g)	52	15	6	2.50
Cream, light	1 tbsp (15 g)	32	18	6	3.00
Cream, heavy	1 tbsp (15 g)	53	13	5	2.60

Food	Portion Size	Calories Per Portion	K Content (mg)	Na Content (mg)	K/Na Ratio (K Factor)
Ice cream	1 cup (133 g)	257	241	84	2.90
Ice milk	1 cup (131 g)	184	265	105	2.50
Milk, skim	1 cup (245 g)	88	355	127	2.80
Milk, powdered skim	1 cup (245 g)	88	355	127	2.80
Milk, whole	1 cup (244 g)	161	342	122	2.80
Yogurt, skim milk	1 cup (245 g)	123	350	125	2.80
Goat milk	1 cup (244 g)	163	439	83	5.30
Human milk	1 cup (244 g)	188	124	39	3.20

NUTS AND SWEETENERS; MISCELLANEOUS

Food	Portion Size	Calories Per Portion	K Content (mg)	Na Content (mg)	K/Na Ratio (K Factor)
Almonds	100 g	598	773	4	190.00
Falafel	3 patties (51 g)	170	298	150	1.99
Honey	100 g	304	51	5	10.00
Hummus (made from garbanzo beans)	1 cup (246 gm)	420	427	599	0.71
Maple syrup*	5 tbsp (100 g)	252	176	10	17.60
Nondairy creamer	½ oz (14 g)	22	5	7	0.71
Peanut butter	100 g	589	627	605	1.00
Peanuts, unsalted	100 g	582	701	5	140.00
Pecans	100 g	687	603	trace	600.00
Potato chips	1 oz (28 g)	150	380	170	2.2
Soy milk	1 cup (240 gm)	140	450	120	3.75
Sugar, brown	5 tsp (70 g)	364	161	17	9.5
Sugar, white	½ cup (100 g)	385	1	—	—
Tahini (sesame butter)	1 tsp (15 g)	89	62	17	3.60
Tofu (raw)	½ cup (124 g)	94	150	9	16.70
Walnuts, English	100 g	651	450	2	225.00

PREPARED FOODS

Food	Portion Size	Calories Per Portion	K Content (mg)	Na Content (mg)	K/Na Ratio (K Factor)
Burrito, beef, (Taco Bell)	184 g	431	320	1311	0.25
Chicken chow mein, canned	100 g	38	167	290	0.58
*Chicken chow mein, frozen dinner, (Banquet)**	12 oz (340 g)	282	241	2268	0.11

Food	Portion Size	Calories Per Portion	K Content (MG)	Na Content (MG)	K/Na Ratio (K Factor)
Chicken, drumstick (Kentucky Fried Chicken)*	57 g	152	122	269	0.59
Corned beef hash	100 g	181	200	540	0.37
Fried shrimp (Arthur Treacher)*	115 g	381	99	537	0.18
Hamburger (Burger King)*	110 g	272	240	505	0.46
Hamburger (McDonald's)*	102 g	255	142	490	0.27
Lasagna, cheese, frozen (Stouffers)*	10+ oz (298 g)	385	580	1200	0.48
Pizza, sausage	100g	245	114	647	0.18
Salisbury steak, 3-course frozen dinner (Swanson)*	16 oz (454 g)	490	545	1680	0.32
Turkey pot pie	100 g	197	114	369	0.31
VEGETABLES (UNPROCESSED WHEN NOT SPECIFIED)					
Alfalfa sprouts	1 cup (33 g)	10	26	2	13.00
Asparagus	4 spears (100 g)	26	278	2	140.00
(cooked, no salt)	100 g	20	183	1	180.00
Beans, black	1 cup (172 gm)	227	611	1	611.00
Beans, green	100 g	25	151	4	38.00
(canned)	100 g	18	95	236	0.40
Beans, kidney (dry)	100 g	343	984	10	98.00
(cooked from dry)	100 g	118	340	3	110.00
(canned)*	⅔ cup (100 g)	90	264	300	0.88
Beans, lima	100 g	111	422	1	420.00
Beans, navy (dry)	100 g	340	1196	19	63.00
Beans, pinto (dry)	100 g	349	984	10	98.00
Beans, yellow wax	100 g	22	151	3	50.00
Bean sprouts	½ cup	16	77	3	25.67
Beets	100 g	32	208	43	4.80
(canned)	100 g	34	167	236	0.71
Broccoli	100 g	32	382	15	25.00
Brussels sprouts	100 g	45	390	14	28.00
Cabbage	100 g	24	233	20	12.00
(cooked)	100 g	20	163	14	12.00

Food	Portion Size	Calories Per Portion	K Content (mg)	Na Content (mg)	K/Na Ratio (K Factor)
Carrots	100 g	31	222	33	6.70
Cauliflower	100 g	27	295	13	23.00
(cooked)	100 g	22	206	9	23.00
Celery	100 g	17	341	126	2.70
Chick-peas (boiled) (garbanzo beans)	1 cup (164 gm)	269	477	11	43.36
Corn, sweet	1 ear (140 g)	70	151	1	151.00
(canned)	100 g	83	97	230	0.42
Cucumber	100 g	15	160	6	27.00
Eggplant	100 g	19	150	1	150.00
Green pepper	100 g	22	213	13	16.00
Lentils (dry)	100 g	340	790	30	26.00
Lettuce, iceberg	100 g	13	175	9	19.00
Lettuce, leaf	100 g	18	264	9	29.00
Mushrooms	100 g	28	414	15	28.00
(canned)	100 g	17	197	400	0.49
Onions, cooked	100 g	29	110	7	16.00
Peas, cooked	1 cup (160 g)	114	314	2	160.00
Peas, canned	100 g	77	96	236	0.41
Pickles, dill	100 g	11	200	1428	0.14
Potato, baked	1 medium (202 g)	145	782	6	130.00
Sauerkraut (canned)	100 g	18	140	747	0.19
Soy beans (dry)	100 g	403	1677	5	340.00
Spinach	100 g	26	470	71	6.60
Squash, acorn	100 g	55	480	1	480.00
Squash, zucchini	100 g	12	141	1	140.00
Sweet potato, baked	100 g	114	243	10	24.00
Tomato	1 medium (135 g)	27	300	4	75.00
(canned)	100 g	21	217	130	1.67

References: Values per 100 g are from Watt, B. K., and A. L. Merrill, *Composition of Foods*, Agriculture Handbook No. 8, U.S. Dept. of Agriculture, U.S. Government Printing Office, Washington, D.C., 1975. Values in common units are from Adams, C. F., *Nutritive Value of American Foods in Common Units*, Agriculture Handbook No. 456, U.S. Dept. of Agriculture, U.S. Government Printing Office, Washington, D.C., 1975. Values marked with asterisk (*) are from Pennington, J. A. T., and H. Nichols Church, *Food Values of Portions Commonly Used* (14th Ed.), Harper & Row, New York, 1985. This book is recommended for those readers who wish additional information on food values. We thank Harper & Row and the authors, J. A. T. Pennington and H. Nichols Church, for allowing us to use their copyrighted material.

If you are eating mainly foods that are typed in boldface in the table, you probably don't need to calculate your K Factor. But if you eat some major "regular type" or italicized items, your K Factor could drop below 3.

Here are two examples of calculating your K Factor. First let's consider a cheese sandwich lunch in Table 5. We can calculate the K Factor of this lunch by making a table of the ingredients (remember, K = potassium, Na = sodium):

TABLE 5

CALCULATING A LUNCH K FACTOR

ITEM	K (MG)	NA (MG)	K FACTOR (K/NA)
2 slices commercial whole-wheat bread	136	264	0.52
1 slice unsalted Swiss cheese	15	6	2.5
1 tablespoon unsalted, eggless mayonnaise (data from label)	34	13	2.6
2 leaves lettuce (10 g)	18	1	18
1 glass skim milk (8 oz)	355	127	2.8
1 apple	152	1	150
Totals	710	412	
Meal's K Factor			1.7

Notice that in this version of lunch, the K Factor is 1.7, even though commercial salted bread was used. If unsalted whole wheat bread had been used, dropping the two-slice amount of sodium from 264 to about 2 mg, the lunch's K Factor would have been 4.6. However, although 1.7 is definitely submarginal, the K Factor for the day could still be kept above 4 by eating a healthy breakfast and dinner.

But suppose you were to sneak in a commercial dill pickle. After all, every ingredient but the bread has a K Factor well above 2. The commercial dill pickle should do little harm, right? Let's take a look in Table 6.

TABLE 6

LUNCH WITH PICKLE ADDED: K FACTOR

ITEM	K (MG)	NA (MG)	K FACTOR (K/NA)
2 slices commercial whole-wheat bread	136	264	0.52
1 slice unsalted Swiss cheese	15	6	2.5
1 tablespoon unsalted, eggless mayonnaise	34	13	2.6
2 leaves lettuce (10 g)	18	1	18
1 glass skim milk (8 oz.)	355	127	2.8
1 apple	152	1	150
1 large commercial dill pickle	200	1428	0.14
Totals	910	1840	
Meal's K Factor			0.49

Quite a bit of harm was done just by that pickle! The huge amount of sodium in the pickle shot the sodium total so high that the K Factor for the whole lunch is now only 0.49! You really sabotage the entire meal just by eating one pickle. Now it would be extremely difficult to bring the day's K Factor above 4, even with a very good breakfast and dinner.

The important point here is that you cannot just estimate the overall K Factor by averaging the individual K Factors. You have to divide the *total* potassium by the *total* sodium in order to determine the overall K Factor.

Now let's consider an entire day. Suppose it looks like Table 7.

TABLE 7

K FACTOR FOR ENTIRE DAY

ITEM	K (MG)	NA (MG)	K FACTOR (K/NA)
Breakfast	1572	204	7.7
Lunch	1065	1016	1.0
Snack	159	1	159.0
Dinner	3137	156	20.1
Totals	5933	1377	
Day's K Factor			4.3

Notice that the overall K Factor for the day is a healthy 4.3.

But suppose it's Friday and you decide to celebrate by having a commercial pizza for dinner instead of the lentil casserole and squash dinner you had originally planned. Table 8 shows what happens to the K Factor for the day.

TABLE 8

FRIDAY K FACTOR WITH BEER AND PIZZA

ITEM	K (MG)	NA (MG)	K FACTOR (K/NA)
Breakfast	1572	204	7.7
Lunch	1065	1016	1.0
Snack	159	1	159.0
½ sausage pizza (200 g)	228	1294	0.18
Two 12-oz beers	256	12	21.3
Totals	3280	2527	
Day's K Factor			1.3

In Table 9, the beer and pizza dinner, considered by itself, turns out to have a very unhealthy K Factor of 0.37

TABLE 9

BEER AND PIZZA DINNER: K FACTOR

ITEM	K (MG)	NA (MG)	K FACTOR (K/NA)
½ sausage pizza (200 g)	228	1294	0.18
Two 12-oz beers	256	12	21.3
Totals	484	1306	
Meal's K Factor			0.37

The pizza-beer fling brought the K Factor for the entire day down to 1.3, from the original menu plan value of 4.3. By changing the canned chunky chicken soup for lunch to low-salt soup, you could bring the K Factor up to 1.8. Since 1.8 is a much healthier K Factor than most people eat, you might allow yourself a pizza once in a rare while if your other meals for the day are very healthy ones. (A better alternative, though, is to make your own pizza, without adding table salt [or sodium chloride], using less cheese, and putting on green peppers, onions, and/or mushrooms instead of sausage. Use unsalted tomato paste and spice it up with herbs!)

ESTIMATING YOUR K FACTOR FROM URINE SAMPLES

Space is provided on your progress sheet for recording and calculating your K Factor. But even if the K Factor in your food is high enough, you might blow it by getting sodium from another source, such as drinking water from a water softener or from an over-the-counter drug. Or perhaps you are eating lots of foods that aren't in the table and you're not sure about the K Factor.

Well, there is another way to keep track of your K Factor, although it's somewhat inconvenient. You can collect your urine for a 24-hour period and take it to your doctor or medical laboratory for a potassium and sodium analysis.

To collect a 24-hour urine sample, you'll need a clean, 1-gallon *plastic* bottle. In it you must collect every drop of urine you produce over a 24-hour period. Here's how to do it.

When you get up in the morning, completely empty your bladder into the toilet as usual. That way you get rid of the previous day's urine and start fresh for the new day. From then on, you need to collect all your urine in the bottle. It will be hard to remember. If you're at home, place the bottle on the toilet seat to remind yourself. If it's a workday, keep the bottle (in a bag if you wish) somewhere where it will remind you, and tie a string on your finger. Continue to collect every drop of your urine through the evening and night. When you get up the next morning, completely empty your bladder *into the bottle.* You now have a 24-hour urine sample.

Take this sample to your doctor or medical lab to have it analyzed to determine how much sodium and potassium you excrete in your urine over a 24-hour period. This will be approximately equal to the amount you are eating per day. (Actually it's a little less, since small amounts are lost in the stool and in the sweat. If you sweated a lot during the 24-hour period, make a note of it, as the lab may want to correct for the estimated loss of sodium and potassium in your sweat; see Chapter 16.)

Since your eating habits are likely to be different on weekdays than on weekends, we recommend you collect samples for analysis from each of these periods.

MONITORING YOUR BLOOD POTASSIUM

One simple step that you can take to help determine if your body is deficient in potassium is to ask your physician to have your blood potassium level measured.

Unfortunately, however, this doesn't always give you the information you need. If the level is between 4 and 5 milliequivalents per liter (mEq/L) (the upper limit of normal), you still may or may not have enough potassium in your body. Why can't you be certain? What you need to know is the level of potassium in your cells, not your blood, and it is possible to have sufficient amounts in the blood but not in the cells.

On the other hand, if the blood level is low (below 4 mEq/L), you may have a problem. The level of potassium in the blood seldom drops unless your body cells are deficient. If it is below the accepted "normal" limit of 3.5 mEq/L, you can be sure the cell level is low as well.

Thus, a blood test cannot assure you that your K Factor is high enough, but it can provide you with an indication that it may be too low.

KEEP TRACK OF YOUR EXERCISE

On the progress chart, space is provided for you to enter the number of times each week you have vigorously (and continuously) exercised for at least 20 minutes, for 20 to 30 minutes, and for over 30 minutes.

Your pulse rate, taken upon awakening, is an easy measure of your progress in the exercise program. Take your pulse before sitting up or getting out of bed. Count the pulses in your wrist or neck for 30 seconds and multiply by 2.

Please review Chapter 11 for recommendations about exercise.

KEEP TRACK OF YOUR WEIGHT

Because of variations in the amount of water in your body during the day, it is best to check your weight at the same time each day, without clothes. Be sure the scale is accurate.

If your weight is normal, a weekly check will ensure that you don't start to gain. But if you use the principles we have outlined for choosing and preparing your food (see Chapter 10) and get at least some regular exercise (see Chapter 11), you shouldn't have any trouble maintaining normal weight.

If you are overweight, our program should help you reduce gradually. If it doesn't, cut your calories by a quarter and be especially careful to eat as little fat as possible (see Chapter 12). A loss of about one or at most two pounds per week is realistic *and* better than the more rapid loss that you could get by severe calorie restriction. If it seems you need to make a conscious effort to reduce calories in ways other than by reducing your dietary fat intake, get the advice of your doctor or a nutritionist before restricting your calories to less than 1200 per day.

KEEP TRACK OF YOUR BLOOD PRESSURE

Measuring your own blood pressure at home is easy, and you really should do it if you want to make sure it is getting down to within the "normal" range. Furthermore, keeping track of your own progress is an excellent way to stay motivated in curing your hypertension. The feedback you get will encourage you to get or keep your K Factor high, your dietary fat low, your weight normal, and your exercise patterns regular.

Figure 20 provides a diagram of the circulatory system, showing how a blood pressure cuff is used to measure the blood pressure inside the artery in your arm.

FIGURE 20

THE CIRCULATORY SYSTEM AND A BLOOD PRESSURE CUFF

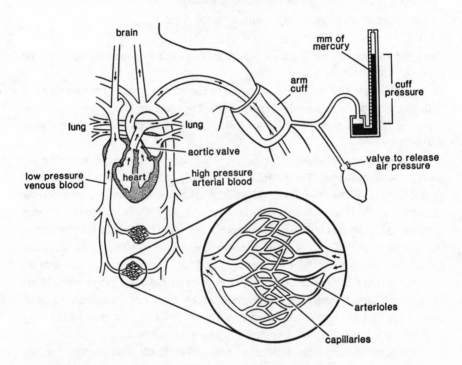

The small-diameter arterioles the blood has to pass through before reaching the capillaries should remind you of the nozzle in our hose drawing in Figure 11 of Chapter 4.

GETTING THE RIGHT EQUIPMENT

First you need the right equipment for measuring your own blood pressure: some kind of *blood pressure cuff* and, if the cuff does not have a built-in listening device, a *stethoscope*. You can obtain both devices in a blood pressure kit or buy them separately.

The Blood Pressure Cuff

The blood pressure cuff is made of cloth with a rubber bladder sewn inside. This bladder is attached by rubber tubing to (1) a rubber bulb with a one-way valve, so that repeatedly squeezing the bulb pumps air into the bladder, (2) an adjustable release valve for letting the air out of the bladder, and (3) a device for measuring the air pressure inside the bladder. The measuring device itself can be one of the following:

- A mechanical dial
- A column of mercury in a calibrated glass tube
- An electronic pressure sensor with a digital display

The most inexpensive cuffs are the dial type (you can buy a reasonably good one for under $30).

If you buy the dial type, you will need to check its accuracy by comparing it with your doctor's cuff (see the next section). The mercury type, more expensive and more likely to break, is more reliably accurate; it is probably the type your doctor has.

The new electronic automatic type has a built-in microphone, eliminating the need for a stethoscope. The systolic and diastolic blood pressure appear on a digital display. Some cost under $100. My colleague Dr. Webb purchased an electronic digital blood pressure monitor by mail order for $49.95 and has found it to be very accurate and reliable. It displays not only systolic and diastolic pressures but also pulse rate. The air pressure release valve has two positions: a slow release (which you adjust with a screwdriver to 2 or 3 mm Hg per second) and a rapid release. The May 1987 issue of *Consumer Reports* (pages 314–319) reported tests of 36 home blood pressure monitors, both mechanical and electronic. Most of these were found to be easily usable and provided readings that varied only slightly from those obtained simultaneously by a trained person.

Cuffs come in three sizes. Before you rush out to the medical supply store, use a tape measure to determine the circumference of (distance around) the midsection of your upper arm. This is the only way you can decide which size to get. Table 10 lists the sizes.

TABLE 10

CHOOSING THE CORRECT CUFF SIZE

ARM CIRCUMFERENCE	CUFF SIZE
6.5 to 10 inches	Small adult cuff
9.5 to 12.5 inches	Standard adult cuff
12.5 to 16.5 inches	Large adult cuff

It is important to get the right size cuff because the wrong one will give you incorrect readings. Since it's a nuisance to keep more than one size cuff on hand, even doctors sometimes make the mistake of using the wrong size. For example, suppose you have a large muscular (or fat) arm, measuring 15 inches around. A standard cuff is not wide enough to transfer the full amount of pressure that is inside the cuff to the tissues surrounding the artery in your arm. You would need to pump in more air to collapse the artery, so that the reading you get will be too high—as much as 30 mm Hg too high. Thus, there are some people who are being treated for high blood pressure who probably don't really have it; they just have big arms!

The Stethoscope

The stethoscope brings the sounds of blood pulsing through your arm's artery to your ears through rubber or plastic tubing. A stethoscope costs only about $5, and some blood pressure kits come with one. There are two types. One has a bell-shaped end for collecting the sound; the other has a thin plastic diaphragm. Either type will work, but we prefer the bell-shaped type.

CHECKING THE ACCURACY OF YOUR EQUIPMENT

Considering that there are all kinds of cuffs, it is important to make sure you are getting the same readings your doctor is getting. Check the accuracy of your equipment against your doctor's mercury type, especially if you have the dial type. You can connect the two with a Y-shaped tubing connector. Sometimes the two cuffs can have a discrepancy of as much as 5%. You can correct for this if you know about it. Your readings will be misleading if you don't.

If you have the electronic type, there is the possibility of error from variations in the position of the microphone. When the microphone is not over the artery, you usually get diastolic pressure readings that are too high (or you may get an error signal). Again, you should compare your instrument's reading with the reading your doctor obtains.

TAKING THE MEASUREMENT

You should be completely relaxed, both mentally and physically, before your blood pressure is measured. You should be in a warm, quiet room, seated in a comfortable chair beside a table. All your muscles should be as relaxed as possible, and you should not talk. You may be pleasantly surprised to find that your blood pressure measured at home is lower than the reading obtained in your doctor's office. If you know that your equipment measures the same as your doctor's, or if you have corrected for any discrepancy, your lower home reading probably occurs because you aren't nervous or worried, as you may have been in the doctor's office. (Chapters 4 and 17 explain how your sympathetic nervous system, activated by being nervous or worried, constricts your arterioles, thus raising your blood pressure.) In the less likely event that your home readings are higher than your doctor's, you should schedule an appointment and take in your cuff to figure out why.

To measure your pressure at home, rest your arm on a table while you are sitting (so that the middle of the cuff will be even with the level of your heart, thus eliminating "hydrostatic" pressure). Your palm should face up. Wrap the cuff around your bare arm and fasten it so that it is snug but not tight. The lower edge should be about one inch above the bend of your elbow (to allow room for the stethoscope over the artery). The arrow on the cuff should be pointing approximately to where your artery is—aimed slightly toward your torso from the middle of the upward surface of your arm, just above the bend at your elbow. Find out exactly where it is by feeling the pulse with your fingers. If you have an electronic cuff, place the circle showing the location of the microphone directly over the artery where you feel your pulse.

If you do not have an electronic cuff, place the end of your stethoscope on your skin over the artery just below the cuff. Apply very light pressure on the head of the stethoscope, just barely firm enough to make even contact with your skin.

By squeezing the bulb, inflate the cuff to a pressure about 40 mm Hg higher than your last systolic reading in order to collapse the artery completely. You will not hear any sound through the stethoscope at this time because all blood flow to your lower arm has been cut off.

Now gradually (at a rate of 2 or 3 mm Hg per second) let the air out of the bladder by turning the screw at the end of the bulb to open the pressure release valve. Or, if you have a two-position air release valve, make sure it is in the slow release position before you pump up the cuff.

When you can hear a beating sound (as little spurts of blood begin to open up the artery again), take a reading of the pressure. This is your systolic blood pressure. (The electronic cuff gives you this reading automatically.)

As the air pressure in the cuff continues to drop, you will continue to hear rhythmic beating sounds in the stethoscope. (Some electronic types make a beeping sound.) The artery is now open when the heart beats, but it is still collapsing between beats because the cuff pressure is greater than the diastolic blood pressure.

As soon as the beating sounds first disappear (the artery is open continuously), take your second pressure reading. This is the diastolic blood pressure. (Again, the electronic cuff gives you this reading automatically.) After diastolic pressure is reached, you may switch to rapid air release to relieve the pressure on your arm. You have now measured your blood pressure.

Repeat the measurement after 5 minutes. Take your blood pressure on at least two different days a week and record the average of the readings on the progress chart.

KEEP TRACK OF YOUR DIETARY FAT

In addition to keeping track of your K Factor, you will also need to watch the amount of fat you eat. As we discussed in Part Three, this will help you lose weight as well as reduce atherosclerosis and decrease your chances of having a heart attack or of developing cancer.

The daily progress chart provides space to record the amount of fat, carbohydrate, and protein in the food you eat. Since fat has about 9 calories per gram, you can calculate what percentage of your calories is from fat with the following formula:

$$\frac{9 \times Fat}{Calories} \times 100$$

For example, if the label on a package of ice cream says there are 9 grams of fat and 160 calories per serving, you would do the following calculation:

$$\frac{9 \times 9}{160} \times 100 \quad or \quad \frac{81}{160} \times 100 \quad or \quad 0.51 \times 100$$

or 51%. You now know that 51% of the calories in the ice cream come from fat. Try this calculation out on some dairy product substitutes. You may be surprised when you find that most nondairy "creamers" and some nondairy ice cream substitutes are loaded with fat.

As we have said, you should keep your daily fat consumption down to less than 20% of your calories. The rest of your calories should come from carbohydrates and protein.

The currently recommended minimum protein consumption is 56 grams per day. You will stay healthy and keep your kidneys happy if most of your calories come from complex carbohydrates such as pasta or potatoes.

USING THE PROGRESS CHART

At the end of this chapter is a sample progress chart together with a blank chart for you to photocopy. The first line of the chart is for recording your blood pressure. I suggest that you measure it twice each day on at least two days each week, and measure it at least twice in a row each time. In the chart, record the average of all the readings.

When you enter your K Factor, you will usually have to estimate your average for the week from your diet. This will be easy while you are following the menu plan. During the transition week the K Factor averages 1.9, and during Days 8 through 14 of the recommended plan the average is 4.9. If you have a determination of the K Factor in your urine done during a particular week, use that value and indicate with a "U" on the chart. Where the chart says drugs, write the names of prescription drugs you're taking, and use a horizontal arrow to indicate the time span.

A central theme of this book is participation with your doctor, and of course, I have already participated by writing the book. But to close the circle, *you* are being offered the chance to participate also.

Your help to continue building a data base on the results of the K Factor program would be appreciated. If you wish to participate, after completing 24 weeks and recording the results on the chart, return a photocopy of your chart along with any shopping tips or other suggestions you might have. If you miss a week here and there, leave that week blank. In order to help verify the report, either print or type your name and address and sign it, or, if you wish anonymity, have your physician sign it and include his or her printed name and address. Then mail the form to:

K Factor
P. O. Box 19
Rochester, VT 05767

AGE 50 **INITIAL WEIGHT** 168 **HEIGHT** 6'0" **SEX** MALE

WEEK	1	2	3	4	5	6	7	8	9	10	11	12
Blood Pressure (systolic/diastolic)		138/87								127/82		
Pulse upon awakening		64								58		
Weight		166								163		
Number of "workouts" (aerobic exercise)												
less than 20 minutes		2								2		
20 to 30 minutes												
greater than 30 minutes		1								2		
K Factor (K/Na ratio)		0.5								4.4		
Serum K		3.8								4.1		
Drugs		Diuril							→			

AGE ▭   INITIAL WEIGHT ▭   HEIGHT ▭   SEX ▭

WEEK	1	2	3	4	5	6	7	8	9	10	11	12
Blood Pressure (systolic/diastolic)												
Pulse upon awakening												
Weight												
Number of "workouts" (aerobic exercise)												
less than 20 minutes												
20 to 30 minutes												
greater than 30 minutes												
K Factor (K/Na ratio)												
Serum K												
Drugs												

PART FIVE

ADDITIONAL
CONSIDERATIONS

CHAPTER 14

Why the Emphasis on Drugs?

One of the most highly developed skills in contemporary Western civilization is dissection: the split-up of problems into their smallest possible components. We are good at it. So good, we often forget to put the pieces back together again.

Alvin Toffler[1]

We often miss the forest for the trees. Antihypertensive drugs have been a success—but only a partial one. Their most obvious and significant success has been reducing (but not eliminating) strokes due to hypertension. The trade-off is that the drugs must be taken for life, frequently make the patient feel bad, and cost the country several billions of dollars each year. Thus, the drug approach to treating high blood pressure can hardly be called an unqualified success. Given what we now know, this isn't too surprising. As long as we didn't have much insight into the mechanism of hypertension, drugs could be developed to treat only the blood pressure rather than the underlying problem.

Now that the evidence is clear that hypertension involves much more than elevated blood pressure, it's time to put the pieces together again. But first let's ask how a whole society, professionals and laypersons alike, could have gone so far down a path that cost so much money yet missed the most important goals: optimum health and long life.

In the 1950s, the decade of the "miracle drugs," the time was ripe for acceptance of drugs as the answer to any condition for which the cause wasn't known. Not only didn't we realize the extent of the problem in primary hypertension, we were mystified as to its cause (except for a few rare pioneers like Dr. Lewis Dahl).

This is revealed in the term itself: Health professionals use the term *primary* to describe a condition for which they don't know the cause; if they know its cause, they call it *secondary*.

A personal example illustrates this almost automatic reliance upon drugs. In 1956, between my junior and senior year in medical school, I had a summer job in a drug company with a group doing research on a drug that inhibited the absorption of cholesterol from the intestine into the blood. The idea was to help prevent heart attacks. At the time, the thought entered my mind that it might be easier simply to eat foods that didn't contain cholesterol. Had I known that only animal products (meat, milk, and egg yolks), not fruits or vegetables, contain cholesterol, this thought might have been more than a passing one, but I had been told that changing the diet just wasn't a practical way to treat people, since they wouldn't follow the recommendations. So, like so many others, I fell back in line and returned to research on a drug to treat a nutritional problem! The moral: When everyone is marching in a given direction, not only is it hard to go the other way, it's difficult to *even see the other path.*

Is there an explanation for our almost unquestioning belief in the efficacy of drugs to treat all health problems?

WHY WERE WE ON THE WRONG PATH?

In my view, our avoidance of lifestyle responsibilities and (until recently) near-total reliance upon drugs to deal with hypertension has been an ultimate result of some fundamental assumptions of Western—especially American—culture. As Pogo used to say, the problem is not them (the medical establishment and the pharmaceutical companies), but us—all of us.

The following are the main points:

• Historically, our culture has regarded science as a means to dominate nature rather than to understand it. In the process, we have cut ourselves off not only from the nature outside of ourselves but from our inner human nature. The latter separation has helped disempower us; and in this obsession with domination and control, we have dismissed anything we can't see as unreal—and "visionary." The spiritual aspect of science—exhibited by such figures as Kepler, Newton, and Einstein—has been dismissed as "impractical." Rather than emphasizing science as a means of *understanding,* our culture has taken the position that "knowledge is power." The resulting alienation, lack of vision, and emphasis on control has had disastrous results for the health of human beings and indeed for the whole planet.

There have been several corollaries of these cultural biases:

- Technology, which is really the application of science, is often confused with science itself; our schools teach "science and technology" rather than science. Our culture idolizes technology. This idolatry inspires a blind faith that the presumed benefits of technology will ultimately outweigh any undesirable side effects. We have made technology and the domination of nature the myth of our time.

- Drugs, such as the "miracle drug" diuretic pill that reduces blood pressure, are decidedly high-tech and glamorous. Nutritional solutions such as Kempner's rice-fruit diet are low-tech and less glamorous.

- A lot of money is behind drugs. Pharmaceutical companies naturally want to see a good return on their sizable investment, and they therefore bombard doctors with intensive marketing efforts.

- Patients themselves demand drugs. The American public by and large wants a pill to cure anything that ails them.

- Doctors are wary of malpractice suits and are therefore wary of prescribing outside the accepted, conventional treatments—until recently consisting primarily of antihypertensive drugs—lest they be liable if something goes wrong.

- In general, doctors know very little about nondrug programs. For example, in medical schools there still is little, if any, training in either nutrition, exercise physiology, or biophysics. Moreover, there has been a growing tendency to diminish education in such systems, or "holistic" disciplines such as physiology and biophysics, to make way for more emphasis upon reductionist "molecular" approaches naturally emphasizing drugs.

- It is difficult to accept a nondrug solution if there is no overall understanding of the problem—a master concept, or paradigm—within which we can see how a nondrug treatment, such as nutrition, can work. Without such a conceptual understanding, we often fail to recognize the truth when we do see it.

- In our approach to hypertension, we have failed to heed the warning of the thirteenth-century thinker Roger Bacon, who identified four explicit sources of erroneous deduction:

  1. Undue regard for established doctrines and authorities
  2. Habit
  3. Prejudice
  4. The false conceit of knowledge

Let's look into this in more detail.

THE TECHNOLOGY MYTH

Like other people, doctors and scientists are products of their culture. American society places a high value on pragmatism—on the visible and the tangible. Even in the highly theoretical science of physics, American scientists are more pragmatic and somewhat less inclined toward theoretical approaches than are their European counterparts. Because of this empirical bias, we tend not to believe in anything we can't see, dissect, or isolate in a test tube. Energy fields, like that represented in this book by the "sodium battery," can't be seen (although they can be measured), nor can they be isolated in a test tube. But molecules and drugs are something we can see *and* isolate in a test tube.

Furthermore, the American culture has also emphasized activism, optimism, and a belief we inherited from the seventeenth-century thinker Francis Bacon: that nature can be, and should be, dominated. This cultural background, this Baconian view, has until recently reinforced our notion that technology can fix all our problems. So in the past few decades, drugs have often seemed like the perfect fix.

Our society has been mesmerized by technology, which we often confuse (even in our schools) with science. The overuse of the phrase "science and technology" has led, in the minds of many, to the mistaken belief that the two are the same. We have forgotten that science is the discovery of *insight* into nature, whereas technology is only an *application* of science. Unless we keep our focus upon the *insight* that science can give into the *whole system* (as emphasized in the "new" paradigm of the science of complexity and chaos,) the application of science—technology—could produce an effect opposite to what we desire. Examples abound, ranging from the use of lead in paint and gasoline, the widespread application of DDT, and the use of chlorinated fluorocarbons to the use of drugs to treat everyone with high blood pressure.

From what you have already read in this book, you can see why I (along with a growing number of physicians) take the view that depending principally upon drugs for the treatment of hypertension, especially borderline cases, does not take into account the whole picture. The emphasis on drugs results in part from a blind faith in technology and from our belief that the purpose of science is to bend nature to our will—to dominate it rather than to understand it, cooperate with it, and find ways to live in harmony with it.

THE MYTH THAT CONTROLLING NATURE WITH TECHNOLOGY IS BETTER THAN WORKING WITH NATURE

Consistent with the Baconian view that total control over nature is possible was the development, around the turn of the century, of the chemist Paul Ehrlich's "magic bullet" concept. Ehrlich, sometimes called the father of the pharmaceutical industry, sold the notion that we could have drugs that not only would find their way, as if by magic, to the desired site in the body, but, like bullets, would not affect anything other than the desired target. We could thus control not only the rest of nature but ourselves also—the ultimate in better living through chemistry!

In an article on the ethics of hypertension, scholars at Columbia University have commented on this cultural bias toward technology and the resultant use of drugs to treat borderline cases of hypertension:

> It is, we believe, an instance in the medical domain of the more general phenomenon of technological optimism—the disposition to employ technologies in the belief that the benefits that flow from them will outweigh whatever unforeseen and undesirable effects ensue, and that these effects will themselves be manageable by existing or potential technological means. . . . Among physicians, technological optimism is conjoined with and bolsters a disposition toward therapeutic activism. When making decisions under conditions of uncertainty (whether [blood] pressure will rise or fall without treatment), physicians prefer to take the risk of treating when intervention may not be called for to the potential error of not treating when treatment is needed.[2]

Whether or not they are magic, drugs are certainly "high tech." So in a culture mesmerized by technology, reliance upon drugs was a natural first reaction.

As an example of "the belief that . . . whatever unforeseen and undesirable effects ensue . . . these effects will themselves be manageable by existing or potential technological means," we now have drugs to treat the side effects of antihypertensive drugs.

THE USE OF DRUGS TO TREAT HYPERTENSION PRESENTED AN OPPORTUNITY FOR PROFIT

The reliance upon antihypertensive drugs presented the opportunity to make a lot of money. And it's understandable that the pharmaceutical companies looked upon this as an opportunity to not only increase the "bottom line" but to provide a useful treatment for one of our nation's most common medical problems. Although obtaining the data is difficult, it is clear that pharmaceutical companies gross several billion dollars per year from sales of antihypertensive drugs. As opposed to basic science journals (most of whom are not supported by any commercial advertising) some medical journals frequently carry advertisements promoting the use of drugs for treating hypertension.

PATIENTS DEMAND DRUGS

In a culture where we have disempowered ourselves, it's not surprising to find people looking for solutions from outside themselves. Accordingly, patients *demand* drugs. If they have the flu, many of them demand a shot or a pill even if they've been told it won't do any good. In this busy world, Americans who don't feel well tend to say, "Give me a pill to make me feel better." The poor doc is bombarded not only by salespeople from drug companies but by patients demanding pills. So have some understanding for the predicament of the doctors.

Taking drugs can be a way to avoid taking charge of your life. It's part of a societal trend to surrender personal responsiblity to powers outside of ourselves. On the other hand, prevention is a mentality that is consistent with personal responsibility, independence, and empowerment.

SUIT-HAPPY, PILL-HAPPY AMERICANS

Once incorporated not only into the education but into the culture in which doctors find themselves, the tendency toward "therapeutic activism" is bolstered by legal considerations. A lot of doctors in private practice are skeptical about using these drugs to treat hypertension, but they're often afraid not to give them. Regardless of the treatment—or lack of treatment—used for any condition, it is still possible for patients to get worse or even die. Life is never certain. But it's a good bet that (especially before the Joint National Committee began recommending lifestyle changes) many physicans have had nightmares of a lawyer saying, "You mean, doctor, that the deceased had hypertension and you didn't even prescribe medicine?"

In our present culture, the best way for a doctor to protect himself or herself against unjustified malpractice suits is to follow conventional, accepted methods of treatment*—even if the doctor has reason to believe that other alternatives may be better. Americans are so "suit happy" that doctors are often afraid to try anything new or different.

THE NUTRITIONAL APPROACH—HIGH SCIENCE, LOW TECH, AND NO GLAMOR

But what about the dietary approaches that had been successfully demonstrated as early as the 1930s and 1950s? Why hadn't they caught on? It frequently happens

---

*The growing tendency of the Joint National Committee over the past eight years to recommend consideration of non-drug approaches should help physicians in this regard.

that the early pioneers of a new idea are ignored. Nowhere is this more striking than in the use of a dietary approach for high blood pressure treatment.

By 1957, when the first potent drugs for hypertension were introduced, the ability of dietary changes to lower elevated blood pressure had been demonstrated time and again. Such early pioneers as Ambard and Beaujard in France, and Allen, Addison, and Priddle in the United States, had demonstrated that either decreasing sodium or increasing potassium in the diet could reverse and perhaps cure high blood pressure. And Dr. Walter Kempner of Duke University had shown hundreds of times that his rice-fruit diet could return blood pressure to normal. These pioneering investigators—and more recently Dahl, Page, Tobian, and others—had the right idea, but they couldn't get anyone to listen. Reflecting their frustration, here is Dr. Lewis Dahl discussing, in 1972, Kempner's rice-fruit diet and his own studies of a high-K-Factor diet:

> For reasons that are difficult to fathom, there appeared a great deal of antipathy to Kempner's reports as well as irrational disbelief in the effectiveness of the diet . . . I have often felt that we became heirs to the antipathies originally directed at Allen and later at Kempner. We decided, nonetheless, to try to detect the dietary factor that made this diet effective. For those of you who are unfamiliar with the diet, let me define it as a *low sodium, or a high potassium,* [emphasis mine] or a high carbohydrate, or a low protein, or a low fat,* or a high fluid diet. In its pristine form it is made up mostly of rice and fruit including juices, but certainly with no added salt (NaCl).[3]

Why were these successful dietary approaches so widely rejected? For one thing, in the 1950s nutrition was virtually unmentioned in medical schools (and even today is usually given lip service). Thus, as Dr. Dahl pointed out, until the thiazide diuretics were introduced, very few physicians thought sodium had much to do with hypertension. As a result, Dr. Dahl suggested, most low-sodium diets were "prescribed haphazardly and unenthusiastically."[4]

With the introduction of the diuretic chlorothiazide in 1957, both patients and physicians found its antihypertensive effects more convenient than dietary approaches. In some quarters, skepticism about the role of dietary sodium persists today. But Dr. Lou Tobian has pointed out that every time these physicians use a diuretic, they "cast a vote for sodium" as a cause of hypertension, since these drugs act by causing the body to lose sodium through the kidneys.

---

*It is amazing how prescient Dahl was. There he was, back in 1972, recognizing the basic dietary principles for a healthy diet that tends to prevent not only hypertension and heart disease, but also some types of cancer as well!

But why were dietary changes prescribed "haphazardly and unenthusiastically"? Most physicians have neither the time nor the background to educate their patients about nutrition and exercise. As far back as 1963, the American Medical Association's Council on Foods and Nutrition stated that "medical education and medical practice have not kept abreast of advances in nutrition." In spite of the fact that nutrition is involved in both the cause and the treatment of diabetes and cancer as well as hypertension, the majority of medical schools still do not require a course dealing specifically with nutrition. Since nutrition is not usually part of their education, future physicians tend to ignore dietary approaches and view them as suspect and "unscientific." Accordingly they aren't prepared to believe in the importance of nutrition in hypertension, let alone to realize that the necessary changes are *not*, in fact, "so complex as to discourage all but the most persistent." Instead, they are trained to believe in drugs, and they learn how to get patients to use them.

THE LACK OF A CONCEPTUAL MODEL

But why did even most nutritionists miss the importance of the K Factor? Let me suggest that even more important than the lack of emphasis upon nutrition in training doctors was the fact that until recently, there was no model, or concept, to explain how raising the ratio of potassium to sodium in the diet could reduce blood pressure.

Thomas Kuhn, a leading historian of science, has emphasized the essential importance of a "paradigm," or general conceptual framework, in the perception and evaluation of familiar information. Without a concept—some idea of how things work that enables us to believe they can work—we often do not "see" the reality behind the facts.

A good example is provided by Semmelweiss's discovery that death rates dropped when doctors who worked in the morgue washed their hands before examining women in the lying-in hospital. Although such washing greatly reduced mortality in the lying-in hospital, the procedure was not widely accepted. Only with the birth of the science of bacteriology and the recognition that germs, or bacteria, can "carry" disease did the logic of Semmelweiss' recommendation become apparent. When this was recognized, the practice urged by Semmelweiss rapidly became the standard.

So probably the reason that the dietary effects discovered by Allen, Addison, Kempner, and others (see Chapter 6) were ignored is that in their time, there was no clearly accepted concept, or model, of how sodium and potassium work in the body. So it is not surprising that only a very few suspected that an imbalance between potassium and sodium produces a fundamental *imbalance within body cells* that can not only elevate blood pressure but affect the metabolism of carbohydrate and fats in the body. If you don't understand something, it's natural to ignore it. So sodium and potassium seemed unimportant; one seemed the same as the other, and their relation to hypertension must have seemed as relevant as the tooth fairy.

WE IGNORED ROGER BACON'S WARNING

For a time it could be argued that the approach to hypertension had not only been influenced by "undue regard for established doctrines and authorities" but by forty years of "habit" and by "prejudice" against the power of nutrition.

Yet it is not easy to let go of an "established doctrine" that has been around so long that it has become a "habit." The hope still lingers that some *new* miracle drug will provide the answer. For example, one reads in the literature that newer drugs are "a reason for *optimism* that carefully tailored therapy will *ultimately diminish*"[5] all the dire consequences of hypertension (emphasis mine).

Nevertheless, the "false conceit of knowledge" is giving way to a complete reexamination, and the situation is changing on many fronts. We are well on our way into a new state of awareness. The drug approach has failed to reduce the most frequent tragic result of hypertension, coronary artery disease, and has reduced the tragic occurrence of strokes due to hypertension by only about a half. A growing awareness of the importance of nutrition and exercise has made us more open to other approaches. Most importantly, years of basic biomedical research have finally given us a model, or concept, for understanding the role of potassium, sodium, calcium, and magnesium in the cell (see Chapter 4).

It was this model, with its prediction that added potassium could help lower blood pressure, that led some of us basic scientists into the study of hypertension. Moreover, the model presents us with a means to understand the newly recognized similarities between hypertension and adult-type diabetes (NIDDM). In fact, the model *predicted* that there would be a relation between diabetes and hypertension[6] and thus provides us with some good leads as to how weight loss and exercise can help restore blood pressure to normal. Finally, and perhaps most importantly, the model indicates that elevated blood pressure is not the fundamental problem— something now well confirmed—but is instead a *consequence* of an imbalance at the level of the living cell. Fortunately, in many people, this imbalance can be corrected by the natural means of proper nutrition, exercise, and weight loss.

SUMMARY

Pogo was right! The problem is not them (the medical establishment and the pharmaceutical companies), but us—all of us. Our culture biased us toward the use of drugs. And after the thiazide diuretics were introduced in 1957, dietary approaches seldom received much attention. The pill had won—but we hadn't.

Moreover, the nutritional approach to primary hypertension was, until recently, ignored not only because future doctors were not educated about nutrition but even more because of the lack of a concept that made it seem realistic. And the bias toward drugs was inevitable in a society that believed that technology could "fix" anything.

But now we realize that drugs affect only some of the *consequences* of this cellular imbalance, such as retention of sodium or increased activity of the sympathetic nervous system, without correcting the imbalance itself.

Drugs may be "magic bullets," but in the case of primary hypertension, they don't quite hit the mark. Fortunately, there *is* a magic bullet—it's called potassium.*

---

*Here I am taking literary license to oversimplify in order to make the point. As already developed in this book, it is the *relation*, or *balance*, between potassium and sodium that is critical. Moreover, other minerals such as magnesium may play a role.

CHAPTER 15

Additional Evidence: Low Dietary K Factor– A Main Cause of Primary Hypertension

If you're still skeptical—good! That means you're thinking for yourself. You're being scientific. But apply your skepticism equally to any view of hypertension. Don't swallow anything (drugs or bananas) without some thinking and consulting with your doctor.

In our cultural environment, primary hypertension *acts* as though it is inherited. A large percentage of people (about 25% to 30%, depending upon the population group) *appear* to inherit a genetic weakness in their ability to handle a diet overloaded with sodium chloride and deficient in potassium, magnesium, or calcium. Because of the imbalance of these minerals in the typical American diet, hypertension is almost inevitable in those with the genetic weakness. This apparent inevitability has helped to reinforce dependency, as opposed to participation, between the patient and doctor—with a lifetime of drugtaking being the only option. But these people are not predestined to hypertension—provided they eat properly and maintain their weight through aerobic exercise. On a low-sodium, high-potassium diet, only about 1% of people will develop hypertension (the rare cases seen in the cultures with diets low in sodium and high in potassium). Apparently this 1% has a very strong inherited tendency for hypertension, although some of them probably have kidney or adrenal gland disease.

A number of other studies also lead to the conclusion that bad genes are not the main culprit. For example, recall that Table 2 in Chapter 5 listed two groups from Tel Aviv, the only difference between them being diet. The vegetarian group (whose diet had a high K Factor) had a very low incidence of hypertension compared to the other group. So the evidence is clear that whether or not those people with a genetic tendency actually get hypertension depends upon their lifestyle, particularly their diet.

We have already summarized evidence that leads to the conclusion that in hypertension, the most important aspect of diet is the K Factor. This evidence included not only the population studies but also medical studies, animal studies, an understanding of the importance of the proper balance between potassium and sodium in the living cell, and the realization that obesity and lack of exercise can compromise the body's ability to balance potassium and sodium.

At this point, I want to reemphasize that a central theme of this book is that when one is considering living systems, it is *never* enough to look at one thing at a time. I have emphasized this with respect to sodium. But although the balance between potassium and sodium seems to be a key factor, I pointed out in Chapter 8 that other substances, such as chloride, magnesium, and calcium, are also involved. Therefore, the K Factor is an approximation that will one day be replaced by something more complete and more accurate.* But at the present state of research, it appears to be not only the best guide we have, but also one that adequately provides a practical guideline for preventing and curing hypertension.

Now you will see additional evidence that supports the conclusion that the balance between potassium and sodium plays a key role in determining whether those with the inherited tendency will develop primary hypertension as they get older.

1. THE LEVEL OF POTASSIUM IN THE BLOOD PLASMA IS CORRELATED WITH HYPERTENSION

As you will recall from Chapter 4, the sodium-potassium pump requires an adequate amount of potassium in the fluid *outside* the cell in order to maintain the proper balance between potassium and sodium *inside* the cell. Since potassium in the fluid outside body cells is in equilibrium with plasma potassium, a decrease in the level of plasma potassium would be expected to decrease activity of the sodium-potassium pump in these cells. This in turn would increase the level of

---

*As an example, my present *guess* is that something like $(K + \frac{1}{2}Mg + \frac{1}{4}Ca)/Na$ would be a somewhat better approximation.

calcium *inside* the cell, causing contraction of the small resistance arteries and therefore raising blood pressure. Thus, a low level of plasma potassium would be expected to contribute to high blood pressure.

In general, physicians have not commented upon a difference in the level of potassium in the blood plasma of hypertensive individuals compared to the level of those with normal blood pressure. However, in a study of 1,462 middle-aged women in Sweden, serum potassium levels in hypertensive women, whether treated or untreated, were significantly lower than in women with normal blood pressure.[1] In another study of ninety-one patients with primary hypertension, a graph of both plasma potassium and total body potassium showed a significant tendency for both diastolic and systolic blood pressures to increase as the plasma potassium levels decreased.[2] These correlations were clearest in younger patients. In people without hypertension, the plasma potassium level was *not* related to blood pressure. This study also found that as the total amount of sodium in the body increased, blood pressure increased.

In a study in London of 3,578 men and women not taking antihypertensive drugs, it was observed that both systolic and diastolic blood pressures were significantly "negatively" associated with plasma potassium: that is, the lower the plasma potassium, the higher the blood pressure tended to be.[3]

Perhaps the most interesting study of serum potassium was of Japanese men in their forties. A total of 1,158 men from six different population groups, with different lifestyles, both urban and rural, were studied. When the average level of plasma potassium of each of the six groups was plotted against the incidence of high blood pressure, a clear tendency for the prevalence of hypertension to increase as plasma potassium decreased was seen.[4]

Data from that paper are summarized in Table 11 and show a steady increase (reported to be statistically significant) in the incidence of hypertension as the serum potassium level decreases; the apparent exception of line 3 is within the level of statistical error. The interpretation of this table is not clouded by possible effects of antihypertensive drugs, since none of the subjects were taking these agents. As you can see, this study found that as the dietary K Factor (K/Na ratio) increases, hypertension decreases.

TABLE 11

HYPERTENSION IN JAPANESE MEN
COMPARED TO SERUM POTASSIUM AND DIETARY K FACTOR

REGION	INCIDENCE OF HYPERTENSION (%)	AVERAGE SERUM POTASSIUM (mEq/L)	AVERAGE DIETARY POTASSIUM/SODIUM RATIO (mg K/mg Na)
A	10.3	4.26	0.197
B	12.0	4.24	0.192
C	13.3	4.29	0.213
D	19.9	4.11	0.187
E	24.9	4.02	0.168
F	33.3	3.85	0.141

In a governmnent-sponsored nationwide study of a very large number of hypertensive patients it was found that when medication was not being used, serum potassium was lowest in groups with the highest blood pressure regardless of age, sex, or race (both blacks and whites were studied). The hypertensive patients taking medication tended to have even lower serum potassium levels— still another finding that raises questions about the use of drugs to treat high blood pressure.[5]

"NORMAL" VALUES FOR PLASMA POTASSIUM MAY BE TOO LOW

Until recently, most authorities did not recognize that serum potassium tends to be depressed in people with hypertension. Accordingly, the "normal" range of serum potassium is based upon large populations, about 20% of whom have high blood pressure. The four recent studies just quoted indicate that this 20% has lower levels of serum potassium than does the rest of the population. This suggests we reconsider the "normal" range of serum potassium. The lower limit of the "normal" level (of 3.5 mEq/L) probably needs to be revised upward.

2. TOTAL BODY POTASSIUM IS
DECREASED IN UNTREATED PRIMARY HYPERTENSION

Since a decrease in plasma potassium slows the sodium-potassium pump, decreasing the amount of potassium inside body cells, a lower plasma potassium level indicates a decreased total body potassium. Therefore, we would expect that the total body potassium of people with primary hypertension would be decreased.

This prediction has been confirmed by a study in which total body potassium was measured in fifty-three patients with untreated primary hypertension and in sixty-two healthy people with normal blood pressure who were used as controls.[6] The total body potassium was an average of 13% lower in the people with untreated primary hypertension than in people with normal blood pressure (with the same amount of body fat). This decrease is statistically significant. The potassium content of small samples of muscle removed from these people confirmed that the decrease was not due to differences in amount of body fat. Analysis of these samples also revealed that the calcium content of the muscle tissue was greater in the subjects with primary hypertension.

As was discussed in Chapter 4, if these changes in potassium and calcium occur in the smooth muscle cells surrounding the arterioles, the tension of these cells would increase, with a resulting constriction of the arterioles and consequent rise in blood pressure. Recently, Drs. Joseph Veniero and Raj Gupta of Albert Einstein College of Medicine have used nuclear magnetic resonance (NMR) to demonstrate that indeed, there is a significant decrease in potassium inside the cells of the major artery of experimental rats with hypertension.[7]

Another study showed that among ninety-one people with hypertension who were not taking drugs, there was a negative correlation between total body potassium and blood pressure—in other words, the lower the total body potassium, the higher the blood pressure.[8] A follow-up on this study reported that both systolic and diastolic blood pressure increases as the ratio of potassium to sodium (K/Na ratio or K Factor) decreases, and that the chances of this relationship being due to chance range between one in a hundred and one in a thousand.[9] This follow-up study also concluded that plasma and total body potassium are probably important in the early stages of primary hypertension and that changes of body sodium may become important later.

3. CORRELATION OF URINARY K/NA RATIO WITH HYPERTENSION

The content of sodium and/or of potassium in a 24-hour urine collection can be a fairly good reflection of the dietary intake. We would expect that as the urinary K Factor rises, the incidence of high blood pressure would fall.

IN JAPAN

This proved to be the case in a Japanese study in which Dr. Naosuke Sasaki of Hirosaki University studied blood pressure, urinary sodium and potassium, and apple consumption.[10] He noticed that in one apple-growing district of Japan, those who ate even one to three apples (which are high in potassium) each day had lower blood pressure than those who ate no apples. When examining middle-aged farmers from four different regions, Dr. Sasaki also found a definite correlation between their blood pressure and urinary K/Na ratio, which reflects the dietary K Factor. This is illustrated in Table 12 and shows that as the average urinary K/Na ratio decreases, both average diastolic and systolic blood pressure rise.

TABLE 12

BLOOD PRESSURE AND URINARY K/NA RATIO
IN FARMERS FROM FOUR REGIONS OF JAPAN

REGION	AVERAGE DIASTOLIC BLOOD PRESSURE (MM HG)	AVERAGE SYSTOLIC BLOOD PRESSURE (MM HG)	AVERAGE URINARY RATIO OF K/NA (MG K/MG NA)
A	78.6	131.4	0.293
B	80.9	139.3	0.252
C	85.9	149.7	0.229
D	86.6	152.5	0.223

IN THE UNITED STATES

In a 1979 study conducted by Dr. W. Gordon Walker and his colleagues[11] at Johns Hopkins School of Medicine, the average urinary K/Na ratio of the 274 volunteers with diastolic blood pressure less than 90 mm Hg was 0.88, while the ratio in urine of the 300 volunteers with hypertension (diastolic pressure greater than 90) was 0.71. There was no correlation with sodium excretion; the decrease in urinary K/Na ratio in the hypertensives was almost entirely due to a decrease in potassium in the urine, and, therefore, presumably in the diet. This finding is especially important because none of the subjects was taking drugs of any kind. Therefore the difference in urinary K/Na ratio cannot be attributed to antihypertensive drugs, such as diuretics, which can cause the body to lose potassium.

IN AMERICAN BLACKS COMPARED TO WHITES

It is well known that blacks have a much higher incidence of hypertension than whites. What is not as widely appreciated is that the dietary K/Na ratio, as reflected by the urinary K/Na ratio, is also lower in blacks than in whites. In one study of women in their early twenties, the urinary K/Na ratio was 0.42 in blacks as compared to 0.62 to whites.[12]

One study begun in 1961 randomly selected both blacks and whites living in Evans County, Georgia.[13] As in almost all American studies, the blacks had a significantly higher incidence of hypertension than did the whites. Surprisingly, black men actually had about 27% *less* sodium in their diet and about 20% less in their urine than the whites. However, the white men had over twice as much potassium in their diet and nearly that much more potassium in their urine. Thus in spite of a decrease in consumption of sodium as compared to whites, the dietary K Factor and the corresponding urinary K/Na ratio of blacks was less than that of the whites. Averaging the men and women together, the urinary K/Na ratio was 0.33 for blacks and 0.44 for whites.

In a study of 662 black and white female high school students in Jackson, Mississippi, there was only a weak correlation between urinary sodium excretion and blood pressure, but a highly significant relation between the urinary K/Na ratio and blood pressure. Those young women with lower urinary K/Na ratio clearly had higher blood pressure.[14] (This study was also mentioned in Chapter 5.) In another study of hypertensive patients, the strong correlation between urinary K/Na ratio and hypertension was not observed, but Dr. Herbert Langford of Jackson, Mississippi, has suggested that the lack of correlation was probably due to the fact that most of the patients were taking antihypertensive medication, which had already lowered their blood pressure.[15]

In African Blacks

In a study of one group of Africans, those living in cities had a urinary K/Na ratio of 0.46 and significantly higher blood pressure than those living in villages, whose urinary K/Na ratio was 0.63. The difference was most striking in the men. The urban men had an average blood pressure of 140/88 mm Hg and a urinary K/Na ratio of 0.50, while the village men had an average blood pressure of 129/78 and a urinary K/Na ratio of 0.89.[16]

In Europeans

Finally, of 694 randomly selected people in a Belgian village, there was no significant relationship between blood pressure and urinary excretion of sodium.[17] However, there was a significant rise in blood pressure associated with *decreased* potassium excretion in the urine.

4. THE K FACTOR AND HYPERTENSION IN EXPERIMENTAL ANIMALS

In Nashville, Tennessee, a physician, Dr. George Meneely, and his colleague Con Ball had been studying the toxic action of table salt, NaCl, on laboratory rats. In 1958, they published the results of studies of the toxic effect of sodium chloride and the protective effect of potassium chloride on the life span of 825 rats.[18] It was probably this group that first suggested the use of the dietary K Factor as an indicator of the likelihood of having hypertension. They found some very surprising results. When rats were fed a diet with high levels of sodium chloride with a K

Factor of only 0.11, the extra sodium resulted in a decrease in average life span from the normal of about 24 months to only 16 months. When the dietary K Factor was increased to 0.8 by addition of potassium chloride while the levels of sodium chloride in the food were kept constant, the average life span increased by 8 months—back to the normal life span of rats without high blood pressure! [Into this technical scientific paper, the authors slipped the following comment: "There may, too, have been some potash (potassium) in the fountain of youth."]

Dr. Lewis K. Dahl and co-workers studied a strain of rats that become hypertensive on a high-sodium diet and confirmed that increasing the K Factor in the diet diminished the rise in blood pressure produced by giving salt. These salt-sensitive rats were divided into six different groups, and each group was placed on a different diet. Each diet contained the same high amount of sodium, but each had a different amount of potassium.[19] The results are summarized in Table 13.

The protective effect of adding potassium to increase the K Factor can be clearly seen. At 12 months (other data indicated that the mean blood pressure had reached nearly its highest level by then), the blood pressure of the different groups steadily decreases as the dietary K Factor increases. This effect is also evident at 6 months and begins to be evident at 1 month. Of even more significance, the authors also reported that the life span of the rats on the diets with higher K Factor was much longer than the others.

A second part of this study showed that not only is the K Factor important, but the *absolute* amounts of sodium and potassium also affect blood pressure. For example, when the K Factor was kept constant at either 0.57 or 1.7, increasing the amount of both sodium *and* potassium threefold resulted in a substantial (about 20 and 15 mm Hg, respectively) rise in blood pressure. Therefore, attention must be given not only to the K/Na ratio of our diet but to the *amount* of sodium in the foods listed in the table in Chapter 13 as well.

TABLE 13

AVERAGE MEAN BLOOD PRESSURES (MM HG)* OF RATS ON A CONSTANT HIGH-SODIUM DIET

MONTHS ON DIET	K/NA RATIO (MG K/MG NA)					
	0.17	0.34	0.42	0.57	0.85	1.7
1	116	109	115	119	110	108
6	166	145	140	143	135	125
12	170	164	162	160	152	137

*Mean blood pressure = diastolic pressure plus ⅓ the difference between systolic and diastolic pressure.

In another animal study, rats were divided into three groups and given food that was identical except for a different K Factor for each group.[20] When the K Factor was lowered from the control value of 1.86 to 0.45 by the addition of sodium, the average systolic blood pressure rose significantly.When a small supplement of potassium was also added along with the sodium, thus raising the K Factor back up to 0.61, blood pressure did not rise nearly as much. This study also found that the animals made hypertensive by a low K/Na ratio had a moderate increase in the amount of adrenaline (a hormone that raises blood pressure) excreted in their urine. When the K Factor was raised from 0.45 to 0.61, by addition of a small amount of potassium, the excretion of adrenaline decreased about 20%.

This effect of increased dietary K Factor on blood pressure has also been demonstrated in other animals with hypertension.[21]

HOW INCREASING DIETARY K WORKS

Increased potassium intake lowers blood pressure toward normal in persons with high blood pressure but has less effect on persons with normal blood pressure. This suggests that extra potassium in the diet does not change normal mechanisms of blood pressure regulation but instead restores damaged mechanisms toward normal.

Several mechanisms have been suggested to account for the ability of potassium to lower blood pressure in people with hypertension. The effect of potassium to relax the smooth muscle surrounding the arterioles is probably both directly and indirectly mediated.

DIRECT EFFECT

A high-potassium diet has been shown to increase the potassium level in the blood serum by 10% to 15%, almost 0.6 mEq/L (see Table 11, earlier in this chapter) and the clinical trials of the high-K diet described in Chapter 6). Since even a very small rise in potassium in the fluid bathing the body cells will increase the activity of the sodium-potassium pumps, this should lower blood pressure by causing relaxation of the small arteries.

A direct effect of potassium has been demonstrated by Dr. F. J. Haddy, who showed that infusion of potassium directly into arteries causes them to relax, thus allowing increased blood flow.[22] In the presence of ouabain, a drug that specifically inhibits operation of the sodium-potassium pump, potassium did not produce this relaxing effect. When the sympathetic hormone adrenaline is used to cause contraction in strips of arteries taken from rats, potassium also causes relaxation. This relaxing effect is consistently greater in arteries taken from rats with the genetic tendency to have hypertension than from normal rats. Addition of ouabain blocks the ability of potassium to relax these strips of arteries.[23] These results indicate that potassium relaxes the smooth muscle cells by stimulating the sodium-potassium pump, as was described in Chapter 4.

At plasma concentrations that might be found with a high-potassium diet, potassium also has a direct relaxing effect upon arterioles, resulting in less resistance to blood flow.[24] Therefore, this relaxing effect of potassium is probably part of the explanation for the ability of extra dietary potassium to lower blood pressure toward normal.

The potassium level in the fluid bathing the body cells is very close to the same level found in the watery part (serum) of the blood. Thus, it is significant that at least five studies have found that plasma potassium is decreased by 5% to 15% in patients suffering from untreated primary hypertension, as we described earlier in this chapter.

All these findings are consistent with the major working hypothesis of this book that considers *an increase in sodium (and thus a decrease in potassium) inside the cell to be a main part of the cause of primary hypertension.* This was discussed in Chapter 4. In fact, several other scientists and I became interested in the problem of hypertension because of our own research upon regulation of the sodium-potassium pump and the known effect (mentioned in Chapter 4) of even small increases in potassium outside the cell to stimulate the sodium-potassium pump and thus keep sodium inside the cell at a low level.

INDIRECT EFFECTS

Besides the probable direct effect of potassium upon the sodium-potassium pump in the walls of the small arteries, there is strong evidence that potassium also exerts some of its effect upon blood pressure by affecting the kidneys, by changing blood hormone levels, and by affecting sympathetic nerve activity.

Extra potassium in the diet causes increased excretion of sodium by the kidney,[25] which in turn leads to a decrease in the amount of sodium in the body and might decrease the release of natriuretic hormone from the brain (see Chapter 17). This would allow the sodium-potassium pump to reduce the level of sodium inside the cells and increase the voltage across their surface membrane. Both effects act to keep intracellular calcium at a low level, thus relaxing the smooth muscle cells.

Not only does the addition of potassium to the diet of people with primary hypertension significantly decrease blood pressure, but in at least one study, this decrease was shown to be correlated with a decrease in the level of noradrenaline in the blood.[26] In other words, with added dietary potassium, the sympathetic nervous system became less active, since noradrenaline is released from sympathetic nerve endings.

Potassium may also have an effect upon the sympathetic nerves that go directly to the arterioles and cause contraction and narrowing of these small resistance arteries.[27] This effect of potassium may be due to stimulation of the sodium-potassium pump in the sympathetic nerve cells, which would decrease their activity by increasing the voltage across their surface membrane, causing fewer impulses to be sent to the arterioles and allowing them to relax.

HYPERTENSION IN THE OBESE

It has already been emphasized that being obese greatly increases your chances of developing primary hypertension. In all populations that have been studied, over-weight people have an increased likelihood of high blood pressure.[28] In the HANES I study, the correlation of blood pressure with body weight was one of the strongest factors.

In clinical trials, loss of only a third to a half of excess body weight has been shown to reduce blood pressure significantly.[29] Moreover, very-low-calorie diets will decrease blood pressure in only 3 to 4 days in almost all obese people.[30] This is long before there is any sizable loss of body fat. This clearly indicates that in the obese, high blood pressure is not due to the mechanical effects of body fat or, as was previously thought, to the increase in small blood vessels associated with excess fat. Rather, the increase in blood pressure must be due to a change in physiogical *function* in obese people.

Chapter 7 outlined the fact that obesity results in increased levels of insulin (commonly known as a sugar hormone). In the late 1960s, the work from my laboratory, which indicated that insulin increases the activity of the sodium-potassium pump, prompted Dr. Jean Crabbe, in Belgium, to study the effect of insulin upon the sodium-potassium pump in the kidney. The work of Dr. Crabbe's group[31] and then that of Dr. Ralph DeFronzo[32] of Yale University Medical School has since conclusively demonstrated that elevation of blood insulin levels results in increased reabsorption of sodium by the kidney, causing the retention of more sodium in the body. For a review, see Sims[33] or Moore.[34]

The elevation of blood levels of insulin by obesity may be a form of compensa-tion for the fact that in obese people, the enlarged fat cells have fewer receptors for the insulin molecule (for a given area of surface membrane). Dr. Ethan Sims[35] of the University of Vermont has pointed out that this elevation of blood insulin in obesity would be expected to cause the kidney to retain body sodium, producing essentially the same effect as too much sodium in the diet. He quotes the conclu-sion of an international meeting on hypertension and obesity held at Florence, Italy, in 1980: "Hyperinsulinemia and related disorders are common features of the syndromes of obesity. There is now much evidence that insulin promotes retention of sodium by the kidney, and this may be a major contributor to hypertension in the obese subgroup of patients."

Dr. Sims points out that modified fasting, which lowers blood insulin, rapidly "brings about an impressive decrease in blood pressure." In the experience of Dr. Wayne Gavryck, a former student and physician friend of mine, when hypertensive patients who are obese are given a very low-calorie diet (400 calories per day), the blood pressure almost always drops significantly within 7 days. Exceptions are uncommon, and the blood pressure is usually down within 3 to 4 days.[36] This procedure also decreases blood pressure in many who are not obese, again demonstrating that it is not fat per se that causes the elevated blood pressure but altered physiology.

Also supporting the idea that insulin has an effect upon sodium excretion in obese hypertensives are the two studies quoted earlier in which high blood pressure was treated by weight reduction.[37] In both these studies about 75% of the people developed normal diastolic blood pressure without drug treatment when calories were restricted. And while caloric intake was restricted, sodium excretion in the urine was significantly increased in spite of the fact that there was no evident change in dietary sodium.

Insulin also affects blood pressure by acting on the hypothalamus, a part of the brain, causing it to step up the activity of the sympathetic nervous system,[38] which then elevates blood pressure by causing constriction of the arterioles, as was discussed in Chapters 4 and 17.

Noradrenaline, which is released by nerves in the sympathetic nervous system, not only plays a direct role in development of hypertension in the obese individual but also affects sodium and potassium balance.[39] Besides reducing plasma insulin levels, in obese people with high blood pressure, weight loss results in a fall in plasma levels of noradrenaline, renin, angiotensin II, and aldosterone[40]—all hormones that tend to increase blood pressure.

EXERCISE AND HYPERTENSION

The effect of too little exercise, like obesity, probably relates to the body's regulation of potassium and sodium. Physical training of overweight middle-aged persons strikingly reduces the blood level of insulin even when there is no change in body fat, while at the same time increasing the number of insulin receptors on skeletal muscle.[41] This drop in blood insulin level should allow the kidney to excrete more sodium, which could help reduce elevated blood pressure. Physical training also has effects on other hormones, such as adrenaline, that affect blood pressure.

DIABETES AND HYPERTENSION

Chapters 3 and 7 referred to the intimate relation between the adult type of diabetes (NIDDM) and hypertension. Both conditions share several features of "Syndrome X," including insulin resistance, high blood levels of insulin, and abnormal blood cholesterol levels.

WHY DOESN'T POTASSIUM ALWAYS LOWER ELEVATED BLOOD PRESSURE?

First of all, it usually does. If you reflect upon it, something that takes 10 to 20 years to develop can hardly be expected to be reversed in 10 to 20 days.

Why there are some exceptions isn't known for sure, but we can make an educated guess. In fact, from what researchers have discovered about the structure of small arteries, we would expect that increasing potassium would result in a relatively rapid drop in blood pressure only in the early stages of hypertension. But this should not be used as an argument against increasing the dietary K/Na ratio as a means of treating established primary hypertension. Remember extra potassium extends the life of laboratory animals and of humans even when it doesn't lower blood pressure.

Thiazide diuretics produce a more rapid drop in blood pressure, but initially this is due to a decrease in cardiac output resulting from dereased blood volume, an effect that hardly seems optimal. Only after a considerable delay do these diuretics result in a reduction of resistance to blood flow.[42]

Part of the delay in lowering blood pressure by potassium most likely is due to the structural changes that occur in the arteries of people and animals with hypertension. You will recall that the abnormal levels of insulin and of angiotensin are probably part of the reason that the small arteries become "muscle-bound."

In addition, the elevated blood pressure itself can contribute to this condition. When the blood pressure is increased by mechanically constricting an artery in experimental animals, the result is an increased thickness of the wall of the artery upstream from the constriction. The mechanism for part of this is similar to the development of increased mass of other body muscles. The increased blood pressure causes increased strain, or tension, on the smooth muscles circling the artery. We know that resistance exercises, either isometric or isotonic, increase the tension of the skeletal muscles and cause hypertrophy, or bulging, of the muscles. Similarly, we would expect the increased tension of the smooth muscles, caused by the high blood pressure, to cause hypertrophy. It does, and this causes part of the increased thickness of the artery wall seen in hypertensive people.

Once established, the thickened arterial walls may remain even if the primary cellular imbalance in sodium, potassium, and calcium is corrected by stimulation of the sodium-potassium pump. Therefore, once hypertension has been present for a sufficient period of time, increasing dietary potassium would not be expected to decrease blood pressure, at least for some time.

However, with proper therapy over sufficient time, even this hypertrophy of the smooth muscles might be expected to decrease somewhat. When the stress on *any* muscle is decreased, the muscle gradually becomes smaller. For example, easier workouts allow the enlarged muscles of the weight lifter to decrease back toward normal size. Also, prolonged bed rest results in decrease in the size and strength of leg muscles. Therefore, the time required for elevated blood pressure to respond to an increase in the dietary K/Na ratio would be expected to be longer in those people whose high blood pressure has gone untreated for a longer time. The effect of the dietary change should be quickest, within several days to a few weeks, in those who have had hypertension only a very short time. In someone who has had untreated hypertension for a much longer period, it might take a few months for the blood pressure to drop.

Unfortunately, if the hypertension has been present for a sufficiently long period, increasing the dietary K/Na ratio, or even the use of drugs, may not decrease the blood pressure very much. We have a pretty good idea why this should be the case. In experimental animals, continued elevation of the blood pressure eventually leads to an increase in collagen in the wall of the artery after the smooth muscles of the arteries hypertrophy. Collagen is a tough structural material; it is collagen that makes meat from an old cow tough to chew. Once the collagen has increased in the wall of the arteries, relaxation or even decrease in the size of the smooth muscles would not allow the artery to expand its interior so the blood can flow more easily. The tough collagen would not allow it. At this point, it is improbable that dietary changes or even drugs would produce much lowering of the blood pressure. This is consistent with what is observed clinically.

Nevertheless, it is important to keep in mind that restoring a normal balance within the body may strengthen arteries, decrease cholesterol, and thus decrease strokes and heart attacks even if the blood pressure doesn't come down.

THE WHOLE PICTURE

Finally, it is important to re-emphasize that the reductionist view of looking at only one factor at a time ignores the reality of the systems, or holistic, functioning of the human body.

Taking this larger view, we can see the reciprocal relation between potassium and sodium *both* at the level of the whole body *and* at the level of the cell.

At the level of the whole body, potassium is a diuretic for sodium, and vice versa. In other words, an increase in dietary potassium will result in an increased loss of sodium through the kidneys. Likewise, an increase in dietary sodium will result in an increased loss of potassium through the kidneys. Conversely, a *decrease* of dietary sodium leads to a decreased loss of potassium through the kidneys with a resulting increase in body potassium and in plasma potassium concentration, and also decreases the content of sodium in blood vessels.[43] These are precisely the same effects produced by increasing dietary potassium. Moreover, reducing weight or increasing exercise produces changes within the body that facilitate the replacement of sodium by potassium.

At the level of the cell, we can also see the reciprocal relation between potassium and sodium. Of course, the sodium-potassium pump moves sodium *out* of the cell in exchange for potassium coming *into* the cell. But, as you will recall from Chapter 4, this exchange is not one-for-one, so you may wonder if decreasing potassium inside the cell will *always* result in an increased level of sodium in the cell.

In Chapter 4 I mentioned that the concentration of potassium plus sodium inside the cell must *always remain constant*. The reason for this is that sodium and potassium make up almost all of the osmotically active particles in the cell that carry a positive charge. A fundamental law of physics* requires that the cell *must* be in osmotic equilibrium with its external environment (and thus with the blood plasma). Since the osmotic pressure of the blood plasma is remarkably constant, it follows that the total concentration of potassium and sodium inside the living cells of your body must be constant in spite of of what we do to ourselves.

Therefore, if the concentration of potassium inside the cell goes down, the concentration of sodium *must* go up—the laws of physics allow no exceptions. And from Chapter 4, you will remember that if the concentration of potassium inside the cell goes down while the concentration of sodium goes up, this amounts to the "sodium battery" being run down.

Most of the potassium in the body is inside its cells. So now we know that if the amount of potassium in your body goes down, the level of sodium inside the cells of your body must go up. In other words, if your body doesn't have enough potassium, the "sodium battery" of its cells will unavoidably be run down. And that, as was carefully explained in Chapter 4, causes all sorts of things to go wrong (including an increase in calcium concentration inside the cell), which can lead to the set of problems we now know as hypertension.

Nature gives us no choice; we *must* have enough potassium for our body cells to work properly.

SUMMARY

Many lines of evidence point to the importance of increasing the amount of potassium and decreasing the amount of sodium in your diet (maintaining a high-K-Factor diet) in order to prevent or reverse high blood pressure. People who do eat a high-K-Factor diet have lower blood pressure and tend to have a higher concentration of potassium in the blood plasma, and less sodium inside body cells. High blood levels of insulin tend to increase the activity of the sodium-potassium

---

*The law of osmotic equilibrium is a consequence of Walter Gibbs' free energy function. This, in turn, is a necessary consequence of two laws of the universe: the First Law of thermodynamics and the Second Law of thermodynamics. You may recall from Chapter 4 that this latter law is also known as the Entropy Law.

pump in the kidneys, causing retention of sodium, but losing weight or exercising helps to restore normal plasma insulin levels. This and other evidence summarized earlier suggests that decreasing dietary sodium and increasing dietary potassium, losing weight, and exercising more are in many ways *doing the same things* in the body. Changing only one component is doing only part of the job.

One might say that sodium and potassium balance each other. The push-pull effect of increasing potassium while decreasing sodium is hard to ignore. One pushes while the other pulls. One is the yin and the other the yang. To have an effect, *both* must be changed. Thus, it is important to keep an eye on the K Factor in the diet *and* to eliminate factors such as obesity and lack of exercise that prevent the body from maintaining a normal balance between potassium and sodium.

PART SIX

SALT, BLOOD PRESSURE REGULATION, AND DRUG ACTION

CHAPTER 16

How Important Is Salt?

"Ye are the salt of the earth"—the well-known quote from the Bible (Matthew 5:13)—not only has poetic and theological meaning but is literally true.

We are what we eat. We eat plants and animals. The animals that we eat in turn eat plants. So, in effect, all the substances in our bodies ultimately come from plants. And the plants themselves get all their minerals—their salts—from the earth.

As was explained earlier, the most abundant mineral inside our body's cells is potassium, so it's not surprising that we need a fair amount of potassium in our food. Fortunately, because both plants and animals contain plenty of potassium, we can easily obtain enough in our food—as long as we don't boil it out.

Animals also need a certain amount of sodium in order for their muscles and nerves to work properly and to keep their "sodium battery" charged, as was discussed in Chapter 4. Carnivores—animals that eat other animals—obtain an adequate amount of sodium in their diet from the fluid surrounding the cells of their prey, as well as the prey's blood, both of which are rich in sodium.

Plant cells, unlike animal cells, contain very little sodium. Plants do not have the sodium requirement that animals have; they do not possess nerve or muscle cells, nor do they have a "sodium battery."

The reason we humans, and many other animals, don't need nearly as much sodium as most of us get turns out to be our body's fantastic ability to conserve sodium.

THE BODY'S ABILITY TO CONSERVE SODIUM

Our ancestors were plant eaters living on a low-sodium diet. In order for these prehumans to survive, they had to develop mechanisms to retain sodium in their bodies and still eliminate water. We have inherited these sodium-conserving mechanisms in our kidneys and in our sweat glands. We'll discuss how the kidneys work and their amazing ability to keep sodium in the body in the next chapter.

Sweat glands work like miniature kidneys. Although it is not widely recognized, our sweat glands are also capable of conserving sodium by secreting large amounts of sweat that almost completely lacks sodium.

In a 1949 study[1] at the University of Michigan Medical School, Dr. Jerome Conn found that when men ate a low-salt (low sodium chloride) diet and worked in a hot environment, their perspiration had only 0.1 grams of sodium chloride (about 40 mg of sodium) in a whole liter (more than a quart) of sweat. The men lost only an additional 0.05 grams of sodium chloride (about 20 mg of sodium) per day in their urine. In total, they lost only about 0.75 grams of sodium chloride (amounting to 300 mg of sodium) per day—which is about 7% of the amount the average American consumes. Thus these men were able to maintain a balance between the amount of salt they were eating and the amount they were losing in their sweat and urine, even though they were losing over seven quarts of sweat a day!

In contrast, when Dr. Conn put the men to work in the same hot environment and had them eat a typical American diet containing 11 grams of sodium chloride (amounting to 4,400 mg of sodium), they lost about 7 grams of sodium chloride in their sweat (1 gram per each of 7 liters). The other 4 grams were lost mostly in their urine; a small amount was lost in their feces. The sweat of the men eating the typical American high-salt diet contained ten times as much sodium as the sweat of the men when they were on the low-salt diet. Thus it appears that the reason we Americans put out a very salty sweat is that our bodies are trying to get rid of the excess salt we have eaten.

If you're sweating a lot, you don't need extra salt, but you do need to drink extra water. In *Eat to Win*, Dr. Robert Haas recommends the following drink for sweating athletes: To every 1 cup of water add 2 tablespoons of fresh orange juice and ⅓ teaspoon of table salt. This will have a K Factor of about 1. We believe it would be even better to cut the salt to ⅙ teaspoon or less, bringing the K Factor up to 2 or more.

MANY GROUPS OF PEOPLE DO QUITE WELL WITHOUT ADDED SALT

In view of the fact that both our kidneys and our sweat glands can get rid of water without losing much sodium, it isn't surprising that people can live quite well without adding salt to their food, even in a very hot climate. In fact, South American Indians, Africans, and Asians living near the equator have been eating a low-sodium diet for thousands of years. As was pointed out in Chapter 5, the people who still eat a diet of unprocessed natural foods, with no added salt, have almost no hypertension: Less than 1% of these populations develop hypertension, and blood pressure does not increase with age. You will recall that these low-blood-pressure groups ranged from the Carajas Indians of Brazil to the Papuans of New Guinea.

Actually, the low-blood-pressure groups live in a variety of climates, and they eat a variety of diets. For example, the diet of the Yanomano Indians is primarily vegetarian, a major component of their diet being plantain (a cooking banana). In contrast, the diet of the Greenland Eskimos—at least in the 1920s, when they were studied by Dr. William Thomas[2]—was completely carnivorous. It consisted of walrus, seal, polar bear, caribou, Arctic hare, fox, birds, and fish—all usually eaten raw and never with any added salt. (Unsalted meats have K Factors of 4.5 or more.)

The Greenland Eskimos' diet was fairly low in fat, since it was carefully removed from the meat for use as fuel. Wild animals do not have fat marbled between the muscle cells, as do fattened beef cattle. (As was described in Chapter 8, excess fat in our food can contribute to high blood pressure, atherosclerosis, heart attacks, and cancer.) Not only were the Greenland Eskimos free of high blood pressure, but they enjoyed general good health even into old age.

The Labrador Eskimos examined in the same study, however, were in very poor health. Their diet was augmented with dried and canned foods, which they purchased from the Hudson's Bay Company in exchange for furs. The latter foods contained added salt and were deficient in vitamin C.

HOW MUCH SODIUM DO WE REALLY NEED?

The Fifth Joint National Committee Report recommends that the daily dietary intake of sodium be kept under 2,300 mg. However, there is considerable reason to believe that the amount of sodium we need is actually lower.

Some of the low-blood-pressure groups of people who eat primarily vegetarian diets have been getting along fine for thousands of years on sodium intakes ranging from 50 mg to 230 mg per day.[3] Some of Dr. Lewis Dahl's patients with hypertension lived on diets containing 50 mg to 300 mg of sodium per day for up to fifteen years with no ill effects.[4] Dr. Walter Kempner's rice-fruit diet has also been used for years by many patients, and this diet provides only 50 mg to 60 mg of sodium per day.[5] Thus, there is considerable evidence that the required amount of sodium is well below the 1,100 mg figure, probably as low as 100 mg to 300 mg. Recently, the National Academy of Sciences has recommended a minimum of 500 mg of sodium per day.

OUR APPETITE FOR SALT

So why do so many people think we need extra salt? Some people say we need extra salt because they think animals do. This misconception probably arises from the well-known fact that cows like to lick salt blocks. However, they do this not so much because their vegetarian diet contains very little sodium as because of the amount of sodium they lose in the very large amount of milk they produce. Holstein cows, for example, can produce as much as 30,000 pounds of milk per year, about 15 times the amount required to nurse a calf. This is about 10 gallons per day and up to 40% of the weight of the cow per week! Because a lactating cow loses so much sodium in her milk, she requires about 30 grams of supplemental salt per day.[6]

In contrast, dry cows (those not producing milk) or beef steers are equally healthy whether or not they are given supplemental salt,[7] and the same is true for other domestic animals.[8] And although wild herbivores such as deer have been reputed to travel great distances to go to natural salt licks, it is difficult to substantiate this belief. For example, Dr. A. R. Patton analyzed mud sent in by forest rangers from areas in the Montana Rockies where wild animals congregate to lick the soil. The rangers called these sites salt licks, but Dr. Patton did not find sodium in any of the mud samples. What he did find, however, was iodine,[9] an element needed to make thyroid hormone.

Probably the major reason we have been conditioned to use so much salt is the history of our culture. About four thousand years ago, trade routes were developed that made sea salt available even to people living far from the sea. Salt came into common use for seasoning and for preserving food. It was also an important item of commerce. In the Bible it is written: "And every oblation of thy meat offering shalt thou season with salt" (Leviticus 2:13). This was written about thirty-five hundred years ago. The word *salary* is derived from the Latin word *salarium* ("salt money"), which was used to pay the Roman soldiers. We still use the expression "Is he worth his salt?" But the four thousand years during which there has been easy access to salt is only one-thousandth of the period of time that human life has existed on this planet.

Thus the "recent" abundance of salt has probably not had time to significantly affect the evolution of humans, especially because the major harmful effect that excess salt produces in some people—high blood pressure—does not usually have lethal effects until after a person has passed child-bearing age.

The fact that we do not need much sodium in our diet is indicated by the low sodium content of human milk (37 to 39 mg per cup, with a K Factor of 3.2 to 3.5).[10] Many modern babies are nourished with cow's milk, however, which has over three times as much sodium as does human milk. Considering that the foods available to children after they are weaned typically have added salt, it is hardly surprising that our palates become habituated to the taste of salt. The result: Any food without added salt doesn't taste right.

Some scientists believe that the major part of our craving for salt is acquired as a dietary habit. We have been taught, or conditioned, to like salt. In fact, one study reported that many people said that after they had been on a low-sodium diet for a few weeks, they actually began to prefer unsalted food.[11] Some of my friends and I can testify to this from our own experience of developing a taste preference for potassium salts, which most people dislike at first.

SUMMARY

Since our kidneys and sweat glands are designed to hold on to sodium, we do not need to eat very much in our food. Our modern food habits, however, have caused us to develop a craving for salt. This craving has resulted in a major health problem—hypertension—in our modern society, where salted foods and foods with much of their natural potassium removed are readily available and extremely popular.

Fortunately, though, most of our craving for salt is a learned habit. And habits can be broken!

How the Kidneys, Hormones, and Nervous System Work Together to Control Blood Pressure

Blood pressure depends on both the output from the heart (the volume of blood pumped per minute) and the peripheral resistance to the flow of blood. Blood pressure is regulated by three main systems: the kidneys, the endocrine system (hormones), and the nervous system. In other words, these three systems are able to control heart output and peripheral resistance.

THE KIDNEYS AND BLOOD PRESSURE

There are several ways the kidneys influence blood pressure. One is thought to be regulation of the volume of blood and other fluids in the body, which could affect both heart output and peripheral resistance. Another is control of the amounts of sodium, potassium, and calcium in the body. We have already discussed how these minerals affect the degree of contraction of the smooth muscle cells in the arterioles.

It has long been known that some diseases of the kidney can cause hypertension. When it is due to an identifiable disease, this type of hypertension is called secondary (see Chapter 1). One example of secondary hypertension involving the kidney occurs when there is an obstruction of the artery to a kidney. This causes an excessive secretion by cells in the kidney of the hormone renin, the effects of which we describe later in this chapter.

THE CONNECTION BETWEEN THE KIDNEYS, SODIUM, AND BLOOD PRESSURE

Blood pressure can be affected by the kidneys even when they are not obviously diseased. An example of this type of hypertension was discovered in laboratory rats by Dr. Lewis Dahl.[1] Through selective breeding, Dr. Dahl and his co-workers developed two strains of rats: salt-insensitive rats that do not develop high blood pressure regardless of what they eat, and salt-sensitive rats that do develop high blood pressure but only when they are raised on a high-salt (NaCl) diet.

In order to excrete the same amount of sodium, the kidneys of the salt-sensitive rats require a higher blood pressure than do those of the salt-insensitive rats. One way of looking at this is that the high blood pressure may be the salt-sensitive rat's way of getting rid of the extra sodium it gets when on a diet high in sodium. It is likely that something similar may be operating in some humans who inherit a tendency for high blood pressure.

The ability of the kidneys to affect blood pressure is dramatically demonstrated by kidney transplant experiments. When kidneys from salt-sensitive rats with high blood pressure are transplanted into rats with normal blood pressure, these recipient rats also develop high blood pressure.[2] On the other hand, when kidneys from rats with normal blood pressure are transplanted into hypertensive rats, the latter develop normal blood pressure.[3] Similar observations have been made in humans: When a good kidney is transplanted into a person with severe kidney disease and hypertension, the blood pressure often returns to normal.[4] In fact, among older investigators, the phrase "hypertension follows the kidneys" was a guideline.

The pioneering work of Dr. Arthur Guyton of the Department of Physiology and Biophysics of the University of Mississippi School of Medicine in Jackson has provided us with a larger perspective from which to view the kidneys and hypertension. Dr. Guyton and his colleagues used a *systems** approach in which they modeled on a computer all the factors, including the kidneys, that affect blood pressure.[5] The results of these computer simulations were eye-opening. Regardless of constriction of the resistance blood vessels, blood pressure would remain

---

*In contrast to a purely molecular approach, which is reductionist, a systems approach attempts to take into account all aspects of the whole system. In the biological sciences in the United States, systems approaches have temporarily gone out of vogue—perhaps in part because such approaches require considerable understanding of mathematics and computer modeling.

elevated over a long period of time *only* if there was a change in the response of the kidneys to blood pressure.

At first, this appears to fly in the face of common sense, which focuses our attention upon the peripheral resistance of the circulatory system. But remember, the blood pressure is the product of both the peripheral resistance and the output from the heart. To prove the point that in the long run it is not peripheral resistance that decides blood pressure, Dr. Guyton points to the example of fistulas* that shunt blood directly from arteries to the veins. Such direct shunting of blood away from the peripheral resistance arteries can decrease total peripheral resistance several fold. This of course results in an immediate drop in blood pressure. Yet within several days, the arterial blood pressure will regain the same value as before, *in spite of the huge decrease in peripheral resistance.*

Obviously, for the blood pressure to return to its previous value, something has changed the output of the heart. What could account for this?

Among other factors, the output of the heart depends upon the total volume of the blood.[†] But it is the kidneys that regulate the total amount of water in the blood, and thus the volume of the blood. All other things being equal, the higher the blood pressure, the faster the rate at which the kidney will remove water (and sodium) from the blood. This relation between blood pressure and volume of water excreted by the kidneys is what Guyton calls the renal function curve. And since changes in this curve affect blood volume, such changes also inevitably affect blood pressure.

The computer simulations conducted by Dr. Guyton's group demonstrated that of all the systems regulating blood pressure, it is the renal function curve that—over a long period of time—is dominant. Regardless of what other factors—hormones, changes in sympathetic nerve activity—might change blood pressure, their effects will be relatively temporary. In the long term (days, weeks, months, and years) the effects of these other systems will be overridden by the renal function curve of the kidney. In the final analysis, it will be the renal function curve that will decide the long-term blood pressure. In this regard, Dr. Guyton likens the kidney to a servomechanism that regulates arterial blood pressure.

---

*Fistulas are abnormal connections in the body—in this case direct connections between arteries and veins. Fistulas are often produced by mechanical damage such as gun-shot wounds or accidents.

[†]As the blood volume increases, more blood pools in the veins leading to the heart, with the result that during its relaxation phase (diastole) the heart fills with more blood. Since the heart contains more blood at the end of diastole, during its contraction phase (systole) the heart pushes more blood out into the aorta and thence to the rest of the arterial system. In other words, the output of blood from the heart increases.

Guyton's focus upon the renal function curve of the kidney as the key long-term determiner of blood pressure has generally been ignored in recent investigations of hypertension. But it is important to point out that this concept not only has never been disproved, it is entirely consistent with all known facts, its logic is compelling, and computer simulation suggests it is an inescapable conclusion.

In view of the strong evidence in favor of Guyton's concept, one might well ask just *why* it hasn't been more accepted. I suspect the main reason is that Guyton's idea is counterintuitive. In fact, when I first heard of it, it shocked me. After all, it had become a mental habit to associate elevated blood pressure with elevated resistance. Perhaps this explanation can help you accept the concept better: If—for whatever reason—the kidneys are not able to excrete all the sodium consumed in the daily diet (this amounts to a shift in the renal function curve), sodium will begin to replace potassium in the body. In this situation, one of two things will inevitably happen: Either the blood pressure will rise (by whatever means) to force more blood through the kidney and thus increase excretion of sodium, or sodium will continue to replace potassium in the body until, as with Lot's wife, there's nothing left but a pillar of salt.

As an interesting sidelight to Guyton's work, in the first half of the twentieth century physiologists used to focus attention upon the role of the kidneys in hypertension. They realized that anything, such as constriction of the arteries to the kidney, that decreased blood flow through this organ (which in Guyton's terminology would change the renal function curve) would result in less excretion of sodium and thus of water by the kidney. In order for the kidneys to get rid of this excess sodium and water, it would be necessary, or *essential,* for the body to raise the blood pressure—hence the origin of the term "essential hypertension."*

HOW THE KIDNEYS WORK

The kidneys work by filtering a huge amount of fluid out of the blood and then reabsorbing most of it back into the blood. Only what the body doesn't need is left in the final urine.

Each of us has two kidneys inside the abdomen next to the back muscles. Each kidney consists of about one million tiny functional units that are called nephrons. The structure of a typical nephron is shown in Figure 21.

---

*Although this term makes historical—indeed perhaps even physiological—sense, I personally don't like because there is nothing "essential" about hypertension. You don't have to get it, and you and I certainly don't want to get it. As a result, in this book I have been using the other term, primary hypertension, to refer to the type that most commonly (in 95% to 98% of the cases) afflicts people.

FIGURE 21

THE STRUCTURE OF A NEPHRON

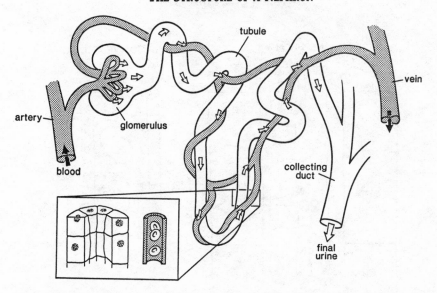

Fig. 21. Simplified diagram of the structure of a nephron: the unshaded tube. The blood vessels are shaded. The watery part of the blood is "filtered" into the glomerulus at the head end of the nephron. As this "preformed urine" passes along the nephron tubule, most of the water and dissolved substances are reabsorbed out of the tubule back into the blood.

A very large volume of fluid enters the nephrons at the glomeruli, where the arterial blood pressure forces (filters) the fluid part of the blood through ultrafine pores. These pores are so small that they allow only salts and other small molecules, such as water and glucose, to pass through; they prevent the blood cells and proteins from entering the nephrons. The resulting ultrafiltrate of the blood ("preformed urine") contains about the same concentration of small molecules and of sodium and other ions as does the blood fluid.

In an average adult, about 50 gallons of this preformed urine are formed each day. Fortunately, the nephrons reabsorb most of this fluid back into the bloodstream; otherwise we would produce 50 gallons of urine per day! Normally all the glucose and amino acids are reabsorbed back into the blood, and more than 99% of the sodium is reabsorbed.

Most of the energy for the reabsorption of sodium comes from the sodium-potassium pump described in Chapter 4. Water follows the reabsorbed substances passively by the process of osmosis. A simplified diagram of how most of the sodium and potassium are reabsorbed from one portion of the nephron tubule is shown in Figure 22.

FIGURE 22

NEPHRON CELL MOVEMENT

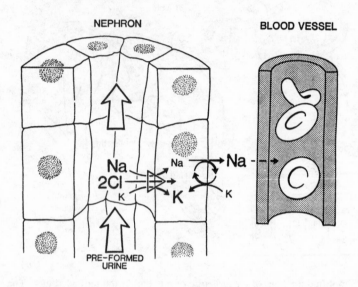

Fig. 22. The movement of Na, K, and Cl (chloride) through the wall of the nephron. Only some of the most important pathways for these ions are shown. The circle on the outer nephron membrane is the metabolically driven sodium-potassium pump described in Chapter 4. The triangle represents a "piggyback" pump that carries Na, K, and Cl together into the nephron cell. The electrical voltages across the cell membranes are not shown.

The inner and outer membranes of the tubule cells are different. The net effect of the ion movements is the movement of sodium, potassium, and chloride (along with water) from the nephron passageway back into the blood. The "Na-K-Cl pump" (the "triangle" in Figure 22), is a recently discovered "piggyback" membrane pump that moves one potassium ion, one sodium ion, and two chloride ions simultaneously across the cell membrane into the nephron cell from the nephron passageway, using energy from the sodium battery that was described in Chapter 4. In addition, the Na^+/H^+ exchange pump is also involved in reabsorption of sodium and excretion of acid by the kidney.

Because the membrane of the tubular cell that faces outward pumps sodium out and potassium into the cell, and because of membrane leakiness, the net effect of all of the membrane transport systems is primarily to move sodium and chloride from the inside of the nephron (that is, from the preformed urine) to the blood.

In the piggyback pump system just described, sodium must be transported back into the body together with chloride; therefore the amount of sodium that can be reabsorbed back into the body from the ultrafiltrate in the tubule is partly limited by the amount of chloride present. For this reason, a low-chloride diet helps the body get rid of sodium in the urine, while a high-chloride diet helps keep sodium in the body. Thus, table salt (in which *all* the sodium comes packaged with chloride) is generally the *worst* form of sodium to have in your diet.

The sodium in unprocessed food isn't quite so bad. In meat, for example, about 15% of the sodium is combined with organic anions rather than chloride. In unprocessed foods, relatively little potassium is complexed with chloride (for example, about 20% in potatoes). Rather, in both plant and animal cells, potassium is associated primarily with a variety of organic negative ions rather than with chloride (Cl⁻). So you can see that the best way to get potassium is in unprocessed foods. Mother Nature has it prepared just right for us.

In summary, the kidneys are good at conserving sodium for the body and at the same time excreting large amounts of potassium into the urine. So it's understandable that we don't need much sodium (only about 100 or 200 mg) but do need a lot of potassium in our diet. Since the kidneys can excrete so much potassium into the urine, the amounts in natural unprocessed foods certainly are not dangerous unless severe kidney disease is present.

REGULATION OF THE KIDNEYS BY HORMONES

ANTIDIURETIC HORMONE

The volume of urine output is regulated by several factors. One of these is *antidiuretic hormone* (ADH), which is secreted by the pituitary gland at the base of the brain. The rate of secretion of ADH depends on blood volume and especially the concentration of salts in the blood. The hormone is carried by the bloodstream to the kidneys, where it causes a reduction in the volume of urine production.

Deficient ADH secretion is known as diabetes insipidus. The people who have this relatively rare condition produce up to 20 liters of urine each day. Because it is so dilute, physicians in the old days noticed that the urine of these patients has an insipid taste, hence the name of the condition. (The more common diabetes is called diabetes mellitus because of the sugar in the urine; *mellitus* means sweet.)

The volume of urine output is also tied to the rate at which the kidneys excrete sodium, which is largely under the control of the hormones EDLS, aldosterone, natriuretic factors, and insulin.

ENDOGENOUS DIGITALIS-LIKE SUBSTANCE (EDLS)

The normal role of the hormone EDLS is to help the body rid itself of excess sodium. Either increasing dietary sodium (which would be equivalent to decreasing the K Factor), or giving steroid hormones that cause retention of sodium, increases EDLS levels in the blood. The increased level of EDLS then causes the kidneys to excrete more sodium in the urine.

EDLS is secreted by a region at the base of the brain called the hypothalamus and also perhaps by the adrenal cortex. EDLS acts by inhibiting the sodium-potassium pumps in the kidney tubules (and in other cells throughout the body). This slows sodium reabsorption, allowing more sodium to be lost in the urine. Researchers have suggested that if the blood level of this natriuretic factor rises sufficiently (for example as it does when you eat a lot of sodium), it may inhibit the sodium-potassium pumps located in the smooth muscle cells in the arterioles throughout the body. This would cause the "sodium batteries" of these cells to run down. Some scientists believe that this is what causes many cases of primary hypertension, since the discharged sodium batteries would result in constriction of the arterioles.[6] As you already know, this would result in increased peripheral resistance, causing the blood pressure to rise.

INSULIN

Insulin is best known for its ability to regulate blood sugar levels and for its role in diabetes mellitus. Although the finding is not yet in the textbooks, insulin is also one of the most potent sodium-retaining hormones.

After our laboratory discovered that insulin stimulates the sodium-potassium pump,[7] a colleague, Dr. Jean Crabbe from the University of Louvain Medical School in Belgium, visited our laboratory and discussed this. Back in Belgium, Dr. Crabbe and his co-workers demonstrated that insulin stimulates the sodium-potassium pump in the kidney so much that, at about twice the normal blood level, insulin can cause almost total reabsorption of sodium from the preformed urine back into the blood.[8]

This effect of insulin partly explains why obese people tend to retain sodium in their body and thus frequently develop high blood pressure. It also explains why people who have been on a very-low-calorie diet or on a total fast (which lowers blood insulin) develop retention of fluid after taking a lot of carbohydrate in their first full meal. The carbohydrate sharply raises their blood sugar, which, in turn, causes the pancreas to release lots of insulin into the blood. This increase in blood insulin then stimulates the sodium-potassium pumps in the kidneys to cause retention of sodium ions (Na^+). Since water always follows Na^+, their kidneys also retain fluid, causing body tissues to swell and causing a temporary weight gain of several pounds.

ALDOSTERONE

Aldosterone, sometimes considered the primary salt-retaining hormone, is se-creted into the blood by the adrenal glands, which sit on top of each kidney. At high levels of aldosterone secretion, almost no sodium is lost in the urine or sweat. In Addison's disease, there is a deficiency in the secretion of aldosterone. This results in the excessive loss of sodium from the body, a hunger for salt, decreased blood volume, and—as you would by now expect—*low* blood pressure.

The opposite symptoms occur in Conn's syndrome (also called primary aldosteronism), which is caused by an adrenal-gland tumor that secretes excess aldosterone. The resulting retention of sodium and water causes high blood pressure. High blood pressure due to primary aldosteronism cannot be cured either by drugs or by raising the K Factor but must be corrected by surgical removal of the tumor.

Aldosterone also causes the kidneys to excrete more potassium. The fact that a high blood level of aldosterone leads not only to retention of sodium in the body and to loss of potassium but also to elevated blood pressure presents one more piece of evidence that excess sodium or too little potassium in the body can cause hypertension.

ANGIOTENSIN AND RENIN

The rate of secretion of aldosterone is controlled partly by the blood level of another hormone called angiotensin—specifically, angiotensin II—which is in turn controlled by an enzyme called renin, which is secreted into the blood by specialized cells in the kidney.

Renin secretion by the kidney is increased by sympathetic nerve activity and/or by low arterial blood pressure in the kidneys and/or decreased level of potassium in the blood plasma. In addition to causing increased secretion of aldosterone, angiotensin II also acts directly on the smooth muscle cells of the arterioles, causing them to contract and raising blood pressure. Moreover, as already discussed in Chapter 4, elevated levels of angiotensin II stimulate the Na^+/H^+ exchange pump and thus increase the tendency for developing "muscle-bound" arteries.

We mentioned earlier in this chapter that a few cases of human hypertension* result from the increased renin secretion (and thus higher levels of angiotensin) caused by an obstruction of the artery leading to a kidney.

The action of renin is summarized in the chart on page 292:

---

*Since these cases of hypertension are secondary to a known cause, in this case narrowing of the renal artery, they are called secondary hypertension as opposed to the more common primary hypertension that is the concern of this book. In this particular type of secondary hypertension, the answer not only isn't drugs or even nutrition, it is surgery to correct the narrowing of the artery. All types of "secondary" hypertension together comprise only about 2% to 5% of the total cases of hypertension.

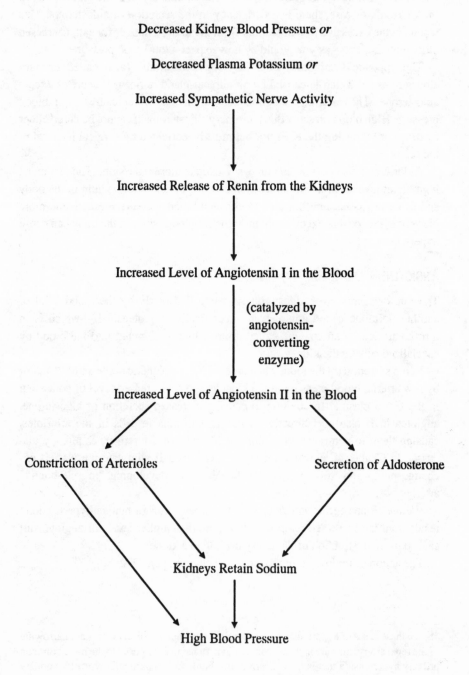

Decreased Kidney Blood Pressure *or*

Decreased Plasma Potassium *or*

Increased Sympathetic Nerve Activity

Increased Release of Renin from the Kidneys

Increased Level of Angiotensin I in the Blood

(catalyzed by angiotensin-converting enzyme)

Increased Level of Angiotensin II in the Blood

Constriction of Arterioles

Secretion of Aldosterone

Kidneys Retain Sodium

High Blood Pressure

High-Renin and Low-Renin Hypertension

One of the first physicians to approach the treatment of hypertension by focusing upon the physiology involved was Dr. John Laragh of Cornell University Medical School in New York. Dr. Laragh's research group actually played a key role in clarifying the importance of the renin-angiotensin system by discoverng the ability of angiotensin II to stimulate secretion of aldosterone by the adrenal gland.[9]

Dr. Laragh logically decided that if drugs were to be used to treat primary hypertension, they should be based upon an ability to specifically act upon the body's regulatory systems that elevate blood pressure. Since the renin-angiotensin system plays a crucial role in blood pressure regulation, he decided to focus upon this system by measuring blood levels of renin in patients with primary hypertension. The results were provocative. In contrast to a fairly narrow range of renin levels found in people with normal blood pressure, in people with hypertension Dr. Laragh's group found that only about 55% had renin levels in the usual range whereas 15% had clearly elevated renin levels and the remaining 30% had lower than usual levels.[10] This wide spectrum of renin levels in these people emphasizes that primary hypertension has several different ways to manifest itself.*

Actually, as Dr. Laragh was the first to point out, those with lower than usual renin levels actually have "normal" levels, considering the fact that their blood pressure is elevated. Therefore, the other 70% can be lumped together into a category called high-renin hypertensives.

This distinction is significant for several reasons. Perhaps the most important is that low-renin patients were found to suffer fewer strokes and heart attacks than the high-renin group. This was true even though the low-renin group often had higher blood pressure than the high-renin group. This was one of the first clues that, as we now know, the problem in hypertension involves much more than just elevated blood pressure. The hypothesis that the damage was due more to the high renin levels than to the elevated blood pressure was borne out by experiments in which injection of renin into animals resulted in severe damage to blood vessels in the kidneys, heart, and brain.[11] Furthermore, kidney damage sometimes results in a sudden increase in renin levels—a situation likely to be accompanied by stroke or heart attack.

Dr. Laragh was quick to point out the significance of this evidence that more than blood pressure is involved, although this seems to have been relatively ignored by others at the time.

---

*However, we will see that just as all roads lead to Rome (hypertension in this case), there is one common denominator—namely, an imbalance between potassium and sodium.

The fact that high levels of renin are involved in many cases of primary hypertension implies that angiotensin II would also be elevated in these people. Since high levels of angiotensin II increase peripheral resistance, it would be logical to try to find a drug that would prevent elevation of this hormone. As you can see from the diagram above, angiotensin I, which produces very little effect on blood pressure, is converted to angiotensin II by the action of angiotensin-converting enzyme (ACE). Squibb pharmaceutical company had purified a component—SQ 20881, or teprotide—of snake venom that specifically inhibits angiotensin-converting enzyme. Dr. Laragh's group injected (it cannot be taken orally) this compound into ninety-three people with primary hypertension and found that it quickly lowered blood pressure. Moreover, as expected, the greatest drops in blood pressure were observed in those people who had the highest levels of renin.[12]

As a direct result of this research, a compound, captopril, that inhibits angiotensin-converting enzyme and can be taken by mouth was finally developed. Thus, we had the first ACE-inhibitor (which is discussed in the next chapter) for use in treating hypertension.

NATRIURETIC FACTORS

Natriuretic factors are recently discovered substances that increase the rate of sodium excretion by the kidneys. The word *natriuretic* comes from *natrium,* for sodium, and *uresis,* meaning "excretion in the urine." Increased consumption of sodium or an increase in the blood volume stimulates the secretion of these factors into the blood.

One natriuretic factor is a peptide, or small protein, manufactured and released from a small "ear," or auricle, which sticks out from the atrium of the heart. Accordingly it is called the atrial natriuretic factor, or ANF. In contrast to EDLS, it does not inhibit the sodium-potassium pump but instead increases sodium excretion by another means.

Until recently, it was thought odd that the heart would have this part, which apparently served no useful function in the body. Now it has been shown that stretching out the auricle of the heart by increased blood volume causes it to secrete atrial natriuretic factor. The atrial natriuretic factor then causes the arterioles in the kidney to enlarge, allowing more preformed urine to be filtered and thus more sodium and water to be lost in the urine. ANF also dilates other blood vessels. ANF is the only hormone known to effectively lower blood pressure, and has been proposed as a new drug for that purpose.

OTHER HORMONES

Other hormones, whose functions are still poorly understood, are secreted by the kidneys and are probably very important. It is now recognized that a class of hormones called prostaglandins are secreted by cells in the kidneys. Prostaglandins appear to help the kidneys excrete sodium. This may account for the reduction in blood pressure that occurs when safflower oil is added to the diet (see Chapter 8), since linoleic acid (the major component of safflower oil) is necessary for the synthesis of prostaglandins.

REGULATION OF BLOOD PRESSURE BY THE NERVOUS SYSTEM

Our blood pressure is regulated from minute to minute by nerves. At specific locations in the walls of the large arteries, special sensors "measure" blood pressure by responding to the amount of stretch in the walls of the arteries. An important location of these sensors is the *carotid sinus*, which is in the arteries that run up the neck to supply the head with blood.

When blood pressure increases for any reason, these sensors send nerve signals to the blood-pressure regulating center located in the lower portion of the brain. In response to the nerve signals, the blood-pressure regulating center sends out nerve signals that slow the heart and dilate the arterioles. The lower output of blood by the heart and the lower peripheral resistance to blood flow both result in lowering the arterial blood pressure back toward normal.

By rubbing the carotid sinus area on the side of your neck near your voice box, you can stimulate these receptors and cause a quick (but temporary) reduction of your blood pressure.

Another example of this reflex occurs when you suddenly sit or stand up after lying down. Gravity pulls the blood downward, lowering the blood pressure in the carotid sinus in your neck. If the carotid sinus reflex didn't act promptly, sending out nerve impulses (over sympathetic nerves) to increase heart output and constrict the arterioles, you would faint from the decreased flow of blood to your head. In fact, fainting when standing up is one of the side effects of some of the blood pressure medicines that act by inhibiting the sympathetic (adrenergic) nervous system, as will be described in the next chapter.

The sympathetic nervous system is the portion of the autonomic (involuntary) nervous system that has as its main function the preparation of our bodies for emergency situations. The sympathetic (adrenergic) nervous system sends nerve signals to the blood-pressure regulating center, telling it to raise the blood pressure, which the center accomplishes by sending signals over sympathetic nerves that go to the heart and blood vessels. This system becomes active when we are frightened, preparing us to run away or to fight by increasing our heart rate and reducing the blood flow to the stomach, intestines, and skin.

Some cases of primary hypertension appear to be associated with increased sympathetic nervous system activity. This could be partly the result of a decrease in the voltage across the surface membrane of the sympathetic nerve cells caused by accumulation of sodium and depletion of potassium inside the cell, which could be helped by dietary changes. The decreased membrane voltage of the sympathetic nerve cells would cause them to fire off nerve signals more often, thus raising blood pressure. Increased sympathetic nervous system activity can also result from the psychological stress caused by our reaction to unpleasant situations.

In obese people, the stimulation of sympathetic nerves by elevated insulin levels may be a compensatory mechanism to limit weight gain. It has been suggested that hypertension is a side effect of this mechanism.[13]

PUTTING IT ALL TOGETHER

Dr. David Young (like Dr. Guyton also of the Department of Physiology and Biophysics of the University of Mississippi School of Medicine in Jackson) has studied the regulation of potassium in the body. Again, as with blood pressure, the interaction between blood hormones and the kidneys hold the key. Like Dr. Guyton, Dr. Young has used the systems approach to model the regulation of potassium in the body and its interaction with the kidneys and with blood pressure.

In the long term, aldosterone appears to be the key hormone regulating the excretion of potassium by the kidneys. The two main factors governing excretion of aldosterone by the adrenal glands are blood levels of angiotensin II and of potassium*—both of which stimulate excretion of aldosterone. The effects of these two factors, blood levels of angiotensin II and of potassium, multiply each other. As a result, when blood levels of angiotensin II are elevated, even small changes in blood levels of potassium produce big changes in aldosterone concentration.[14] This means, for example, when plasma potassium is at 3.5 mEq/L (which often occurs in people with hypertension—see Chapter 15), even a five- or sixfold increase in angiotensin II will produce only a modest increase in the blood level of aldosterone.

The rate of filtration of the watery part of the blood into the "preformed urine" is called the glomerular filtration rate, or GFR for short. The GFR is increased as a result of an elevation of blood pressure and/or an elevation of blood potassium level.[15] Increasing the GFR (by increasing the rate of flow of "preformed urine" into the distant end of the kidney tubule) tends to decrease release of renin into the blood.[16] Thus, in high-renin hypertension, increasing the blood level of potassium would be expected to lower the elevated renin level toward normal.

In fact, increasing blood potassium *does* decrease release of renin into the blood.[17] Thus, increasing dietary potassium in people with high-renin hypertension would be expected to lower blood levels of renin, and thus of angiotensin II,

---

*You may remember from a previous chapter that I use the more vernacular "blood levels of potassium" instead of the more scientifically accurate "plasma potassium level."

thus not only decreasing peripheral resistance but also shifting the renal function curve in such a way as to lower blood pressure.

People with low-renin hypertension are considered "salt-sensitive" and, in contrast to those with high-renin hypertension, have an increased blood volume caused by too much sodium in their blood. In fact, their depressed blood levels of renin are due precisely to the fact that they have too much sodium in their blood.* As Dr. John Laragh points out, their low-renin levels are actually normal for their situation.[18] In other words, their renin-angiotensin system is responding normally to an elevated "salt" (sodium chloride) intake. In other words, they are salt-sensitive. Saying that these people are salt-sensitive is equivalent to saying that decreasing the sodium chloride in their diet will lower their blood pressure.

So in either high-renin or in low-renin hypertension, increasing dietary potassium or decreasing dietary sodium (either of which is equavilant to increasing the dietary K Factor) would, on the basis of physiological principles, be expected to eventually lower blood pressure.

Especially relevant to the theme of this book is the result of Dr. Young's computer simulation model. This model predicts that potassium intake higher than that typical of the usual American will result in sodium being excreted from the body and will decrease angiotensin II levels—both of which will combine to result in a decrease in blood pressure. Even more striking is the fact that Dr. Young's computer simulation indicates that even if normal regulation of aldosterone levels is lost, maintaining the proper ratio of dietary potassium to sodium (what is called the K Factor in this book) will maintain the desirable balance between potassium and sodium within body cells and thus maintain blood pressure in the healthy range.[19]

Even more exciting is the fact that the computer model predicts that the "gray area" for potassium to sodium is (on the basis of number of atoms of each) between 1:3 and 3:1. Translating these ratios into the K Factor gives a range between 0.57 and 5.1. In other words, in Dr. Young's model, if the dietary K Factor is above approximately 5, one will almost never have a decreased potassium/sodium balance in the body, and if it is below approximately 0.6, one will almost always have a decreased potassium/sodium balance. As outlined earlier in this book, a proper balance between potassium and sodium inside the body's cells is necessary for healthy blood pressure.

Dr. Young's result is in remarkable quantitative agreement with the "gray area" range derived in this book, whereby a K Factor above 4 almost always prevents hypertension whereas the chance of developing hypertension increases dramatically as the K Factor drops below about 0.8 to 1.0 (see Chapters 5 and 15).

---

*It is generally agreed that slight increases in the plasma sodium level inhibits renin release.[20]

The fact that more than one line of evidence (correlations of the dietary K Factor in different populations with incidence of hypertension, composition of human milk, clinical studies, and computer simulation) gives not only the same qualitative prediction, but also nearly the same *quantitative* prediction is a very encouraging sign that the dietary K Factor does indeed play a key, if not *the* key, role in preventing or causing hypertension.

SUMMARY

The kidneys, the endocrine system (hormones), and the nervous system all play important roles in regulating blood pressure. Since our lives depend on maintaining our blood pressure, it is not surprising that so many systems have evolved to take care of this important function.

In spite of this complexity, computer simulation of a model taking all the most important systems into account has demonstrated that a dietary K Factor above 5 will almost always keep potassium and sodium within the body in proper balance. On the other hand, the computer simulation indicates that a dietary K Factor below about 0.6 will almost always result in an imbalance within the body. In previous chapters, you have seen that such an imbalance will almost inevitably eventually lead to hypertension.

CHAPTER 18

Antihypertensive Drugs

This chapter briefly describes how antihypertensive drugs reduce blood pressure. Table 14 lists the most common antihypertensive drugs. All these drugs also have many less common side effects that are not listed here. More drugs are being developed every month; if you don't find yours listed here, consult with your doctor.

TABLE 14

ANTIHYPERTENSIVE DRUGS

TYPE	GENERIC NAME	TRADE NAMES	COMMON SIDE EFFECTS
DIURETICS			
Thiazide diuretics	Chlorothiazide	Diuril Aldochlor* Diupress	Low plasma potassium due to urinary potassium loss, muscle weakness or cramping, faintness on stand-
	Chlorthalidone	Hygroton Regroton Novothalidon Tenoretic Uridon	ing, impotence, increased blood triglycerides, increased blood cholesterol, increased blood uric acid, low plasma magnesium
	Hydro-chlorothiazide	Maxzide* Aldoril Dyazide*	

Warning: If you are currently taking one of the adrenergic inhibiting drugs, do not *suddenly* stop taking it, as this could cause a heart attack or sudden death. In fact, any change in your current medication should only be done in consultation with your physician.

---

*Many of the trade-name drugs combine two or more generic drugs into one pill; thus some trade names appear twice.

TYPE	GENERIC NAME	TRADE NAMES	COMMON SIDE EFFECTS
Potassium-sparing diuretics	Spironolactone	Aldactone Aldactazide	Hyperkalemia, enlargement of male breasts, breast pain, menstrual irregularities, intestinal problems, lethargy
	Triamterene	Dyremium Maxzide* Dyazide*	Hyperkalemia, nausea, weakness, leg cramps
Other diuretics	Furosemide	Lasix	Potassium loss, nausea, vomiting, diarrhea, headache, weakness
ADRENERGIC (SYMPATHETIC) INHIBITING DRUGS			
Central-acting adrenergic inhibitors	Clonidine	Catapres Combipres	Drowsiness, fatigue, dry mouth, constipation, dizziness, sexual dysfunction, insomnia, rebound hypertension
	Methyldopa	Aldoclor* Aldomet Aldoril*	Headache, weakness, nausea, dry mouth, drowsiness, fatigue, constipation, dizziness, sexual dysfunction
Sympathetic nerve ending blockers	Guanethidine	Ismelin Esimil	Diarrhea, weakness, stuffy nose, failure to ejaculate, slow heart rate
	Rauwolfia alkaloids	Harmonyl Raudixin	Sexual dysfunction, stuffy nose, depression, lethargy
	Reserpine	Diupress* Serpasil	Faintness on standing up, diarrhea, weakness, stuffy nose, failure to ejaculate, slow heart rate, depression
Alpha-adrenergic blockers	Phenoxy-benzamine	Dibenzyline	Dizziness on standing, stuffy nose, fast heartbeat, failure to ejaculate
	Phentolamine	Regitine	Dizziness on standing, weakness, failure to ejaculate, stuffy nose, fast heart beat, nausea, vomiting, diarrhea

*Many of the trade-name drugs combine two or more generic drugs into one pill; thus some trade names appear twice.

Type	Generic Name	Trade Names	Common Side Effects
	Prazosin	Minipress	Dizziness on standing, weakness, drowsiness, headache, failure to ejaculate, stuffy nose, fast heartbeat, nausea, vomiting, diarrhea, may decrease blood cholesterol
Beta-adrenergic blockers	Metoprolol Nadolol Propanolol	Lopressor Corgard Inderal Inderide	Slow heartbeat, nausea, appetite loss, fatigue, depression, insomnia, nightmares, decreased ability to exercise, elevated blood triglycerides, sexual dysfunction
VASODILATORS			
Vasodilators	Hydrazaline	Apresoline Dralzine Unipres	Headache, fast heartbeat, nausea
	Minoxidil	Loniten	Fast heart beat, fluid retention, excess hair growth, breast pain
NEWER DRUGS			
Angiotensin inhibitors	Captopril Saralasin	Capoten Lopirin Sarenin	Rash, dry cough, danger of hyperkalemia, may increase fetal mortality during pregnancy
Calcium channel blockers	Diltiazem Nifedipine	Anginyl Cardizem Adalat Nifedin	Headache, dizziness, nausea, edema
	Verapamil	Calan Cordilox Isoptin Vasolan	Flushing, edema, hypotension, constipation

Sources: See reference 1.

DIURETICS

THIAZIDE DIURETICS

Diuretics (commonly called "water pills") are drugs that stimulate the kidneys to produce a larger volume of urine. Thiazide diuretics accomplish this by causing the kidneys to reabsorb less sodium back into the blood and thus to excrete extra sodium. Water accompanies this extra sodium in the urine, leading to the increased urine volume.

Thiazide diuretics decrease blood pressure in two ways: First, the loss of sodium and water leads to a decrease in blood volume, which in turn reduces blood pressure by decreasing output of blood from the heart. Soon after this, the heart output returns to normal, but the blood pressure stays down because the loss of sodium from the body results in a decrease in the peripheral resistance to blood flow (by mechanisms described in Chapter 4).

In people whose kidneys are no longer functioning—patients on artificial kidney machines—thiazide diuretics have no effect on blood pressure.[2] Since diuretics do not affect the amount of sodium removed by the artificial kidney machine, this suggests that the decreased peripheral resistance induced by the thiazide diuretics is due to the loss of sodium. As Dr. Louis Tobian has repeatedly pointed out, every physician who uses a thiazide diuretic for treating hypertension is casting a vote for the idea that too much sodium is a key factor in causing essential hypertension.

One way of looking at hypertension is that our bodies sense the presence of too much sodium. The response is to increase the blood pressure, forcing more blood through the kidneys and thus resulting in some of the extra sodium and water being forced out into the urine. By increasing sodium excretion by the kidneys, the thiazide diuretics reduce the sodium in the body enough that the blood pressure no longer has to be elevated to do this.

Unfortunately, the thiazide diuretics also cause the excretion of extra potassium. This can lead to a deficiency of potassium in skeletal muscles,[3] which can cause mild weakness, a fairly common side effect of these drugs. The extra loss of potassium through the kidney can also result in a decrease in the level of plasma potassium.[4] If you are also taking a digitalis compound for your heart, this drop in plasma potassium can be very dangerous, leading to an irregular rhythm of your heart (cardiac arrhythmia).

Of course, the irony of the thiazide diuretics is that potassium deficiency is part of the problem in your developing primary hypertension in the first place. Although we don't yet know all the effects of a deficiency in body potassium, it is established that they include abnormal carbohydrate metabolism, glycosuria (sugar in the urine), disturbed acid-base balance, and kidney disease.[5]

A frequent complication of the thiazide diuretics is elevation of the blood uric acid level. This can precipitate an attack of gout.

As mentioned in Chapter 2 and discussed in Chapter 3, thiazide diuretics also elevate blood levels of cholesterol and other fats, which are known to increase your chances of having a heart attack. Recall from Chapter 2 that treatment of borderline hypertension with thiazide diuretics apparently increases the death rate, with most of the deaths resulting from heart attacks.[6]

Prolonged use of thiazide diuretics results in a decrease not only in blood potassium but also in body magnesium content,[7] which can, in turn, make it difficult for the body to restore its potassium. Moreover, magnesium is needed for the parathyroid glands to respond to calcium. As we've already indicated, a deficiency in calcium can predispose to hypertension.

POTASSIUM-SPARING DIURETICS

The potassium-sparing diuretic spirolactone is thought to block the action of the hormone aldosterone.[8] Remember from Chapter 17 that aldosterone causes the kidneys to conserve sodium by causing more of it to be reabsorbed out of the preformed urine in the nephrons, thus putting it back into the blood. Therefore, when spirolactone is given, this action of aldosterone is blocked, and more sodium (along with water) is lost in the urine.

Aldosterone also stimulates secretion of potassium from the blood into the forming urine in the kidney nephrons. Therefore, spirolactone causes the kidneys to conserve potassium, keeping it in the body instead of excreting it in the urine along with the excreted sodium. For this reason, spirolactone lacks one of the undesirable side effects of the thiazide diuretics—loss of body potassium. You can see that spirolactone will have some of the same beneficial effects on blood pressure as a diet with a high K Factor. The high-K-Factor diet, however, does not have any undesirable side effects, whereas spirolactone use can result in lethargy, enlargement of male breasts, breast pain, menstrual irregularities, or intestinal problems.[9]

The other potassium-sparing diuretic listed in Table 13 is triamterene. Triamterene directly inhibits the transport of sodium out of and the secretion of potassium into the preformed urine in the kidney tubules.[10] Thus, like spirolactone, triamterene promotes the loss of sodium through urination, while conserving potassium. Both these effects will reduce the blood pressure by the mechanisms described in Chapter 4. However, triamterene can cause nausea, leg cramps, or weakness.

OTHER DIURETICS

Furosemide has sometimes been used for treating hypertension as well as for treating congestive heart failure and other conditions that cause fluid accumulation. It acts on the kidney tubules to inhibit the reabsorption of sodium and chloride and, to some degree, potassium. Thus more salts and water remain in the final urine. Getting rid of extra sodium is beneficial for reducing the blood pressure, but the extra loss of potassium may be a harmful side effect, as was discussed in the section on thiazide diuretics.

ADRENERGIC INHIBITORS

There are four types of antihypertensive drugs that inhibit the sympathetic nervous system, whose major function is to prepare the body for "fight or flight" by delivering more blood to the arm and leg muscles. To accomplish this, the sympathetic nervous system causes the heart to pump out more blood by increasing the heart's rate of beating and the strength of its contractions. In addition, the sympathetic nervous system tightens the blood vessels going to the stomach, intestines, skin, and other regions, since it's more important to run away from a tiger than to digest your hamburger or stay cool. Both the increased cardiac output and the increased peripheral blood vessel resistance caused by sympathetic nerve activity will lead to increased blood pressure.

Even when a person is sitting or standing at rest and not frightened, there is a basal level of sympathetic nervous system activity. Thus there is a constant stream of nerve impulses arriving at the arteriolar smooth muscles, causing them to have a "resting" tone or tension. Therefore, a drug that inhibits the sympathetic nervous system will tend to lower the blood pressure by decreasing the basal smooth muscle tone, allowing the arterioles to widen.

CENTRALLY ACTING ADRENERGIC INHIBITORS

Adrenergic inhibitors can be centrally acting or peripherally acting. The centrally acting adrenergic inhibitors block the sympathetic nervous system in the brain or spinal cord. Both types have various undesirable side effects (see Table 14).

Methyldopa

Methyldopa inhibits the outflow of nerve signals from the sympathetic nervous system.[11] Since sympathetic nerve signals generally tell smooth muscle cells in the blood vessels to contract, the inhibition of these signals allows the arteriolar smooth muscle cells to relax, thus lowering peripheral resistance and blood pressure.

Clonidine

Clonidine's major hypotensive effect stems from its action on the blood pressure regulating center in the medulla of the brainstem.[12] It inhibits sympathetic nerve output and stimulates parasympathetic nerve outflow; both these central effects result in a lowering of the blood pressure. *Caution: Sudden withdrawal of clonidine can cause a life-threatening hypertensive crisis.*

PERIPHERALLY ACTING ADRENERGIC INHIBITORS

The rest of the adrenergic inhibiting drugs act primarily at the endings of the sympathetic nerves, where they make functional contact with smooth muscle cells. By functional contact, I mean that this is where the nerve signals are transmitted to the muscle cells, causing them to increase their level of contraction. The nerve endings do not actually physically touch the smooth muscle cells; instead, they are separated by a narrow *synaptic* gap. Thus the electrical nerve signals cannot be directly conducted from the nerve cell endings to the smooth (or heart) muscle cells. To get the signal across the synaptic gap, the electric nerve signal causes the sympathetic nerve endings to release the chemical *norepinephrine* (I will call it by the common name, *noradrenaline*), which is stored in the nerve terminal. The noradrenaline then diffuses across the synaptic gap and attaches to *receptor* protein molecules on the surface of the smooth muscle cells. This attachment causes a pore in the muscle cell membrane to open, allowing calcium to enter the cell, where it activates the contractile machinery. This is illustrated in Figure 23.

Reserpine and the Rauwolfia Alkaloids

Several chemicals called alkaloids may be extracted from the root of the plant *Rauwolfia serpentina,* a climbing shrublike plant that is native to India. The ancient Hindus used these alkaloids for treating snake bites and hypertension.[13] One of these alkaloids, reserpine, has been widely used for treating hypertension since the rediscovery of the rauwolfia alkaloids in the 1950s.

Reserpine and the other rauwolfia alkaloids act by depleting the stores of noradrenaline in the nerve endings. This affects the brain as well as the peripheral nerve endings, but the peripheral effects are considered to be the most important. Because of the depletion of stored noradrenaline, the nerve signals do not release as much noradrenaline and fewer calcium channels open in the smooth muscle membrane, resulting in less tension in the muscle cells. This dilates the arterioles and lowers blood pressure. The effect of reserpine lasts for about a week, so the physician must be aware of the cumulative effect of daily doses.

Guanethidine

Guanethidine, like reserpine, also inhibits the *presynaptic* release of noradrenaline. It does this both by directly inhibiting the release mechanism and by depleting the amount of stored noradrenaline.

FIGURE 23

ALPHA-ADRENERGIC INNERVATION OF ARTERIOLAR SMOOTH MUSCLE

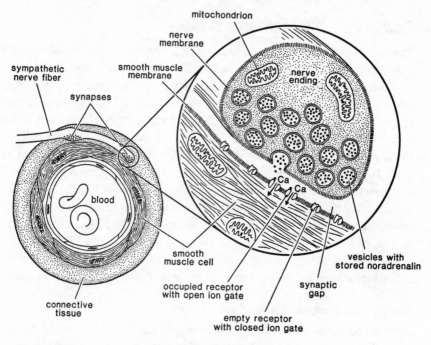

Fig. 23. Diagram of the sympathetic (specifically, alpha-adrenergic) innervation of arteriolar smooth muscle. On the left is a cross section of an arteriole; the circled portion of this is enlarged on the right.

ADRENERGIC BLOCKERS

In contrast to reserpine and guanethidine, which act on the nerve endings, the adrenergic blockers act by inhibiting the postsynaptic receptors on the smooth muscle membrane—that is, they block the membrane from receiving noradrenaline. The postsynaptic receptors normally respond to the noradrenaline released by the nerve endings. There are two major types of noradrenaline receptors: *alpha* receptors and *beta* receptors—and there are "blocker" drugs for each.

Alpha Blockers

Alpha receptors are found on the smooth muscle cells in almost all the body's arterioles. Activation of these receptors by noradrenaline causes the arterioles to constrict. Thus, the alpha blocking drugs—phenoxybenzamine, phentolamine, and prazosin—reduce blood pressure by blocking the transmission of sympathetic nerve signals to the arterioles, allowing the arteriolar smooth muscle to relax and widening the passageway for blood flow. This effect is greatest when you are standing and is minimal when lying down (very few sympathetic nerve signals are sent out when you are lying at rest). The side effects of the alpha blocking drugs result from the fact that alpha receptors are found not only in arteriolar muscle but also in heart muscle, intestinal muscle, and sexual tract muscle. As listed in Table 14, these side effects include fast heartbeat, diarrhea, and failure of ejaculation.

Alpha blockers such as prazosin appear to actually improve blood cholesterol levels.

Beta Blockers

Beta receptors are found on smooth muscle cells in the arterioles of the heart, intestines, and skeletal muscles. These receptors are activated by adrenaline. Adrenaline hormone is released from the inner cells of the adrenal glands when they are stimulated by sympathetic nerve signals. It then circulates in the blood.

In contrast to the alpha receptors just discussed, activation of the beta receptors by adrenaline causes *dilation*, not constriction, of the arterioles that have beta receptors. One would therefore think that a beta blocker such as propranolol, which blocks these dilation receptors, might constrict the arterioles of the heart, intestines, and arm and leg muscles, and thus cause an increase in blood pressure. But because the blood level of adrenaline is normally fairly low and because the drugs have other effects, beta blockers do reduce blood pressure.

The exact mechanisms by which the beta blockers reduce blood pressure are not known for certain, but one mechanism appears to be inhibition of the kidneys' secretion of renin into the blood. Ordinarily the secretion of renin is stimulated by activation of beta receptors on the secretory cells in the kidneys. As described in the preceding chapter, renin causes an increased production of angiotensin in the blood. Angiotensin II has two actions that raise the blood pressure: It causes arteriolar smooth muscle to contract, and it acts on the adrenal gland, causing the outer cells to secrete more aldosterone into the blood. Aldosterone in turn acts on the kidneys to cause sodium and water to be retained by the body and potassium to be lost in the urine. Thus beta blockers, by inhibiting this process, may actually help improve the body's K Factor.

Another mechanism by which beta blockers might reduce blood pressure is reduction of the amount of noradrenaline that is released from sympathetic nerve terminals. This could occur because there are beta receptors on the nerve terminal membrane that, when activated, cause more noradrenaline to be released. Propranolol and the other beta blockers block this noradrenaline release.

Because a major function of the sympathetic nervous system is to prepare the body for "fight or flight," increased activity of this system occurs in situations of stress, either temporary or ongoing. It is the increased activity of the sympathetic nervous system that causes the heart to beat faster and increases the rate of sweating and other symptoms in people who are under intense stress. One study in the *American Journal of Medicine*[14] described the use of a beta blocker to prevent stage fright in performers. This emphasizes the fact that people who are on beta blockers may not show the symptoms and outer signs of stress even though they may be experiencing it internally.

One of the limitations of beta blockers is that elevated blood pressure in blacks often does not respond as well to these drugs as in whites. Another problem is that beta blockers decrease output from the heart in virtually everyone. This can severely limit a person's ability to exercise, and of course, exercise should be an important part of the program for most people with hypertension.

VASODILATORS

Hydrazaline and minoxidil both reduce blood pressure by acting directly on the arteriolar smooth muscle cells and causing them to relax. An interesting side effect of minoxidil is that it stimulates hair growth. A solution of the drug is now being applied to the heads of younger bald men to stimulate the regrowth of hair. For this topical (external) application, minoxidil is now called Rogaine.

NEWER DRUGS

ANGIOTENSIN-CONVERTING ENZYME (ACE) INHIBITORS

We have described how propranolol, a beta blocker, can reduce blood pressure by inhibiting renin secretion. This renin inhibition in turn reduces the amount of angiotensin in the blood.

There are also drugs that specifically reduce blood levels of angiotensin II. We've seen that this hormone is involved in producing some of the problems in hypertension. Angiotensin-converting enzyme is required for the conversion of angiotensin I to angiotensin II. This is especially important in high-renin hypertension. Since renin catalyzes the production of angiotensin I, people with high blood levels of renin will also have high levels of angiotensin II *unless* the angiotensin-converting enzyme is inhibited.

Captopril is an ACE-inhibitor that lowers the level of angiotensin II in the blood by inhibiting the renin-stimulated angiotensin II production. Saralasin inhibits the actions of angiotensin on the kidneys and on arteriolar smooth muscle. These angiotensin inhibitors are especially effective in reducing the blood pressure of hypertensive people who have higher than normal blood levels of renin.

ACE-inhibitors such as captopril have been shown to be effective in the treatment of hypertension in people with diabetes.[15] Moreover, captopril lowers blood pressure without decreasing or even actually *increasing* flow of blood to the heart, brain, and kidneys. This is in contrast to some diuretics and beta blockers that reduce blood flow to these vital organs.[16] For example, in contrast to beta blockers, at least one ACE-inhibitor (lisinopril)[17] can lead to improvement in bicycle and treadmill exercise tolerance, at least when used to treat congestive heart failure.

Like all drugs, however, ACE-inhibitors can have their drawbacks. ACE-inhibitors, like beta blockers, often do not work as well in blacks with hypertension as they do in whites. In addition, there is a growing consensus that ACE-inhibitors should not be used during pregnancy. This is based upon the report that in experimental animals, ACE-inhibitors can result in fetal loss as high as 80%.[18] In humans, ACE-inhibitors also increase serious fetal complications including neonatal death and neonatal kidney failure.[19]

CALCIUM CHANNEL BLOCKERS

As pointed out in Chapter 4, the amount of tension in smooth muscle cells is controlled by the concentration of calcium inside these cells. Much of this calcium enters the cells through "slow" calcium channels in the cell membrane, which can be opened by a decrease in the membrane voltage, such as occurs in sympathetically stimulated cells. The calcium channel blockers block these channels so that they cannot open, thus slowing the movement of calcium into cells. In the smooth muscle cells of the resistance arteries, this blunts the rise of calcium, thus reducing their constriction of the channel for blood flow. Calcium channel blockers may also be able to allow the overenlarged heart, which so commonly occurs in hypertension, to recover to a more normal size.[20]

Calcium channel blockers do not appear to have a negative effect upon serum potassium or cholesterol levels.[21] However, these drugs may disturb carbohydrate metabolism in diabetic patients.[22]

SUMMARY

The drugs used for treating hypertension work by a wide variety of mechanisms. Usually these mechanisms merely treat the symptom (high blood pressure) without curing the basic cause.

All these drugs have undesirable side effects because they act at several locations and tend to upset the body's normal balance. The most common side effects include these:

Undesirable changes in blood cholesterol and triglycerides. This is frequent with diuretics and with beta blockers. It appears not to occur with calcium channel blockers nor with ACE-inhibitors, and some alpha blockers, such as prazosin, may change blood cholesterol in the direction we consider desirable.

Undesirable changes in blood plasma potassium levels. Thiazide diuretics frequently lower plasma potassium. Potassium-sparing diuretics and also ACE-inhibitors tend to elevate plasma potassium levels above normal. If drugs raise plasma potassium much above the upper limit of normal, the situation can be *very dangerous,* since this can lead to an irregular beat (arrhythmia) of the heart that is potentially fatal.

Impotence. You may have noticed that most of these drugs include sexual dysfunction in their side effects. When I discussed this with one practicing cardiologist, he commented that it's not surprising that impotence can occur with almost all of these drugs. Here is another case where I had not recognized "2 plus 2 equals 4." When I asked why, he replied that it was obvious: In order for an erection to take place, blood pressure in the penis must rise. Therefore any drug that interferes with the mechanisms that can raise blood pressure locally will inevitably pose the danger of inhibiting erections. This applies to thiazide diuretics, beta blockers, and calcium channel blockers.

In contrast, the eating and exercise program presented in this book corrects the basic imbalance that causes hypertension in the first place. And instead of the drug side effects, which make you feel *worse,* the K Factor program makes you feel *better.* And after all these years, no one has yet reported that fruits such as bananas or even vegetables such as broccoli have caused so much as even one case of impotence!

PART SEVEN

FOR
THE PHYSICIAN

CHAPTER 19

Information for the Physician

The goal of treating patients with hypertension is to prevent morbidity and mortality associated with high blood pressure and to control blood pressure by the least intrusive means possible [emphasis mine].
Fifth Report of the Joint National Committee, 1993[1]

Some physicians have had reservations about the exclusive reliance on antihypertensive drugs for several years. Even in 1983, Dr. Norman Kaplan pointed out that treating borderline and mild hypertensives without drugs would "fly in the face of current dogma and practice."[2] But until 1984 the official medical position of the Joint National Committee on the Detection, Evaluation, and Treatment of High Blood Pressure[3] was that all hypertensives be treated with drugs.

The movement away from drugs has begun. In its 1984 Special Report, even the prestigious Joint National Committee began to recommend that patients with less severe hypertension no longer be started on drug therapy unless they have risk factors. In that report the committee recommended: "For those with diastolic blood pressures in the 90 to 94 mm Hg range who are otherwise at low risk, nonpharmacologic therapy should be pursued aggressively while blood pressures are carefully monitored." Moreover, in its 1988 Report,[4] the Joint National Committee added a new "step" to the previous four. This new step, the first in the new strategy, consists of approaches based upon changing lifestyle. And in a further move in this direction, the 1988 report recommended trying a "step-down" approach to drug therapy in those patients with mild hypertension who after beginning drugs have had normal blood pressure for at least one year. This trend has been continued in the 1993 Report of the Joint National Committee (JNC 5),[5] which now places a much more explicit emphasis upon change in lifestyle in the treatment of hypertension.

This move toward emphasizing the importance of lifestyle was initially prompted in part by the surprising results of the MRFIT study,[6] which demonstrated a dissociation between the effects of drugs upon blood pressure and upon mortality. When stepped-care drug therapy, as opposed to "usual care," was used to lower blood pressure, mortality was unchanged in the group with diastolic pressures between 95 and 100 mm Hg, and it may actually have been increased in the group with diastolic pressures between 90 and 94 mm Hg.

Up to 75% of U.S. citizens suffering from hypertension have diastolic blood pressures between 90 and 104 mm Hg.[7] Thus, perhaps half of the people with hypertension have diastolic blood pressures in the range from 90 to 100 mm Hg and fall into the category of those whose overall mortality rate may not be benefited by drug therapy, according to the MRFIT and British[8] MRC studies.

Not only is a lifetime of drug therapy expensive, but unpleasant side effects are frequent. Many of these side effects are well known, but as Drs. Berchtold, Sims, Horton, and Berger[9] of the University of Vermont School of Medicine have pointed out, there is as yet no way "of knowing or of evaluating possible long-term effects in a population that may be taking drugs for a matter of decades." Although the newer drugs hold promise of fewer serious side effects, we need to heed the caution of the Fifth Joint National Committee Report (JNC 5), which reminds us that long-term controlled clinical trials have not yet produced data on the effects of alpha blockers, ACE-inhibitors, or calcium antagonists on cardiovascular complications and mortality in hypertensive patients.[10]

Since primary hypertension* is due to a genetic predisposition that becomes manifest only as a result of mistakes of lifestyle (especially improper food preparation, lack of exercise, and obesity), the only long-term answer seems to be a return to proper nutrition, exercise, and normal weight as outlined in this book and recommended by JNC 5.

In light of the development discussed in this book, it is reasonable to expect that as time goes by, more and more patients with primary hypertension will eventually be treated without drugs. As recommended by JNC 5, those people being treated with drugs should also change their approach to nutrition and to exercise.

In fact, in view of the evidence presented in this book that almost all cases of

---

*Instead of the term *essential hypertension,* I use the older term *primary hypertension.* I found that some readers got confused by the term *essential* because they felt it implied that if something is "essential" it must be necessary or good.

hypertension are due to mistakes in lifestyle, we all can hope for the day when our entire society corrects its habits of food preparation, and primary hypertension becomes an uncommon problem. Indeed, recognition of this has led the Working Group of the National High Blood Pressure Education Program (NHBPEP) (sponsored by the National Heart, Lung, and Blood Institute) to make this statement:

> ... this is an appropriate time for the National High Blood Pressure Education Program (NHBPEP) in conjunction with other interested parties to initiate a national campaign whose specific goal is the primary prevention of high blood pressure. ... The campaign should inform the public and health care providers about the lifestyles and specific factors which increase the risk of developing high blood pressure. ...[11]

THE GOAL OF HYPERTENSION TREATMENT

The goal is not merely to get the blood pressure down. In its 1993 report (JNC 5) the Joint National Committee reminds us that the ultimate goal is to *"prevent the morbidity and mortality associated with high blood pressure and to control blood pressure by the least intrusive means possible."*

That's what we want to keep in focus. Everything discussed in this book indicates that to best accomplish this, we need to correct the fundamental imbalances at the cellular level that cause the elevated blood pressure, elevated insulin levels, and abnormal blood cholesterol levels that characterize the hypertension syndrome.

RESTORING THE BALANCE

This book has summarized the evidence that primary hypertension not only involves increased insulin levels and deranged cholesterol levels but is most often due to an imbalance between sodium, potassium, calcium, and magnesium in the body. Direct evidence of this imbalance is provided by the observation that *untreated* hypertensives have a significant deficiency in total body potassium (see Chapter 15). This imbalance causes abnormal functioning of body cells, with high blood pressure being just *one* consequence. (Defects in blood vessel integrity including thickening,[12] elevated plasma insulin levels, and abnormal blood cholesterol levels are others.)

The observation is highly important that in human beings, increasing dietary potassium—thus increasing the dietary K Factor—protects against strokes.[13] Dr. Lou Tobian (see Chapter 6) and his group in Minnesota have conducted extensive experiments with hypertensive rats demonstrating that the protective effect of potassium is *independent of changes in blood pressure.* Moreover, it has now been shown that potassium has this same ability to protect human beings against strokes. *The importance of this cannot be overemphasized.*

In confirming the original experiments of Dr. George Meneely and Con Ball, Dr. Tobian's group has gone much further and demonstrated that potassium protects not only against stroke but against kidney disease in hypertensive rats. These results with experimental animals suggest that increasing the K Factor should not only decrease strokes in humans but also help protect them from kidney disease due to hypertension.

In fact, from what we understand about the basic physiology and biophysics involved, this protective effect of potassium, independent of blood pressure, might have been predicted if any of us had thought about it earlier. The effect of potassium upon blood pressure *was* predicted from our knowledge of basic biophysics and physiology (that's what got several of us who have experience in basic research thinking along these lines in the first place).

We now know that the balance of such ions as potassium, sodium, and calcium, as well as the pH inside the cell, plays an important role in regulating several fundamental cell processes, including cell division. Thus, it is not out of the question that the dietary imbalance that causes hypertension in those so genetically predisposed may produce other problems. As one possible example, there is some evidence that a high-sodium diet can increase the probability of stomach cancer.

The mounting evidence that potassium can extend life *regardless of changes in blood pressure* emphasizes that the goal should be much more than just lowering blood pressure. This not only demonstrates the importance of adequate dietary potassium but underscores the fact that blood pressure is a *sign* of the underlying problem and not the whole problem, as we used to think.

The obvious way to achieve our goal is to restore a normal balance within body cells. Although drugs may lower blood pressure and even blood cholesterol, it remains to be seen if they can restore the normal *balance* between sodium, potassium, calcium, magnesium and pH in body cells. The way to restore the proper cellular balance is to eat a diet with that balance while eliminating such factors as obesity and lack of exercise, which prevent the body from maintaining the normal ionic balance. In other words, people should keep themselves physically fit and eat the foods their physiological systems were designed to handle over a million years of human evolution.

Compared with drugs, the relatively innocuous procedure of adjusting the ratio of potassium to sodium in the food we eat to a more "natural" balance, decreasing excess body fat, exercising regularly, and avoiding excess alcohol appears to be the safer approach.

THE "DANGERS" OF POTASSIUM

Isn't a program that significantly increases potassium intake dangerous? Not if the change is made gradually, as outlined in Chapter 10, and kidney function is normal. It has yet to be sufficiently recognized that the gradual change, over a few days, allows *extrarenal* mechanisms[14] (which take potassium up into body cells) as well as *renal* mechanisms (which excrete part of an excess potassium load) to become more effective in "buffering" plasma potassium against elevations.

Physicians tend to be wary of giving anything orally that contains a potassium salt. A typical illustration of this reservation is this statement in a book published in 1978 on the management of essential hypertension: "The indiscriminate use of salt substitutes is to be condemned as a dangerous practice. Indeed, severe toxicity with near-fatal hyperkalemia (high blood potassium) has been reported in a small child who ingested approximately 1 to 1.5 teaspoonsful of a salt substitute from his father's 'medicines.'"[15]

To put this in perspective, even table salt (NaCl) can also be poisonous, especially in small children. For example, in an Associated Press release in U.S. newspapers in March 1984, it was reported that an infant had died as a result of drinking a milk formula that was accidentally contaminated with NaCl.

POTASSIUM IS NOT TO BE FEARED—JUST RESPECTED

Why are many physicians so afraid of potassium? Although it's just a speculation, perhaps the following may make sense: Our first exposure to the use of potassium is in a hospital setting, where it is often given intravenously. As we all know, if the flow of potassium-containing fluid directly into the blood speeds up too much, it is possible to raise the concentration of potassium in the blood to levels that can trigger a cardiac arrhythmia. Understandably, it is drilled into medical students and nurses that (in the hospital setting) potassium can be *very* dangerous. This wariness with regard to potassium may be reinforced by the fact that potassium-containing pills can cause a stomach ulcer.* Every time we physicians have heard about potassium, it's been with a warning—and, for these particular situations, a warning well heeded.

However, we are talking about a *health,* not a *disease* (or hospital) setting. In a

---

*The tendency of potassium pills to cause ulcers is due to the high local concentration of potassium salt in the intestine when the pill dissolves. "Slow-release" pills have greatly reduced this problem. For slow-release potassium pills, the incidence is one small bowel ulcer out of 100,000 patient-years. The ulcer problem can be further reduced by using liquid or effervescent potassium preparations.

health setting, such as the home, where potassium is taken only orally, additional potassium is a different matter, especially when it is taken in natural foods, such as fruits and vegetables. Potassium in natural foods is partly complexed to organic material and therefore is absorbed more slowly into the blood. There is no doubt that normal kidneys can handle the amounts of potassium recommended here if it is taken in as food.

In fact, the high-potassium diet required to prevent or cure high blood pressure is eaten today by precisely those groups of people among whom hypertension is rare. And our ancestors evolved over millions of years on a high-potassium diet.* During that time our kidneys and extrarenal mechanisms developed the means to cope with rather large amounts of potassium compared with what most of us eat now. If potassium in food were dangerous, the human race would have died out long ago. And if the large amount of potassium in many natural foods (a potato or banana, for example) were dangerous to people, vegetarianism would be a dying fad (pun intended).

Provided the guidelines outlined here are followed, and the patient does not have kidney disease, all the evidence indicates that, in contrast to drugs, *this procedure can do no conceivable harm.*

THE IMPORTANCE OF EXTRARENAL POTASSIUM REGULATION

Many physicians are afraid of oral potassium because of the possibility of hyperkalemia. It's widely recognized that this can result from kidney disease, which can involve a decreased ability to excrete potassium. This is an important consideration, but a large part of an acute potassium load is handled by extrarenal mechanisms.

Dr. Ralph DeFronzo of Yale University Medical School has studied this.[16] When 50 mEq of potassium is given intravenously over a period of 4 hours, the rise in blood plasma potassium is only 1 mEq/L, rather than the 3 mEq/L expected if all had remained in the extracellular fluid. Nevertheless, during this time, only 40% of the potassium load is excreted by the kidneys. The remaining potassium is removed from the blood into body cells by extrarenal mechanisms.

The most important of these extrarenal mechanisms involves the elevation of blood insulin by plasma potassium. The elevated insulin level then acts through the mechanism first documented by my research group and that of Dr. Torben Clausen in Aarhus, Denmark,[17] among others, namely, insulin stimulation of the

---

*In this perspective, what is recommended here is not a "high"-potassium diet, but a diet with *normal* levels of potassium; the diet of modern society actually is a low-potassium diet.

sodium-potassium pump. Dr. DeFronzo has called insulin the "most potent hormone for extrarenal potassium regulation."[18] This has practical implications, as demonstrated by the fact that in dogs, diabetes results in a *doubling* of the elevation of plasma potassium level in response to potassium loads.

When body potassium is replenished, the ability to handle a potassium load without spiking plasma potassium is greatly improved. This is known as potassium tolerance. Conversely, if a person is deficient in body potassium, the ability to handle a potassium load is compromised. So potassium deficiency presents a delicate problem. The potassium needs to be restored, but not too fast.

Diminished ability to handle potassium may be explained at least in part by the finding by Dr. Torben Clausen[19] that in rats, potassium deprivation leads to an 80% decrease in the number of sodium-potassium pumps in muscle. Since insulin affects only the rate of each pump, this would blunt the ability of insulin to remove potassium from the plasma during a potassium load.

There are at least two clinical lessons to be drawn from this:

1. In people suspected of having a decreased amount of total body potassium, restoration of potassium through diet, and especially if intravenously, should be done *gradually*. One or two weeks should be enough time, and this has been taken this into account in the nutritional suggestions in Chapter 10 about getting started on the program. The evidence clearly shows that the majority of untreated hypertensives have diminished amounts of total body potassium. If they have been on thiazide diuretics, this condition may have been worsened.

2. Because of a possible relative hypoinsulinemia, most diabetics may have their extrarenal potassium regulatory mechanism compromised. Until further research is done, it is especially important that dietary potassium in diabetics should be increased gradually. In addition, in these patients, the plasma potassium should probably be checked—perhaps as often as every other day—for a couple of weeks until a new steady state is obtained. Of course, insulin dosage should be maintained at adequate levels.

WHAT ABOUT KIDNEY DISEASE?

As you know, potassium supplements in pill or liquid form can be hazardous to persons with decreased kidney function. The also applies to potassium-containing salt substitutes, which patients may take even if you don't advise it. So a urinalysis and serum creatinine for evaluation of kidney function in the initial physical examination is especially important.

If the patient has a kidney problem, a thorough evaluation of kidney function—including glomerular filtration rate (GFR), clearance tests, and so on—should be done. Your approach must be tailored for that patient. Of course, if the patient's serum creatinine *and* serum potassium are elevated, you have some definite signs that the patient's kidneys are having trouble handling potassium. If the kidney disease is so extreme as to require need of a dialysis machine, you should be wary even of high-potassium foods.

But remember, we're not really talking about large amounts of potassium in an absolute sense—just about amounts that are large relative to the deficient levels in our present diet. The amounts required are those found naturally in food before it is processed commercially or prepared in the kitchen. Virtually any patient who can handle lots of vegetables and fruits can be on a high-K-Factor diet! If there is a suspicion of a kidney problem, in spite of the protection of extrarenal mechanisms, it is prudent to suggest that the patient avoid potassium-containing salt substitutes. This is probably overconservative, but the proper K Factor can easily be obtained by food alone if it is properly selected and prepared.

THE DIAGNOSIS OF HYPERTENSION

The new criteria for diagnosing hypertension as defined by JNC 5 are outlined in Table 1 of Chapter 1. The JNC also suggests that to guard against the misdiagnosis of hypertension:

> Hypertension should not be diagnosed on the basis of a single measurement. Initial elevated readings should be confirmed on at least two subsequent visits over one to several weeks (unless systolic blood pressure is 210 mm Hg or greater, and/or diastolic blood pressure is 120 mm Hg or greater), with average levels of diastolic blood pressure of 90 mm Hg or greater and/or systolic blood pressure of 140 mm Hg or greater required for diagnosis.[20]

This caution reflects, among other considerations, a 1987 editorial in the *American Journal of Cardiology,* in which Dr. Norman Kaplan of Dallas, Texas, warned against the misdiagnosis of hypertension due to the influence of the doctor's office upon the patient's blood pressure:

> readings in as many as 80 percent of patients are lower when taken out of the office—This study and many more document the inescapable fact that, for some patients, the doctor's office may be the only place where the blood pressure is high.[21]

Dr. Kaplan refers to this as "white coat hypertension" and estimated that it leads to misdiagnosis in as much as 20% of the people who are labeled hypertensive.

Once hypertension is diagnosed, possible causes of secondary hypertension, such as those outlined in Chapter 9, should be considered before treatment is begun.

RECOMMENDATIONS FOR TREATING PRIMARY HYPERTENSION

With the appearance of the 1984 Special Report, there was a new consensus that those with diastolic blood pressure below 95 mm Hg should be treated by a nondrug approach. The 1984 Special Report also pointed out that such nondrug approaches as weight reduction have value even in people with more severe hypertension who *do* receive drug treatment. The 1988 Report of the Joint National Committee contained a further significant step in the direction toward nondrug approaches. In their 1988 Report,[22] the Joint National Committee added a *new* first step in which "for some patients" nonpharmacological approaches are tried before the four drug steps are entered (see Figure 3 in Chapter 2). Moreover, the 1988 Report recommends that in patients with mild hypertension whose blood pressure has been "controlled" for at least one year, reducing antihypertensive drugs in a stepwise fashion be considered.

The 1993 report (JNC 5)[23] goes further and now recommends that patients diagnosed as having Stage 1 (diastolic pressure 90–99 mm Hg) and Stage 2 (diastolic pressure 100–109) hypertension be vigorously encouraged to make lifestyle modifications for three to six months before resorting to drugs to reduce blood pressure.* Moreover, JNC 5 recommends that if blood pressure has not decreased significantly within that time, lifestyle modifications be continued *even after* drug therapy is begun.

In addition to making lifestyle changes that increase the dietary K Factor, reduce excess weight, increase exercise, and cut down on alcohol, JNC 5 also emphasizes that it is essential for people with hypertension to avoid smoking. Recall the editorial accompanying the 1985 British Medical Research Council study, which concluded:

> In advising hypertensive patients we must continue to emphasize the great importance of stopping smoking, for this may turn out to be a more important therapeutic manoeuvre than the prescription of blood pressure lowering drugs.[24]

The 1993 Report points out that the cost of lifelong antihypertensive therapy, 70% to 80% of which is due to drug costs, represents a significant component of the nation's financial committment to health. Accordingly, the 1993 Report concludes

---

*The 1993 Report of the Joint National Committee states that initial diastolic blood pressure of 120 mm Hg or above, or systolic blood pressure of 210 mm Hg or above, or evidence of target organ damage may require immediate drug therapy.

that "for individual as well as societal reasons, minimizing cost must be an essential component of the health care provider's responsibility."

The information in this book will still help you motivate your patients and educate them, as recommended by JNC 5, about the meaning of their blood pressure readings as well as the lifestyle changes that will provide the greatest— and the least expensive—protection against hypertension. And, as JNC 5 recommends, it seems logical to consider that even when drugs are used, lifestyle modifications, such as the K-Factor approach, should still be employed (except perhaps when the drugs are potassium-sparing diuretics, beta blockers, or possibly ACE-inhibitors—see the following warning), since the aim should include correcting the primary problem, not just lowering blood pressure.

The clear advantage of drugs remains in situations in which you want to get the blood pressure down fast; if a patient walks in the door with severe hypertension, we would all probably agree to use drugs to get the pressure down out of the high danger zone, and worry about nutrition and exercise later.

WHAT IS A DESIRABLE K FACTOR?

You will recall from evidence summarized in Chapters 5 and 7 that any person with a dietary K Factor* of less than about 1.4[†] and a genetic predisposition is a candidate for primary hypertension. As the potassium-to-sodium ratio drops below around 1.0 or 0.8, the probability of getting hypertension—and that it will be severe—rapidly increases. As pointed out in Chapter 5, the dietary K Factor of the average American adult male is only 0.38, right in the high danger zone!

In Chapter 5, it was pointed out that hypertension is rare in populations in which the K Factor was increased to values closer to 2 or more. In clinical trials, only when the K Factor is raised above approximately 3 or 4 (the same value found in human milk) is blood pressure *consistently* restored toward normal. So this would suggest that the dietary K Factor be kept well above 4. But remember from Chapter 15 that increasing the *total* amount of sodium and potassium too much can be bad *even if* the K Factor is above 4. Therefore, not only should the level of potassium be *increased,* but also the level of sodium should be *decreased.* Keep in

---

*The weight ratio of potassium to sodium.

[†]This threshold of around 1.5 is is not absolute but ranges between about 0.6 to 3.0. Moreover, the threshold is a variable that depends upon other parameters discussed in this book including dietary calcium, total amounts of sodium and potassium, and exercise. Nevertheless, it appears that the figures presented here are adequate to provide practical guidelines.

mind that in our country, people consume several times the required amount of sodium. Remember that although the minimum safe daily sodium requirement has been set at 1,100 mg per day, more likely (see evidence in Chapter 16) it is only about 200 to 300 mg per day (500 to 800 mg of NaCl). When food is processed and prepared the way the average American gets it, it contains *several grams* of sodium per day. In the United States, it's almost impossible to get too little sodium. Remember that most Americans have a long way to go: from an average dietary K Factor of 0.38 to a recommended value at least ten times that.

GETTING STARTED

Because of the reduced ability to handle potassium in potassium deficiency, restoring body potassium should be started slowly. As stated in Chapter 10, it is a good idea to eliminate the use of table salt for one week before starting the first, or transition, week of the menu program. During the transition week, the K Factor is increased to about 4. If there is any question about kidney function or insulin deficiency, or if the patient is elderly, you might make some dietary substitutions to increase the K Factor more slowly.

POTASSIUM-CONTAINING SALT SUBSTITUTES

Moderate use of potassium-containing salt substitutes is not unduly dangerous. If a person has normal kidney function, up to 175 mEq per day (6.8 grams/day) of potassium[25] has been reported as not being dangerous for an adult. It is very unlikely that an adult will take more than this amount of potassium salts to add taste to his or her food, since 6.8 grams would be 2¼ teaspoonsful! The greatest danger is probably to young children, who might ingest these salts in excess, as indicated by the McMahon quote earlier in this chapter. Therefore, although the use of salt substitutes is recommended, like many other things, *they should be kept out of the reach of young children.*

POTASSIUM SUPPLEMENTS IN PILL OR LIQUID FORM

Only in cases in which the patient will not adopt the appropriate dietary changes— and especially if thiazide diuretics are also used—might a physician, after evaluation of kidney function and serum potassium level, also want to prescribe potassium in liquid or slow-release form.

If the patient must be on a thiazide diuretic (which may be a dubious choice; see Chapter 18), we're not sure if the K-Factor diet can provide adequate potassium. If during administration of thiazide diuretics, the patient's serum potassium level remains low after a month on the K Factor approach, potassium supplements in pill or liquid may then be indicated. When present, hypokalemia is probably part of the pathophysiological mechanism of primary hypertension. Therefore, it is *especially* important to evaluate periodically the serum potassium levels of patients taking thiazide diuretics.

ADVANTAGES OF INCREASING THE DIETARY K FACTOR WHEN DRUG THERAPY IS USED

Even when drugs are used, especially if they are thiazide diuretics, increasing the dietary K Factor not only will oppose diuretic-induced depletion of body potassium may potentiate the action of these drugs, allowing smaller doses to be used.[26] In fact, a 1991 study from the University of Naples has shown that increasing dietary potassium can allow a *more than 50% reduction* in antihypertensive drug dosage in 81% of patients,[27] thus minimizing side effects. Moreover, about half (38% of the total receiving increased dietary potassium) of these developed normal blood pressure *even when all drugs were discontinued.**

DRUGS THAT MAY MAKE THE K FACTOR DANGEROUS

A note of caution about potassium-sparing diuretics. These are uncharted waters. You will need to use your own judgment. If the patient is on these when dietary potassium is increased, it is probably prudent to follow their plasma potassium carefully. It would seem best to decrease the potassium-sparing diuretics somewhat before, or during, the dietary changes. Of course, another option would be to replace them with another drug during or before the transition to a high-K-Factor diet.

A note of caution about beta blockers. Beta blockers diminish the regulation of serum K during potassium loading. In the presence of beta blockers, plasma potassium can spike during a potassium load.

A note of caution about ACE Inhibitors. ACE inhibitors can cause hyperkalemia,[28] especially in people with reduced renal function or those receiving potassium supplements. Therefore, increasing dietary potassium in patients receiving ACE inhibitors poses the obvious danger of producing a dangerously high level of plasma potassium. Accordingly, it would seem prudent to follow the serum potassium level when increasing dietary potassium in someone on an ACE-inhibitor.

A note of caution about thiazide diuretics. You already know that thiazide diuretics tend to cause loss of body potassium. This is precisely what should *not*

---

*This compares to the development of normal blood pressure without drugs in 9% of controls who received no extra dietary potassium.

happen in the hypertensive patient. From what is known of the role of potassium in the biophysics of the living cell (see Chapter 4), one would expect the thiazides to make the patient more prone to the sequelae of decreased body potassium, including cardiac arrhythmias, sudden death, and perhaps weakened arterial system. Unfortunately, this expectation is borne out by evidence that shows that treatment with thiazides can be especially dangerous in patients with EKG abnormalities.[29] Based upon these considerations, some physicians are moving away from using thiazides for hypertension. Indeed, the trend in that direction was evident in the Joint National Committee's 1988 version of stepped care.[30]

A note of caution about indomethacin. Nonsteroidal anti-inflamatory drugs such as indomethacin and other prostaglandin synthetase inhibitors can produce clinically significant hyperkalemia, especially in people who have renal disease such as glomerulonephritis.

A note of caution about digitalis. Since digitalis inhibits sodium-potassium pumps, it diminishes the ability of the body to prevent hyperkalemia.

Other drugs that may induce hyperkalemia include heparin and cyclosporin.

In the majority of cases where drugs are implicated in hyperkalemia, a condition that compromises the body's ability to regulate potassium is also present. The most common are renal insufficiency, diabetes mellitus, and metabolic acidosis. As was pointed out earlier, diabetes is associated with a decreased activity of the sodium-potassium pumps. This is almost certainly the reason for the decreased ability of diabetics to prevent hyperkalemia.

A note about the importance of serum potassium. In light of basic physiology, it's difficult to understand the resistance some clinicians seem to have to careful monitoring of serum potassium levels even if the patient is on a thiazide diuretic. Remember, people with primary hypertension have deficient body potassium stores even before they are given drugs such as thiazides. Four different studies show that people with hypertension frequently have, as expected on physiological considerations, lowered serum potassium levels. Not enough attention has been paid to these facts.

The level of serum potassium is often, but not always, an indicator of total body potassium. A decrease in serum potassium is correlated in an approximately linear fashion with a decrease in total body potassium; as a rough guide, a drop of 0.25 mEq/L in serum potassium represents roughly a 100 mEq decrease in total (roughly 3000 mEq) body potassium.[31] Because of this, and the key importance of potassium, it would seem a good policy to determine the serum potassium in every untreated hypertensive before starting treatment, whether the treatment is drugs, diet, or both. If the patient is already on drugs, especially if those drugs are thiazide diuretics, a serum potassium should be determined as a benchmark before starting the K-Factor approach.

Based upon the evidence that a low serum potassium level can be part of the pathological mechanism of primary hypertension *and* the fact that the "normal" serum potassium range is probably skewed too low by the inclusion of hypertensives in the data, the following guidelines can be suggested for serious consideration. Though not cast in concrete, they are based upon the presently available information.

If the serum potassium is

- between 4.0 and 5.0 mEq/L, it is probably still a good idea to recheck it twice, say at monthly intervals.
- 4.0 or less (*especially* if it is below the "accepted" lower limit of 3.5), it should be rechecked every two or three weeks until at least two successive readings are between 4.0 and 5.0

If a patient is on thiazide diuretics, the serum potassium level should be monitored closely—probably at least once a month—even if the level is between 4.0 and 5.0 mEq/L. This has not been the usual practice, but it may become so as the importance of potassium is better appreciated (at least until thiazide diuretics are no longer widely used for primary hypertension).

HYPOKALEMIA

Physicians realize the danger of hyperkalemia, but what about hypokalemia? In the context of primary hypertension, debates about hypokalemia usually fail to consider the evidence (summarized in Chapters 4 and 15) indicating that hypokalemia is prevalent even in untreated hypertensives. Moreover, it is probably part of the pathophysiological mechanism contributing to, among other things, the elevation of blood pressure.

CAUSES

Hypokalemia is often associated with hypertension (see Chapter 15). In addition, hypokalemia can be caused by thiazide diuretics, loop diuretics, osmotic diuretics, carbonic anhydrase inhibitors, magnesium deficiency, Cushing's disease, licorice intoxication, primary aldosteronism, and some high-renin hypertension (especially malignant hypertension).

Thiazide diuretics are especially prone to produce hypokalemia with at least a third and perhaps more than 40%[32] of patients on long-term thiazide therapy having plasma potassium concentrations definitely below the normal range.[33] In more than 40% of the cases in which diuretics have caused abnormally low serum potassium, an associated decrease in serum magnesium level occurs. Moreover, in these patients with hypomagnesemia, attempts to correct the hypokalemia are ineffective until normal levels of magnesium are restored.[34]

CONSEQUENCES

Besides making hypertension worse, hypokalemia can decrease glomerular filtration rate, decrease renal concentrating ability, increase sodium reabsorption, increase ammoniagenesis, and cause glucose intolerance. Although the extent of the danger is debated,[35] there is considerable evidence that hypokalemia can cause arrhythmias. In fact, the biophysics of potassium in the cell clearly tells us that hypokalemia would cause some abnormality in membrane voltage and thus make cardiac cells more prone to an abnormality in rhythm.

An increased risk for cardiac irregularities has been correlated with decreases in serum potassium levels of greater than 0.6 mEq/L.[36] Some specialists suspect that some of the sudden deaths described in the MRFIT study may have been due to hypokalemia. In patients with myocardial infarction, a higher frequency of ventricular fibrillation occurs among those with hypokalemia.[37] In these people, the presence of hypokalemia increases the likelihood of clinically important cardiac arrhythmias from 15% to more than 40%.[38] Patients with diuretic-induced hypokalemia have an increased incidence of serious ventricular ectopic activity. Regardless of whether diuretics are the cause of hypokalemia, a serum potassium below 3.5 mEq/L greatly increases the risk of ventricular arrhythmias during myocardial infarction.[39]

Because the activity of the membrane sodium-potassium pump depends upon potassium, hypokalemia is especially dangerous under conditions in which this pump has already been slowed, as in digitalis therapy[40] or hypoinsulinemia.[41]

TREATING OBESE HYPERTENSIVES

Obesity is a major contributor to hypertension. In clinical trials, loss of only a third to a half of excess body weight has reduced blood pressure significantly. The effect of obesity on cellular regulation of potassium and sodium was discussed in Chapters 4 and 7. The importance of obesity in hypertension is reflected by the statement of the Report of the Fifth Joint National Committee[42] that

> In overweight patients with Stage 1 hypertension [diastolic pressure between 90 and 99 and/or systolic between 140 and 159 mm Hg], an attempt to control blood pressure with weight loss and other lifestyle modifications should be tried for at least 3 to 6 months prior to initiating pharmacologic therapy.

Because of the increased risk of diabetes and heart attack associated with any degree of obesity, it is better if body weight (actually body fat) is reduced to a normal level. So it is very important that those who are overweight and have hypertension reduce excess weight by at least half and preferably to a normal level.

Especially since people with either obesity *or* hypertension are more prone to have elevated blood levels of both cholesterol and of insulin, the use of drugs, such as thiazide diuretics and beta blockers, that can adversely change blood lipids, deserves serious thinking in hypertensives who are obese. Moreover, long-term treatment with diuretics and beta blockers apparently increases the risk of development of diabetes.[43]

TREATING DIABETICS WHO HAVE HYPERTENSION

In Chapter 7, you have seen evidence that both hypertension and Type II (NIDDM) diabetes mellitus involve "insulin resistance." This fact is reflected in the 1993 JNC Report, which points out:

> The syndrome of insulin resistance very closely parallels Type II diabetes mellitus. Hypertension, dyslipidemia, hyperinsulinemia, glucose intolerance, and, frequently, upper body obesity comprise this syndrome. Insulin resistance can be improved by weight loss and exercise.

Moreover, in Chapter 4, I presented evidence suggesting that "insulin resistance" may be secondary to deficient stores of body potassium.

Patients who already have diabetes mellitus may be adversely affected by treatment with diuretics and, if the diabetes is insulin-dependent, also by beta blockers.[44] As a result, it has been recommended that if antihypertensive drugs are to be used, patients with NIDDM diabetes and hypertension should be treated with calcium channel blockers, angiotensin-converting enzyme inhibitors (ACE-inhibitors) and prazosin hydrochloride, an alpha blocker, since these have much fewer metabolic side effects than do thiazide diuretics or beta blockers.[45] ACE-inhibitors, such as captopril, have been reported to be effective in treating hypertension in people with diabetes.[46] The JNC 5 points out that alpha$_1$-receptor blockers and ACE-inhibitors may decrease insulin resistance.

EVALUATING THE PATIENT FOR AEROBIC EXERCISE

It's a good idea for the patient to undertake a reduced fat diet before beginning exercise. There should also be a screening for evidence of cardiovascular disease. Although nothing is foolproof, the two best indicators are probably the serum cholesterol and an exercise EKG, although its also important to note family history of heart disease, excess dietary fat, and especially history of smoking.

As an example of the value of proper medical evaluation, at Dr. Kenneth Cooper's Aerobics Center in Dallas, by 1985 more than five thousand participants had been followed; they had collectively run more than six million miles (an average of over a thousand miles per person) with only two cardiac-related events and *no* fatalities. These people had all been screened with an exercise tolerance stress test to maximum heart rate as well as a complete physical exam and medical history.

DECREASING OR WITHDRAWING DRUGS: STEP-DOWN THERAPY

According to the JNC 5 Report:

> Sound patient management should include attempts to decrease the dosage or number of antihypertensive drugs while maintaining lifestyle modificaiton . . . after blood pressure has been effectively controlled for 1 year and at least four visits, it may be possible to reduce antihypertensive drug therapy in a deliberate, slow, and progressive manner.[47]

"In a deliberate, slow, and progressive manner" are key words here. When drugs are reduced, or especially discontinued, in a given patient, the actual change can be dangerous.

NEVER WITHDRAW ANY DRUG SUDDENLY.

This should be emphasized to the patient: *Any* sudden change in the physiological state of a person can be dangerous. For example, sudden withdrawal of clonidine can precipitate a rebound hypertension. If a patient has angina, a sudden withdrawal of beta blockers can precipitate anginal attacks. So drug withdrawal should always be done under your supervision and it should be gradual, in a series of steps.

Since there is relatively little experience in taking hypertensive patients completely off drugs, these thoughts are offered for your consideration: Even when you think a patient should eventually be taken off drugs, unless the patient is taking potassium-sparing diuretics, beta blockers, ACE-inhibitors, indomethacin, or other drugs that can produce hyperkalemia, it is probably best to establish the patient on the nutritional and other lifestyle procedures recommended here for a few weeks and then reevaluate before starting to taper—or "step-down"—the drug dosage.

During the step-down period, the patient should be carefully monitored and the dose of drugs could be decreased in small decrements. On the basis of the biological half-life of drugs and the adaptive processes within the body, the dose should be changed probably no more than perhaps every two to four weeks. By monitoring blood pressure, serum potassium, and other appropriate signs depending upon the drugs and upon the presence of other conditions, such as diabetes, obesity, and so on, you can use your judgment as to whether and when to make the next reduction in drug dosage.

To maximize the success of step-down therapy, it is important to keep in mind this point emphasized by the JNC 5:

> Step-down therapy is especially successful in patients who are also following lifestyle treatment recommendations: a higher percentage maintain normal blood pressure levels with less or no medication.[48]

Remember that Kempner, Priddle, and other pioneers found evidence that blood pressure could be lowered by a proper K Factor even when the diastolic pressure was well over 100 mm Hg. And if you agree with the anthropologists, as I do, that hypertension is a cultural disease of lifestyle, then it should be clear that drugs cannot provide the fundamental long-term answer.

SUMMARY

There are many things a person can do to lower his or her blood pressure and to protect against the tragic consequences of hypertension, such as stroke. For success, a holistic approach is vital. The Fifth Report of the Joint National Committee[49] now recommends that patients diagnosed as having Stage 1 (diastolic pressure 90–99 mm Hg) and Stage 2 (diastolic pressure 100–109) hypertension be vigorously encouraged to make lifestyle modifications for three to six months before resorting to drugs to reduce blood pressure.

The key steps to protecting your patients from hypertension include increasing the dietary K Factor to above approximately 4 (reducing dietary sodium and increasing potassium), starting regular moderate aerobic exercise, losing excess body fat, decreasing alcohol consumption, and perhaps increasing dietary magnesium and calcium. Provided that your patient has normal kidney function, there are no known harmful effects of these measures.

If this program doesn't decrease the blood pressure, don't let the patient get discouraged; encourage him or her to stay with it. It may take weeks or months for blood pressure to respond to the program, especially if the hypertension has been present for several years. JNC 5 points out that "Planned patient education programs may significantly improve adherence to treatment schedules, improve blood pressure control, and decrease hypertension-related morbidity and mortality."[50] To accomplish this, JNC 5 recommends including the patient in decision making, educating family members, and suggesting mutual support groups to enhance motivation. This book would make an ideal text for such educational activities, and, by educating the patient about basic facts, would facilitate communication between doctor and patient.

Remember that increasing dietary potassium, and thus the K Factor, can decrease stroke-related deaths even if the blood pressure doesn't come down. This isn't surprising, since the increased blood pressure is a *sign* of an abnormal balance in the body's cells. Increasing the dietary K Factor to normal will act to correct this imbalance in these cells.

Correcting this imbalance by a proper dietary K Factor, exercise, weight loss, and decreased alcohol consumption can improve health and increase life span, even if blood pressure doesn't return to normal levels. You can't say that about drugs.

References

INTRODUCTION

1. Working Group Report on Primary Prevention of Hypertension. National High Blood Pressure Education Program: National Heart, Lung, and Blood Institute. *Arch. Intern. Med.* 153:186–208 (1993).
2. Moore, R. D., and G. D. Webb. *The K Factor: Reversing and Preventing High Blood Pressure Without Drugs.* New York: Macmillan (1986).
3. See 1.
4. See 1.
5. Rashi, F. Health Care Reform: Medical costs are rising rapidly, and millions of people have no health care coverage. The nation urgently needs a universal insurance program. *Scientific American* 267(5):46–53 (1992).
6. Ginzberg, E. The health swamp. *New York Times.* Nov. 12, 1992, p. A25.
7. Stason, W. B. Costs and quality trade-offs in the treatment of hypertension. *Hypertension* 13(suppl I):I-145–148 (1989).
8. See 1.
9. Fifth Joint National Committee on Detection, Evaluation, and Treatment of High Blood Pressure. *Arch. Intern. Med.* 153:154–183 (1993).
10. See 1.
11. See 9.
12. Prigogine, I., and I. Stengers. *Order Out of Chaos: Man's New Dialogue with Nature.* New York: Bantam Books, 1984.
13. Dahl, L. K. Salt and hypertension. *Am. J. Clin. Nutr.* 25:231–244 (1972).
14. See 9.
15. Plato, *Philebus.*

INTRODUCTION TO PART ONE

1. Nissinen, A., and K. Stanley. Unbalanced diets as a cause of chronic diseases. *Am. J. Clin. Nutr.* 49:993–998 (1989).
2. Working Group Report on Primary Prevention of Hypertension. National High Blood Pressure Education Program: National Heart, Lung, and Blood Institute. *Arch. Intern. Med.* 153:186–208 (1993).
3. The Joint National Committee of Detection, Evaluation, and Treatment of High Blood Pressure. The 1988 report of the Joint National Committee of Detection, Evaluation, and Treatment of High Blood Pressure. *Arch. Intern. Med.* 148:1023–38 (1988); see p. 1033.

4. Tyroler, H. A. Twenty-year mortality in black residents of Evans County, Georgia. *J. Clin. Hypertension.* 3(suppl):9–15 (1987).
5. Zusman, R. M. Editorial: Alternative antihypertensive therapy. *Hypertension* 8:837–842 (1986).
6. Kempner, W. Treatment of hypertensive vascular disease with rice diet. *Am. J. Med.* 4:545–577 (1948).
7. Cade, R., D. Mars, H. Wagemaker, C. Zauner, D. Packer, M. Privette, M. Cade, J. Peterson, and D. Hood-Lewis. Effect of aerobic exercise training on patients with systemic arterial hypertension. *Am. J. Med.* 77:785–90 (1984); and McCarron, D. A., L. E. Hare, and B. R. Walker. Therapeutic and economic controversies in antihypertensive therapy. *J. Cardiovasc. Pharmacol.* 6:S837–40 (1984). The estimate of the amount Americans spend on antihypertensive drugs is based on the average drug cost per year per patient being $500. This is a compromise between the average of $1350 spent by the patients in the Cade et al. study, most of whom were probably taking more than one drug, and the average cost for only one drug of $125 per year reported by McCarron et al. From reference 2 of Chapter 1, we know that 18 million Americans are taking antihypertensive drugs. This calculates out to an estimate of *$9 billion* spent each year by Americans for drugs to treat high blood pressure.
8. Page, L. B., A. Damon, and R. C. Moellering, Jr. Antecedents of cardiovascular disease in six Solomon Islands societies. *Circulation* 49:1132–46 (1974).
9. Multiple Risk Factor Intervention Trial Research Group. Multiple risk factor intervention trial. Risk factor changes and mortality results. *J. Am. Med. Assoc.* 248:1465–77 (1982).
10. Medical Research Council Working Party. MRC trial of treatment of mild hypertension: Principal results. *Br. Med. J.* 291:97–104 (1985); and see accompanying editorial by A. Breckenridge. Treating mild hypertension. *Br. Med. J.* 291:89–97 (1985).
11. See 2.
12. American Heart Association, Vermont Affiliate. Hypertension: One major risk factor for your heart. *Heartline* 5:2 (1985).
13. See 3, p. 1027
14. The Fifth Report of the Joint National Committee on Detection, Evaluation, and Treatment of High Blood Pressure. *Arch. Intern. Med.* 153:154–183 (1993).

CHAPTER 1

1. Working Group Report on Primary Prevention of Hypertension. National High Blood Pressure Education Program: National Heart, Lung, and Blood Institute. *Arch. Intern. Med.* 153:186–208 (1993).
2. The Third Report of the Joint National Committee of Detection, Evaluation, and Treatment on High Blood Pressure. *Arch. Intern. Med.* 144:1045–57 (1984); this definition is continued in the 1988 Report of the Joint National Committee. *Arch. Intern. Med.* 148:1023–38 (1988), and in the Fifth Report of the Joint National Committee. *Arch. Intern. Med.* 153:154–183 (1993).
3. Medical Research Council Working Party. MRC trial of treatment of mild hyperension: Principal results. *Br. Med. J.* 291:97–104 (1985); and Waaler, H. T., and J. Holmen. Systolic and diastolic blood-pressure values indicating equivalent risk. *N. Engl. J. Med.* 325:434–5 (1991).

4. Keli, S., B. Bloemberg, and D. Kromhout. Predictive value of repeated systolic blood pressure measurements for stroke risk: The Zutphen study. *Stroke* 23(3): 347–51 (1992).

5. Society of Actuaries & Association of Life Insurance Medical Directors of America. *Blood Pressure Study 1979.* Society of Actuaries & Association of Life Insurance Med. Directors of America (1980).

6. Ibid.

7. See 3, second reference.

8. MacMahon, S., R. Peto, J. Cutler, R. Collins, P. Sorlie, J. Neaton, R. Abbott, J. Godwin, A. Dyer, and J. Stamler. Blood pressure, stroke, and coronary heart disease. Part 1: Prolonged differences in blood pressure; prospective observational studies corrected for the regression dilution bias. *Lancet* 335:765–774 (1990).

9. The Fifth Report of the Joint National Committee on Detection, Evaluation, and Treatment of High Blood Pressure. *Arch. Intern. Med.* 153:154–183 (1993).

10. The Trials of Hypertension Prevention Collaborative Research Group. The effects of nonpharmacologic interventions on blood pressure of persons with high normal levels: Results of the Trials of Hypertension Prevention, Phase I. *J. Am. Med. Assoc.* 267(9):1213–1220 (1992)

CHAPTER 2

1. Hollenberg, N. K. Cardiovascular therapeutics in the 1980s: "An Ounce of Prevention." *Am. J. Med.* 82(Suppl 3A):1–3 (1987).

2. Kempner, W. Treatment of hypertensive vascular disease with rice diet. *Am. J. Med.* 4:545–77 (1948).

3. See Introduction, reference 7.

4. U.S. Public Health Service. *The 1980 report of the Joint National Committee on Detection, Evaluation, and Treatment of High Blood Pressure.* NIH Publication No. 81-1088 (1980).

5. Kaplan, N. M. Cardiovascular risk reduction: The role of antihypertensive treatment. *Am. J. Med.* 90(suppl 2A):19s–20s (1991).

6. Medical Research Council Working Party. MRC trial of treatment of mild hyperension: Principal results. *Br. Med. J.* 291:97–104 (1985); and see accompanying editorial by A. Breckenridge. Treating mild hypertension. *Br. Med. J.* 291:89–97 (1985)

7. The Joint National Committee of Detection, Evaluation, and Treatment of High Blood Pressure. The 1984 report of the Joint National Committee of Detection, Evaluation, and Treatment of High Blood Pressure. *Arch. Intern. Med.* 144:1045–57 (1984).

8. The Joint National Committee of Detection, Evaluation, and Treatment of High Blood Pressure. The 1988 report of the Joint National Committee of Detection, Evaluation, and Treatment of High Blood Pressure. *Arch. Intern. Med.* 148:1023–38 (1988).

9. The Fifth Report of the Joint National Committee on Detection, Evaluation, and Treatment of High Blood Pressure. *Arch. Int. Med.* 153:154–183 (1993).

10. Baker, C. E. Jr. *Physicians' Desk Reference* (PDR). 34th ed. Oradell, N.J.: Medical Economics Co. (1980).

11. See 3.

12. Zusman, R. M. Editorial: Alternatives to traditional antihypertensive therapy. *Hypertension* 8(10):837–842 (1986).

13. See 3.

14. Carb, J. D., N. O. Borhani, T. P. Blaszkowski, N. Zimbaldi, S. Fotin, W. Williams. Long-term surveillance for adverse effects of antihypertensive drugs. *J. Am. Med. Assoc.* 253:3263–68 (1985).

15. Weber, M. A. Antihypertensive treatment: Considerations beyond blood pressure control. *Circulation* (suppl IV) 80(6):IV-120–IV-127 (1989).

16. Hollenberg, N. K. Management of hypertension and cardiovascular risk. *Am. J. Med.* 90(suppl 2A):2S–6S (1991); and Dyckner, T., and P. O. Wester. Potassium/magnesium depletion in patients with cardiovascular disease. *Am. J. Med.* 82(suppl 3A):11–17 (1987).

17. Hollenberg, N. K. Management of hypertension and cardiovascular risk. *Am. J. Med.* 90(suppl 2A):2S–6S (1991).

18. Weinberger, M. H. Cardiovascular risk factors and antihypertensive therapy. *Am. J. Med.* 84(suppl 4A):24–29 (1988).

19. Bulpitt, C. J., M. J. Shipley, and A. Semmence. Blood pressure and plasma sodium and potassium. *Clin. Sci.* 61:85s–87s (1981); and Usehima, H., M. Tanigaki, M. Ida, T. Shimamoto, M. Konishi, and Y. Komachi. Hypertension, salt, and potassium. *Lancet* 1:504 (1981).

20. Tzagournis, M. Interaction of diabetes with hypertension and lipids—Patients at high risk: An overview. *Am. J. Med.* 86(suppl 1B):50–54 (1989), see p. 52; and Chait, A. Effects of antihypertensive agents on serum lipids and lipoproteins. *Am. J. Med.* 86(suppl 1B):5–7 (1989).

21. Veterans Administration Cooperative Study Group on Antihypertensive Agents. Comparison of propanalol and hydrochlorothiazide for the initial treatment of hypertension. II. Results of longterm therapy. *J. Am. Med. Assoc.* 248:2004–11 (1982); Flamenbaum, W. Metabolic consequences of antihypertensive therapy. *Ann. Intern. Med.* 98:875–80 (1983); and Leren, P., P. O. Foss, A. Helgeland, I. Hjermann, I. Holme, and P. G. Lund-Larsen. Effect of propranolol and prazosin on blood lipids. The Oslo study. *Lancet* 2:4–6 (1980).

22. See 3.

23. See 3.

24. Veterans Administration Cooperative Study Group on Antihypertensive Agents. Effects of treatment on morbidity in hypertension. I. Results in patients with diastolic blood pressures averaging 115 through 129 mm Hg. *J. Am. Med. Assoc.* 202:1028–34 (1967).

25. Veterans Administration Cooperative Study Group on Antihypertensive agents. Effects of treatment on morbidity in hypertension. II. Results in patients with diastolic blood pressures averaging 90 through 114 mm Hg. *J. Am. Med. Assoc.* 213:1143–52 (1970).

26. Smith, W. M. Treatment of mild hypertension. Results of a ten-year intervention trial. *Circ. Res.* 40(suppl 1):I-98–I-105 (1977); and Smith, W. M., S. C. Edlavitch, and W. M. Krushalt. United States Public Health Service hospitals intervention trial in mild hypertension. In *Hypertension—Determinants, Complications and Intervention,* ed. G. Onesti, and C. R. Klimt. New York: Grune and Stratton (1979).

27. Hypertension Detection and Follow-up Program Cooperative Group. Five-year findings of the hypertension detection and follow-up program. I. Reduction in mortality of persons with high blood pressure, including mild hypertension. II. Mortality by race/sex and age. *J. Am. Med. Assoc.* 242:2562–77 (1979); and Hypertension Detection and Follow-up Program Cooperative Group. The effect of treatment on mortality in "mild" hypertension. *N. Engl. J. Med.* 307(16):976–80 (1982).

28. Bonita, R., and R. Beaglehole. Increased treatment of hypertension does not explain the decline in stroke mortality in the United States, 1970–1980. *Hypertension* (suppl I) 13(5):I-69–I-73 (1989).

29. Management Committee: The Australian therapeutic trial in mild hypertension. *Lancet* 1:1261–67 (1980).

30. Helgeland, A. Treatment of mild hypertension: A five-year, controlled drug trial: The Oslo Study. *Am. J. Med.* 69:725–732 (1980); and Leren, P., and A. Helgeland. Coronary heart disease and treatment of hypertension: Some Oslo study data. *Am. J. Med.* 80(suppl 2A):3–6 (1986).

31. Oliver, M. P. Risks of correcting the risks of coronary disease and stroke with drugs. *N. Engl. J. Med.* 306(5):297–98 (1982).

32. Multiple Risk Factor Intervention Trial Research Group. Multiple risk factor intervention trial. Risk factor changes and mortality results. *J. Am. Med. Assoc.* 248:1465–77 (1982).

33. Multiple Risk Factor Intervention Trial Research Group. Mortality rates after 10.5 years for participants in the multiple risk factor intervention trial. *J. Am. Med. Assoc.* 263:1795–1801 (1990).

34. Morgan, T. O., W. R. Adam, M. Hodgson, and R. W. Gibberd. Failure of therapy to improve prognosis in elderly males with hypertension. *Med. J. Aust.* 2:27–31 (1980).

35. Lundberg, G. D. Editorial: MRFIT and the goals of the Journal. *J. Am. Med. Assoc.* 248:1501 (1982).

36. Medical Research Council Working Party. MRC trial of treatment of mild hypertension: Principal results. *Br. Med. J.* 291:97–104 (1985).

37. Breckenridge, A. Editorial accompanying British MRC report. Treating mild hypertension. *Br. Med. J.* 291:89–97 (1985).

38. See 36.

39. See 37.

40. European Working Party: Mortality and morbidity results from the European Working Party on High Blood Pressure in the Elderly trial. *Lancet* 1:1349–1354 (1985).

41. R. Collins, R. Peto, S. MacMahon, et al. Blood pressure, stroke, and coronary heart disease. Part 2. Short-term reductions in blood pressure: Overview of randomized drug trials in their epidemiological context. *Lancet* 335:827–838 (1990).

42. Cruickshank, J. M. Coronary flow reserve and the J curve relation between diastolic blood pressure and myocardial infarction. *Br. Med. J.* 297:1227–1230 (1988).

43. Alderman, M. H., W. L. Ooi, S. Madhavan, and H. Cohen. Treatment-induced blood pressure reduction and the risk of myocardial infarction. *J. Am. Med. Assoc.* 262:920–924 (1989).

44. Working Group Report on Primary Prevention of Hypertension. National High Blood Pressure Education Program: National Heart, Lung, and Blood Institute. *Arch. Intern. Med.* 153:186–208 (1993).

45. See 7.
46. Wilcox, R. B., J. R. A. Mitchell, and J. R. Hampton. Treatments of high blood pressure: Should clinical practice be based on results of clinical trials? *Br. Med. J.* 293:433–437 (1986).
47. See 12.
48. The Joint National Committee of Detection, Evaluation, and Treatment of High Blood Pressure. The 1988 report of the Joint National Committee of Detection, Evaluation, and Treatment of High Blood Pressure. *Arch. Intern. Med.* 148:1023–38 (1988).
49. See 9.
50. Schoenberger, J. A. New approaches to a first-line treatment of hypertension. *Am. J. Med.* 84(suppl 3B):26–31 (1988).
51. Bonita, R., and R. Beaglehole. Does treatment of hypertension explain the decline in mortality from stroke? *Br. Med. J.* 292:191–2 (1986).
52. Stason, W. B. Costs and quality trade-offs in the treatment of hypertension. *Hypertension* 13(suppl I):I-145–I-148 (1989).
53. Kase, C. S. Intracerebral hemorrhage: Common nonhypertensive causes. *Curr. Concepts Cerebrovasc. Dis.: Stroke* XX(4):19–24 (1985).
54. See 28.
55. Ibid.
56. Ibid.
57. See 51.
58. Eilhelmsen, L. Risks of untreated hypertension. *Hypertension* (suppl I) 13(5):I-33–I-34 (1989).

CHAPTER 3

1. Hollenberg, N. K. Management of Hypertension and cardiovascular risk. *Am. J. Med.* 90(suppl 2A):2S–6S (1991).
2. Pollare, T., H. Lithell, and C. Berne. Insulin resistance is a characteristic feature of primary hypertension independent of obesity. *Metabolism* 39:(2)167–74 (1990); Weber, M. A., D. H. G. Smith, J. M. Neutel, and W. F. Graettinger. Cardiovascular and metabolic characteristics of hypertension. *Am. J. Med.* 91(Suppl 1A): 4S–10S (1991); and Ferrannini, E., G. Buzzigoli, R. Bonadonna, M. A. Giorico, M. Oleggini, L. Graziadei, R. Pedrinelli, L. Brandi, and S. Bevilacqua. Insulin resistance in essential hypertension. *N. Engl. J. Med.* 317:(6)350–57 (1987).
3. Moore R. D. The case for intracellular pH in insulin action. In *Molecular Basis of Insulin Action,* ed. M. P. Czech, 145–170. New York: Plenum, 1985.
4. Moore, R. D., and G. D. Webb, *The K Factor: Reversing and Preventing High Blood Pressure Without Drugs.* New York: Macmillan (1986); New York: Pocket Books (1987).
5. Moore, R. D., M. L. Fidelman, and S. H. Seeholzer. Correlation between insulin action upon glycolysis and change in intracellular pH. *Biochem. Biophys. Res. Commun.* 91:905–10 (1979); and Fidelman, M. L., S. H. Seeholzer, K. B. Walsh, and R. D. Moore. Intracellular pH mediates action of insulin on glycolysis in frog skeletal muscle. *Am. J. Physiol.* 242:C87–C93 (1982).
6. Julius, S., K. Jamerson, A. Mejia, L. Krause, N. Schork, and K. Jones. The association of borderline with target organ changes and higher coronary risk: Tecumseh blood pressure study. *J. Am. Med. Assoc.* 264:354–58 (1990).

7. Modan, M., H. Halkin, S. Almog, M. Shefi, A. Eshkol, and A. Lusky. Insulin resistance—a condition linking hypertension glucose intolerance obesity and Na⁺ K⁺ imbalance. *Israel J. Med. Sci.* 20:292 (abstr.) (1984); and Modan, M., H. Halkin, S. Almog, A. Lusky, A. Eshkol, M. Shefi, A. Shitrit, and Z. Fuchs. Hyperinsulinemia. A link between hypertension obesity and glucose intolerance. *J. Clin. Invest.* 75:809–17 (1985).

8. Pell, S., and C. A. D'Alonzo. Some aspects of hypertension in diabetes mellitus. *J. Am. Med. Assoc.* 202:104–10 (1967).

9. See 3, first reference; and Bjorntorp, P., K. de Jounge, L. Sjostrom, and L. Sullivan. The effect of physical training on insulin production in obesity. *Metabolism* 19:631–38 (1970).

10. Welborn, T. A., A. Breckenridge, A. H. Rubinstein, C. T. Dollery, and T. Russell Frazer. Serum-insulin in essential hypertension and in peripheral vascular disease. *Lancet* 1:1336–37 (1966).

11. Olefsky, J. M., J. W. Farquhar, and G. M. Reaven. Reappraisal of the role of insulin in hypertriglyceridemia. *Am. J. Med.* 57:551–60 (1974).

12. Flack, J. M., and J. R. Sowers. Epidemiological and clinical aspects of insulin resistance and hyperinsulinemia. *Am. J. Med.* 91(suppl 1A):11S–21S (1991).

13. Ferrari, P., and P. Weidmann. Editorial review: Insulin, insulin sensitivity and hypertension. *J. Hypertension* 8:491–500 (1990).

14. Reaven, G. M. Insulin resistance, hyperinsulinemia, and hypertriglyceridemia in the etiology and clinical course of hypertension. *Am. J. Med.* 90(suppl 2A):7S–12S (1991).

15. Krauss, R. M. The tangled web of coronary risk factors. *Am. J. Med.* 90(suppl 2A):36S–41S (1991).

16. Denker, P. S., and V. E. Pollock. Fasting serum insulin levels in essential hypertension. *Arch. Intern. Med.* 152:1649–1651 (1992).

17. Welborn, T. A., A. Breckenridge, A. H. Rubinstein, C. T. Dollery, and T. Russell Frazer. Serum-insulin in essential hypertension and in peripheral vascular disease. *Lancet* 1:1336–37 (1966); and Singer, P., W. Godicke, S. Voigt, I. Hajadu, and M. Weiss. Postprandial hyperinsulinemia in patients with mild essential hypertension. *Hypertension* 7:182–86 (1985).

18. Pollare, T., H. Lithell, and C. Berne. Insulin resistance is a characteristic feature of primary hypertension independent of obesity. *Metabolism* 39:(2)167–74 (1990).

19. Ibid.

20. See 13.

21. Reaven, G. M. Banting Lecture 1988. Role of insulin resistance in human disease. *Diabetes* 37:1595–607 (1988).

22. Morgan, T. O., W. R. Adam, M. Hodgson, and R. W. Gibberd. Failure of therapy to improve prognosis in elderly males with hypertension. *Med. J. Aust.* 2:27–31 (1980).

23. Izzo, J. L., and A. L. M. Swislocki. Workshop III—Insulin resistance: Is it the link? *Am. J. Med.* 90(suppl 2A):26S–31S; see also 12.

24. Tzagournis, M. Interaction of diabetes with hypertension and lipids—patients at high risk: An overview. *Am. J. Med.* 86(suppl 1B):50–54 (1989), see p. 52; and Chait, A. Effects of antihypertensive agents on serum lipids and lipoproteins. *Am. J. Med.* 86(suppl 1B):5–7 (1989).

25. Ames, R. P. Negative effects of diuretic drugs on metabolic risk factors for coronary heart disease: Possible alternative drug therapies. *Am. J. Cardiol.* 51:632–38 (1983).

26. Julius, S., T. Gudbrandsson, K. Jamerson, S. T. Shahab, and O. Andersson. The hemodynamic link between insulin resistance and hypertension. *J. Hypertens.* 9:983–86 (1991).

27. Leren, P., P. O. Foss, A. Helgeland, J. Hjermann, I. Holme, and P. G. Lund-Larsen. Effect of propranolol and prazosin on blood lipids: The Oslo Study. *Lancet* 2(8184):4–6 (1980).

28. Velasco, M., E. Hurt, H. Silva, A. Urbina-Quintana, O. Hernandez-Pieretti, E. Feldstein, and G. Camejo. Effects of prazosin and propranolol on blood lipids and lipoproteins in hypertensive patients. *Am. J. Med.* 80(suppl 2A):109–13 (1986).

29. Neusy, A. J., and J. Lowenstein. Effect of prazosin, atenolol, and thiazide diuretic on plasma lipids in patients with essential hypertension. *Am. J. Med.* 80(suppl 2A):94–9 (1986); and Itskovitz, H. D., K. Krug, S. Khoury, and J. L. Mollura. The long-term antihypertensive effects of prazosin and atenolol. *Am. J. Med.* 86(suppl 1B): 82–84 (1989).

30. Leren, P., and A. Helgeland. Coronary heart disease and treatment of hypertension. *Am. J. Med.* 80(suppl 2A):3–6 (1986).

31. The Joint National Committee of Detection, Evaluation, and Treatment of High Blood Pressure. The 1988 report of the Joint National Committee of Detection, Evaluation, and Treatment of High Blood Pressure. *Arch. Intern. Med.* 148:1023–38 (1988).

32. Chiati, A. Effects of antihypertensive agents on serum lipids and lipoproteins. *Am. J. Med.* 86(suppl 1B):5–7 (1989).

33. Lardinois, C. K., and S. L. Neuman. The effects of antihypertensive agents on serum lipids and kipoproteins. *Arch. Intern. Med.* 148:1280–88 (1988).

34. See 26 and 12.

35. See 26.

36. See 12.

37. Man In't Veld, A. J. Calcium antagonists in hypertension. *Am. J. Med.* 86(suppl 4A):6–14 (1989).

38. Weinberger, M. H.. Cardiovascular risk factors and antihypertensive therapy. *Am. J. Med.* 84(suppl 4A):24–9 (1988).

39. See 27.

40. Swislocki, A. L. M., B. B. Hoffman, W. H.-H. Sheu, Y.-D. I. Chen, and G. M. Reaven. Effect of prazosin treatment on carbohydrate and lipoprotein metabolism in patients with hypertension. *Am. J. Med.* 86(suppl 1B):14–8 (1989).

41. Lardinois, C. K., and S. L. Neuman. The effects of antihypertensive agents on serum lipids and lipoproteins. *Arch. Intern. Med.* 148:1280–88 (1988).

CHAPTER 4

1. Smith, T. J., and I. S. Edelman. The role of sodium transport in thyroid thermogenesis. *Fed. Proc.* 38:2150–53 (1979).

2. Moore, R. D. Effect of insulin upon sodium pump in frog skeletal muscle. *J. Physiol.* 232:23–45 (1973); and Gavryck, W. A., R. D. Moore, and R. C. Thompson. Effect of insulin upon membrane-bound $(Na^+ + K^+)$-ATPase extracted from frog skeletal muscle. *J. Physiol.* 252:43–58 (1975).

3. Moore, R. D., J. W. Munford, and T. J. Pillsworth, Jr. Effects of streptozotocin diabetes and fasting on intracellular sodium and adenosine triphosphate in rat soleus muscle. *J. Physiol.* 338:227–94 (1983).

4. Ibid.

5. Blaustein, M. P., and J. M. Hamlyn. Pathogenesis of essential hypertension: A link between dietary salt and high blood pressure. *Hypertension* 18(suppl III)(5):III-184–III-195 (1991).

6. Daniel, E. E., A. K. Grover, and C. Y. Kwan. Isolation and properties of plasma membrane from smooth muscle. *Fed. Proc.* 41:2898–904 (1982).

7. Moore, R. D., M. L. Fidelman, J. C. Hansen, and J. N. Otis. The role of intracellular pH in insulin action. In *Intracellular pH: Its Measurement, Regulation and Utilization in Cellular Functions,* ed. R. Nuccitelli and D. W. Deamer, 385–416. New York: Alan R. Liss (1985); Moore, R. D. The case for intracellular pH in insulin action. In *The Molecular Basis of Insulin Action,* ed. Czech, 145–170. New York: Plenum (1985); and Moore, R. D. The role of intracellular pH in insulin action and diabetes mellitus. In *Current Topics in Membranes and Transport,* Vol. 26: Na^+–H^+ *Exchange, Intracellular pH and Cell Function,* ed. P. Aronson and W. Boron, 263–290. Orlando, Fla.: Academic Press (1986).

8. Madshus, I. H. Regulation of intracellular pH in eukaryotic cells. *Biochem. J.* 250:1–8 (1988).

9. See 5.

10. See 5.

11. Winkler, M. M. Regulation of protein synthesis in sea urchin eggs by intracellular pH. In *Intracellular pH: Its Measurement, Regulation, and Utilization in Cellular functions,* ed. R. Nuccitelli and D. W. Deamer, 325–40. New York: Alan R. Liss (1982).

12. Resnick, L. M. Hypertension and abnormal glucose homeostasis. *Am. J. Med.* 87(suppl 6A):17S–22S (1989); and Levy, J., M. B. Zemel, and J. R. Sowers. Role of cellular calcium metabolism in abnormal glucose metabolism and diabetic hypertension. *Am. J. Med.* 87(suppl 6A):7S–16S (1989).

13. Resnick, L. M., R. K. Gupta, H. Gruenspan, M. H. Alderman, and J. H. Laragh. Hypertension and peripheral insulin resistance: Possible mediating role of intracellular free magnesium. *Am. J. Hypertension* 3:373–79 (1990).

14. One way to test this idea is to add potassium to arteries and see what happens—especially if we block the sodium-potassium pump. If the idea is correct, this should relax the small arteries, but not if the sodium-potassium pump is blocked. When this experiment is done, increasing the level of potassium from 3.6 to 6.0 mEq/L causes the small arteries to relax so they let blood flow through more easily. (See Chen, W. T., R. A. Brace, J. B. Scott, D. K. Anderson, and F. J. Haddy. The mechanism of the vasodilator action of potassium. *Proc. Soc. Exper. Biol. Med.* 140:820–24 [1972]). Not only that, but when the heart drug digitalis, which specifically inhibits the sodium-potassium pump, is added to the small arteries first, potassium no longer makes them dilate! So the evidence seems pretty good that part of the elevation of blood pressure is due to insufficient potassium to directly stimulate the sodium-potassium pump so the sodium battery can remain charged and the muscle cells in the small arteries can stay relaxed.

15. Goggins, G. D., and G. D. Webb. Increased electrogenic pumping and elevated sodium activity in skeletal muscle cells from hypertensive stroke prone rats. *Physiologist* 29:129 (1986); and Goggins, G. D. Intracellular sodium activity and membrane potential in skeletal muscle cells of spontaneously hypertensive stroke-prone rats. M.A. Thesis, University of Vermont (1987).

16. See 5.

17. Blaustein, M. P. Sodium ions, calcium ions, blood pressure regulation, and hypertension: A reassessment and a hypothesis. *Am. J. Physiol.* 232:C165–73 (1977).

18. Jelicks, L. A., and Gupta, R. K. NMR measurement of cytosolic free calcium, free magnesium, and intracellular sodium in the aorta of the normal and spontaneously hypertensive rat. *J. Biol. Chem.* 265(3):1394–1400 (1990).

19. Dowd, T. L., and R. K. Gupta. Multinuclear NMR studies of intracellular cations in perfused hypertensive rat kidney. *J. Biol. Chem.* 267:3637–3643 (1992).

20. Zierler, K. L., and D. Rabinowitz. Effect of small concentrations of insulin on forearm metabolism: Persistance of its action on potassium and free fatty acids without its effect on glucose. *J. Clin. Invest.* 43:950–62 (1964).

21. Ferrannini, E., G. Buzzigoli, R. Bonadonna, M. A. Giorico, M. Oleggini, L. Graziadei, R. Pedrinelli, L. Brandi, and S. Bevilacqua. Insulin resistance in essential hypertension. *N. Eng. J. Med.* 317(6):350–357 (1987).

22. Natali, A., D. Santoro, C. Palombo, M. Cerri, S. Ghione, and E. Ferrannini. Impaired insulin action on skeletal muscle metabolism in essential hypertension. *Hypertension* 17(2):170–178 (1991).

23. Rocchini A., D. Kvesalis, and C. Moorehead. Insulin and renal sodium handling in obese adolescents: A cause of hypertension (abstr.) *Hypertension* 10:358 (1987).

24. Gupta, A. K., R. V. Clark, and K. A. Kirchner. Effects of insulin on renal sodium excretion. *Hypertension* 19(suppl I):I-78–I-82 (1992).

25. Reaven, G. M. Insulin resistance, hyperinsulinemia, and hypertriglyceridemia in the etiology and clinical course of hypertension. *Am. J. Med.* 90(suppl 2A):7S–12S (1991).

26. Livine, A., J. W. Balfe, R. Veitch, A. Marquez-Julio, S. Grinstein, and A. Rothstein. Increased platelet Na^+/H^+ exchange rates in essential hypertension: application of a novel test. *Lancet* 1(8532):533–536 (1987); Schmouder, R. L., and A. B. Weder. Platelet sodium-proton exchange is increased in essential hypertension. *J. Hypertension* 7:325–30 (1989); and Levine, A. A., O. Aharonovitz, and E. Paran. Higher Na^+–H^+ exchange rate and more alkaline intracellular pH set point in essential hypertension: Effects of protein kinase modulation in platelets. *J. Hypertension* 9:1013–19 (1991).

27. Ng, L. L., C. Dudley, J. Bomford, and D. Hawley. Leucocyte intracellular pH and Na^+/H^+ antiport activity in human hypertension. *J. Hypertension* 7:471–75 (1989); and Ng, L. L., D. A. Fennell, and C. Dudley. Kinetics of the human leucocyte Na^+/H^+ antiport in essential hypertension. *J. Hypertension* 8:533–37 (1990).

28. Feig, P. U., M. A. D'Occhio, and J. W. Boylan. Lymphocyte membrane sodium-proton exchange in spontaneously hypertensive rats. *Hypertension* 9:282–88 (1987).

29. Morduchowicz, G. A., D. Sheikh-Hamad, O. D. Jo, E. P. Nord, D. B. N. Lee, and N. Yanagawa. Increased Na^+/H^+ antiport activity in the renal brush border membrane of SHR. *Kidney Int.* 36:576–81 (1989).

30. Izzard, A. S., and A. M. Heagerty. The measurement of internal pH in resistance arterioles: Evidence that intracellular pH is more alkaline in SHR than WKY animals. *J. Hypertension* 7:173–80 (1989).

31. Syme, P. D., L. Arnolda, Y. Green, J. K. Aronson, D. G. Grahame-Smith, and G. K. Radda. Evidence for increased in vivo Na^+–H^+ antiporter activity and an altered skeletal muscle contractile response in the spontaneously hypertensive rat. *J. Hypertension* 8:1027–36 (1990).

32. See 30.

33. See 30.

34. Levine, A. A., O. Aharonovitz, and E. Paran. Higher Na^+–H^+ exchange rate and more alkaline intracellular pH set point in essential hypertension: Effects of protein kinase modulation in platelets. *J. Hypertension* 9:1013–19 (1991).

35. Schmouder, R. L., and A. B. Weder. Platelet sodium-proton exchange is increased in essential hypertension. *J. Hypertension* 7:325–30 (1989).

36. See 30.

37. Red blood cells appear to be the exception.

38. Steinhardt, R. A., and M. M. Winkler. The activation of protein synthesis by intracellular pH. In *Circulation, Respiration, and Metabolism: Current Comparative Approaches*, ed. R. Gilles, 474–82. New York: Springer-Verlag (1985).

39. Madshus, I. H. Regulation of intracellular pH in eukaryotic cells. *Biochem. J.* 250:1–8 (1988).

40. Bobik, A., A. Grooms, S. Grinpakel, and P. Little. The effects of alterations in membrane sodium transport on rat aortic smooth muscle proliferation. *J. Hypertension* 6(suppl 4):S219–S221 (1988).

41. Winkler, M. M. Regulation of protein synthesis in sea urchin eggs by intracellular pH. In *Intracellular pH: Its Measurement, Regulation, and Utilization in Cellular Functions*, ed. R. Nuccitelli and D. W. Deamer, 325–40. New York: Alan R. Liss (1982).

42. Moore, R. D., and G. D. Webb. *The K Factor: Reversing and Preventing High Blood Pressure Without Drugs*. New York: Macmillan (1986).

43. Moore, R. D. Elevation of intracellular pH by insulin in frog skeletal muscle. *Biochem. Biophys. Res. Commun.* 91:900–04 (1979); Moore, R. D., and R. K. Gupta. Effect of insulin on intracellular pH as observed by 31P NMR spectroscopy. *Int. J. Quantum Chem. Quantum Biol. Symp.* 7:83–92 (1980); Moore, R. D. Stimulation of Na^+/H^+ exchange by insulin. *Biophys. J.* 33:203–10 (1981); and see 7, first reference.

44. Grinstein, S., and A. Rothstein. Topical review: Mechanisms of regulation of the Na^+/H^+ exchanger. *J. Membrane Biol.* 90:1–12 (1986).

45. Rosic, N. K., M. L. Standaert, and R. J. Pollet. The mechanism of insulin stimulation of (Na^+,K^+)-ATPase transport activity in muscle. *J. Biol. Chem.* 260(10):6206–12 (1985).

46. Although the sodium battery is partly run down in people with hypertension, insulin should still increase activity of the Na^+/H^+ exchange pump. This is because in most body cells, the sodium battery normally is charged much more than is necessary in order to run this pump. Moreover, insulin apparently stimulates the Na^+/H^+ exchange pump by increasing the ability of the pump to bind, or "pick up," acid inside the cell. This increases the "set point" of this pump to a higher pH inside the cell. See reference 44.

47. See 34.
48. For discussion, see Moller, D. E., and J. S. Flier. Insulin resistance—mechanisms, syndromes, and implications. *N. Engl. J. Med.* 325(13):938–48 (1991); and Lever, A. F. Editorial review: Slow pressor mechanisms in hypertension: A role for hypertrophy of resistance vessels? *J. Hypertension* 4:515–24 (1986).
49. Cruz, A. B., D. S. Amatuzio, F. Grande, and L. J. Hay. Effect of intraarterial insulin on tissue cholesterol and fatty acids in alloxan-diabetic dogs. *Circ. Res.* 9:39–43 (1961).
50. See 48, second reference.
51. Berk, B. C., M. S. Aronow, T. A. Brock, E. Cragoe, M. A. Gimbrone, and R. W. Alexander. Angiotensin II-stimulated Na^+/H^+ exchange in cultured vascular smooth muscle cells. *J. Biol. Chem.* 262:5057–64 (1987); Hatori, N., B. P. Fine, A. Nakamura, E. Cragoe, and A. Aviv. Angiotensin II effect on cytolic pH in cultured rat vascular smooth muscle cells. *J. Biol. Chem.* 262:5073–78 (1987), Brock, T. A., L. J. Lewis, and J. Bingham Smith. Angiotensin increases Na^+ entry and Na^+/H^+ pump activity in cultures of smooth muscle from rat aorta. *Proc. Natl. Acad. Sci. USA* 79:1438–42 (1982).
52. See 51, second reference.
53. For discussion, see 48, second reference.
54. Izzo, J. L., and A. L. M. Swislocki. Workshop III—insulin resistance: Is it the link? *Am. J. Med.* 90(suppl 2A):26S–31S (1991).
55. Resnick, L. M. Hypertension and abnormal glucose homeostasis. *Am. J. Med.* 87(suppl 6A):17S–22S 1989).
56. Ibid.
57. Reaven, G. M. Role of insulin resistance in human disease. *Diabetes* 37:1595–1607 (1988).
58. Nizet, A., P. Lefebvre, and J. Crabbe. Control by insulin of sodium potassium and water excretion by isolated dog kidneys. *Pflug. Arch.* 323:11–20 (1971); Defronzo, R. A., R. Sherwin, M. Dillingham, R. Hendeler, W. Tamborlane, and P. Felig. Influence of basil insulin and glucagon secretion on potassium and on sodium metabolism—studies with somatostatin in normal dogs and in normal and diabetic human beings. *J. Clin. Invest.* 61:472–79 (1978); Gupta, A. K., R. V. Clark, and K. A. Kirchner. Effects of insulin on renal sodium excretion. *Hypertension* 19(suppl I):I-78–I-82 (1992).
59. Rowe, J. W., J. B. Young, K. L. Minaker, A. L. Stevens, J. Pallotta, and L. Landsberg. Effect of insulin and glucose infusions on sympathetic nervous system activity in normal man. *Diabetes* 30: 219–25 (1981).
60. See 57.
61. Stout, R. W. Insulin as a mitogenic factor: Role in the pathogenesis of cardiovascular disease. *Am. J. Med.* 90(suppl 2A):62S (1991).
62. See 3, first reference; and Bjorntorp, P., K. de Jounge, L. Sjostrom, and L. Sullivan. The effect of physical training on insulin production in obesity. *Metabolism* 19:631–38 (1970).
63. Welborn, T. A., A. Breckenridge, A. H. Rubinstein, C. T. Dollery, and T. Russell Frazer. Serum-insulin in essential hypertension and in peripheral vascular disease. *Lancet* 1:1336–37 (1966); and see 57.
64. Modan, M., H. Halkin, S. Almog, M. Shefi, A. Eshkol, and A. Lusky. Insulin resistance—a condition linking hypertension glucose intolerance obesity and Na^+ K^+ imbalance. *Israel J. Med. Sci.* 20:292 (abstr.) (1984); and Modan, M., H. Halkin, S.

Almog, A. Lusky, A. Eshkol, M. Shefi, A. Shitrit, and Z. Fuchs. Hyperinsulinemia. A link between hypertension obesity and glucose intolerance. *J. Clin. Invest.* 75:809–17 (1985).
65. See 21.
66. See 57.
67. See 13.
68. Ambrosioni, E., F. V. Costa, C. Borghi, S. Boschi, and A. Mussi. Cellular and humoral factors in borderline hypertension. *J. Cardiovasc. Pharmacol.* 8(suppl. 5):S15–S22 (1986).
69. Helderman, J. H., D. Elahi, D. K. Andersen, et al. Prevention of the glucose intolerance of thiazide diuretics by maintenance of body potassium. *Diabetes* 32:106–11 (1983).
70. Gordon, P. Glucose intolerance with hypokalemia. *Diabetes* 22:544 (1972).
71. Glynn, I. M. Sodium and potassium movements in human red cells. *J. Physiol.* (Lond.) 124:278–310 (1956); and Sjodin, R. A. The kinetics of sodium extrusion in striated muscle as functions of the external sodium and potassium ion concentrations. *J. Gen. Physiol.* 57:164–87 (1971).
72. Zivin, J. A., and D. W. Choi. Stroke Therapy. *Scientific American* 56–63 (July, 1991). Choi, D. W. Bench to Bedside: The Glutamate Connection. *Science* 258:241–243 (1992). McCulloch, J. Excitatory Amino Acid Antagonists and Their Potential for Treatment of Ischemic Brain Damage in Man. *Br. J. Clin. Pharm.* 34:106–144 (1992).
73. Dyckner, T., and P. O. Wester. Potassium/magnesium depletion in patients with cardiovascular disease. *Am. J. Med.* 82(suppl 3A):11—17 (1987).
74. Avolio, A. P., K. M. Clyde, T. C. Beard, H. M. Cooke, and M. O'Rourke. Low salt diet and improvement of arterial distensibility in normotensive subjects. *Circulation* 72(suppl III): III–39 (abstr.) (1985).
75. Ericsson, F. Intracellular potassium in man. *Scand. J. Clin. Lab. Invest.* 42(suppl 163):1–58 (1982).
76. Veniero, J. C., and R. K. Gupta. NMR measurement of intracellular free potassium in the perfused normotensive and spontaneously hypertensive rat aorta by a multinuclear subtraction procedure. *Am. J. Hypertension* 5:360 (1992).
77. Parker, J. C., and L. R. Berkowitz. Physiologically instructive genetic variants involving the human red cell membrane. *Physio. Rev.* 63:261–313 (1983).
78. See 5.
79. See 5.
80. Christlieb, A. R. Diabetes and hypertensive vascular disease. Mechanisms and treatment. *Am. J. Cardiol.* 32:592–606 (1973).
81. See 30.
82. See 30.
83. See 34.

CHAPTER 5

1. Working Group Report on Primary Prevention of Hypertension National High Blood Pressure Education Program. National Heart, Lung, and Blood Institute. *Arch. Intern. Med.* 153:186–208 (1993).

2. Trowell, H., and D. P. Burkitt. *Western Diseases: Their Emergence and Prevention.* London: Edward Arnold, 1981.
3. Acsadi, G., and J. Nemeskeri. *History of Human Lifespan and Mortality.* Budapest: Akademai Kiado (1970).
4. See 2; and Truswell, A. S., and J. D. L. Hansen. Medical research among the !Kung. In *Kalahari Hunter-Gatherers,* ed. R. B. Lee and I. DeVore. Cambridge, Mass.: Harvard University Press (1976).
5. Page, L. B., A. Damon, and R. C. Moellering, Jr. Antecedents of cardiovascular disease in six Solomon Islands societies. *Circulation* 49:1132–46 (1974).
6. Hicks, C. S., and R. F. Matters. The standard metabolism of the Australian aborigines. *Aust. J. Exp. Biol. Med. Sci.* 11:177–83 (1933); and Nye, L. J., and L. J. Jarvis. Blood pressure in Australian aboriginal, with consideration of possible aetiological factors in hyperplasia and its relation to civilization. *Med. J. Aust.* 2:1000–1001 (1937).
7. Truswell, A. S., B. M. Kennelly, J. D. Hansen, and R. B. Lee. Blood pressures of !Kung bushmen in northern Botswana. *Am. Heart J.* 84:5–12 (1972); and see 3.
8. Lowenstein, F. W. Blood pressure in relation to age and sex in the tropics and subtropics. *Lancet* 1:389–92 (1961).
9. Kean, B. H. The blood pressure of the Cuna Indians. *Am. J. Tropical Med.* 24:341–43 (1944).
10. Thomas, W. A. Health of a carnivorous race. A study of the Eskimo. *J. Am. Med. Assoc.* 88:1559–60 (1927).
11. Donnison, C. P. Blood pressure in the African native. *Lancet* 1:6–7 (1929).
12. Murphy, W. Some observations on blood pressures in humid tropics. *N. Z. Med. J.* 54:64–73 (1955).
13. Whyte, H. M. Body fat and blood pressure of natives in New Guinea: Reflections on essential hypertension. *Aust. Ann. Med.* 7:36–46 (1958).
14. Kaminer, B., and W. P. W. Lutz. Blood pressure in bushmen of the Kalahari desert. *Circulation* 22:289–95 (1960).
15. Connor, W. E., M. T. Cerqueira, R. W. Connor, R. B. Wallace, M. R. Malinow, and H. R. Casdorph. The plasma lipids, lipoproteins, and the diet of the Tarahumara Indians of Mexico. *Am. J. Clin. Nutr.* 31:1131–42 (1978); and Cerqueira, M. T., M. McMurry Fry, and W. E. Connor. The food and nutrient intakes of the Tarahumara Indians of Mexico. *Am. J. Clin. Nutr.* 32:905–15 (1979).
16. Williams, A. W. Blood pressure of Africans. *East Africa Med. J.* 18:109–17 (1941).
17. Morse, W. R., and Y. T. Beh. Blood pressure amongst aboriginal ethnic groups of Szechwan province, west China. *Lancet* 1:966–7 (1937).
18. Oliver, W. J., E. L. Cohen, and J. V. Neel. Blood pressure, sodium intake, and sodium related hormones in the Yanomamo Indians, a "no-salt" culture. *Circulation* 52:146–51 (1975).
19. See 15.
20. See 15, second reference.
21. See 2; and Tobian, L. Salt and hypertension. *J. Med. Assoc. Georgia.* 69:827–34 (1980).
22. See 2.
23. Dr. Mark Cohen, Professor of Anthropology, SUNY, Plattsburg, New York, personal communication.

24. Beaglehole, R., E. Eyles, and I. Prior. Blood pressure and migration in children. *Int. J. Epidemiol.* 8:5–10 (1979); and Cassel, J. Studies of hypertension in migrants. In *Epidemiology and Control of Hypertension.* ed. O. Paul, 41–58. Miami: Symposium Specialists, 1975.

25. Tobian, L. Perspectives on treating hypertension *Am. J. Med.* 81(suppl 4C):2–7 (1986).

26. See 23.

27. See 9.

28. Page, L. B., D. Vandevert, K. Nader, N. Lubin, and J. R. Page. Blood pressure, diet, and body form in traditional nomads of the Qash'qai tribe, southern Iran. *Acta Cardiol.* 33:102–3 (1978).

29. Dr. Mark Cohen, Professor of Anthropology, SUNY, Plattsburg, New York, personal communication; and Denton, D. The most-craved crystal: Why humans consume salt in such excess. *The Sciences* (Nov./Dec.): 29–34 (1986).

30. See 18; and Chagnon, N. A. *Yanomamo, the Fierce People.* New York: Holt Rinehart and Winston, 1968.

31. Sacks, F. M., B. Rosner, and E. H. Kass. Blood pressure in vegetarians. *Am. J. Epidemiol.* 100 (5):390–8 (19).

32. Groen, J. J., K. B. Tijong, M. Koster, A. F. Willebrands, G. Verdonck, and M. Pierloot. The influence of nutrition and ways of life on blood cholesterol and the prevalence of hypertension and coronary heart disease among Trappist and Benedictine monks. *Am. J. Clin. Nutr.* 10:456–70 (1962).

33. Webster, I. W., G. K. Rawson. Health status of Seventh-day Adventists. *Med. J. Aust.* 1:417–20 (1979); and Simons, L., J. Gibson, A. Jones, D. Bain. Health status of Seventh-day Adventists. *Med. J. Aust.* 2:148 (1979); Armstrong, B., A. J. Van Merwyk, and H. Coates. Blood pressure in Seventh-day Adventists vegetarians. *Am J. Epidemiol.* 105:444–9 (1977); Rouse, I. L., B. K. Armstrong, L. J. Beilin. The relationship of blood pressure to diet and lifestyle in two religious populations. *J. Hypertension.* 1:65–71 (1983).

34. Ophir, O., G. Peer (Peresecenschi), J. Gilad, M. Blum, and A. Aviram. Low blood pressure in vegetarians: The possible role of potassium. *Am. J. Clin. Nutr.* 37:755–62 (1983).

35. See 31.

36. Armstrong, B., A. J. Van Merwyk, and H. Coates. Blood pressure in Seventh-day Adventists vegetarians. *Am J. Epidemiol.* 105:444–9 (1977): and Beilin, L. J., I. L. Rouse, B. K. Armstrong, B. M. Margetts, and R. Vandongen. Vegetarian diet and blood pressure levels: Incidental or causal association. *Am. J. Clin. Nutr.* 48:806–810 (1988).

37. See 2 and 21.

38. See 33, first reference.

39. See 32.

40. Sacks, F. M., P. G. Woods, and E. H. Kass. Stability of blood pressure in vegetarians receiving dietary protein supplements. *Hypertension* 6(2):199–201 (1984).

41. Sacks, F. M., and E. H. Kass. Low blood pressure in vegetarians: Effects of specific foods and nutrients. *Am. J. Clin. Nutr.* 48:795–800 (1988).

42. Margetts, B. M, L. J. Beilin, B. K. Armstrong, and R. Vandongen. Vegetarian diet in mild hypertension: Effects of fat and fiber. *Am. J. Clin. Nutr.* 48:801–805. (1988).

43. See 34.
44. Eaton, S. B., and M. Konner. Paleolithic nutrition. *N. Engl. J. Med.* 312:283–9 (1985).
45. See 18.
46. See 7.
47. See 34.
48. Ibid.
49. Grim, C. E., F. C. Luft, J. Z. Miller, G. R. Meneely, H. D. Battarbee, C. G. Hames, and L. K. Dahl. Racial differences in blood pressure in Evans County, Georgia: Relationship to sodium and potassium intake and plasma renin activity. *J. Chron. Dis.* 33:87–94 (1980).
50. Ueshima, H., M. Tanigaki, M. Iida, T. Shimamoto, M. Konishi, and Y. Komachi. Hypertension, salt, and potassium. *Lancet* 1:504 (1981).
51. Leary, W. E. Black hypertension may reflect other ills. *New York Times,* Tuesday, Oct. 22, C3 (1991).
52. The Joint National Committee of Detection, Evaluation, and Treatment of High Blood Pressure. The 1988 report of the Joint National Committee of Detection, Evaluation, and Treatment of High Blood Pressure. *Arch. Intern. Med.* 148:1023–38 (1988), see p. 1033.
53. See 49.
54. Zinner, S. H., H. S. Margolius, B. Rosner, H. R. Keiser, and E. H. Kass. Familial aggregation of urinary kallikrein concentration in childhood: Relation to blood pressure, race and urinary electrolytes. *Am. J. Epidemiol.* 104:124–32 (1976); Luft, F. C., C. E. Grim, N. Fineberg, and M. C. Weinberger. Effects of volume expansion and contraction in normotensive whites, blacks, and subjects of different ages. *Circulation* 59:643–50 (1979); and Watson, R. L., H. G. Langford, J. Abernethy, T. Y. Barnes, M. J. Watson. Urinary electrolytes, body weight, and blood pressure. Pooled cross-sectional results among four groups of adolescent females. *Hypertension* 2(suppl I):I93–8 (1980).
55. Tobian, L., D. MacNeill, M. A. Johnson, M. C. Ganguli, and J. Iwai. Potassium protection against lesions of the renal tubules, arteries, and glomeruli and nephron loss in salt-loaded hypertensive Dahl S rats. *Hypertension* 6(suppl I):I-170–I-176 (1984).
56. Tobian, L. High potassium diets reduce stroke mortality and arterial and renal tubular lesions and sometimes even the blood pressure in hypertension. In *The Regulation of Potassium Balance,* ed. D. W. Seldin and G. Giebisch. New York: Raven Press (1989), see p. 347–368.
57. Tobian, L., J. Lange, K. Ulm, L. Wold, and J. Iwai. Potassium reduces cerebral hemorrhage and death rate in hypertensive rats, even when blood pressure is not lowered. *Hypertension* 7(suppl I):I-110–I-114 (1985).
58. See 56.
59. Kesteloot, H., D. X. Huang, Y. Li, J. Geboers, and V. Joossens.The relationship between cations and blood pressure in the People's Republic of China. *Hypertension* 9 (6):654–9 (1987).
60. See 32; 36, first reference; and Rouse, I. L., L. J. Beilin, B. K. Armstrong, and R. Vandongen. Blood-pressure-lowering effect of a vegetarian diet: Controlled trial in normotensive subjects. *Lancet* 1:5–9 (1983).
61. See 34.

62. Sasaki, N., T. Mitsuhashi, and S. Fukushi. Effects of the ingestion of large amounts of apples on blood pressure in farmers in Akita prefecture. *Igaku Seibutsugaku* 51:103–5 (1959); and Sasaki, N. High blood pressure and the salt intake of the Japanese. *Jap. Heart J.* 3:313–24 (1962).

63. Reed, D., D. McGee, K. Yano, and J. Hankin. Diet, blood pressure, and multicollinearity. *Hypertension* 7:405–10 (1985).

64. Altman, P. L., and D. S. Dittmer, eds. *Biological Handbooks. Blood and Other Body Fluids,* 455–8. Washington, D.C.: FASEB (1961).

CHAPTER 6

1. Kaplan, N., and C. V. Ram. Editorial: Potassium supplements for hypertension. *N. Engl. J. Med.* (March 1): 624 (1990).

2. Khaw, K. T., and E. Barrett-Connor. Dietary potassium and stroke-associated mortality: A 12-year prospective population study. *N. Engl. J. Med.* 316(5):235–40 (1987).

3. Tobian, L. The protective effects of dietary K against the lesions of NaCl-induced hypertension. *Abstracts of Papers of the 149th National Meeting of the American Association for the Advancement of Science* 64 (1983).

4. Tanaka, H., Y. Tanaka, M. Hayashi, Y. Ueda, C. Date, T. Baba, H. Shoji, T. Horimoto, and K. Owada. Secular trends in mortality for cerebrovascular diseases in Japan, 1960 to 1979. *Stroke* 13(5): 574–81 (1982).

5. Tobian, L., J. Lange, K. Ulm, L. Wold, and J. Iwai. Potassium reduces cerebral hemorrhage and death rate in hypertensive rats, even when blood pressure is not lowered. *Hypertension* 7 [suppl I]:I-110–I-114 (1985).

6. Khaw, K. T., and E. Barrett-Connor, 1987. Dietary potassium and stroke-associated mortality: A 12-year prospective population study. *N. Engl. J. Med.* 316:(5)235–40 (1987).

7. Smeda, J. Hemorrhagic stroke development in spontaneously hypertensive rats fed a North American, Japanese-style diet. *Stroke* 20:1212–18 (1989).

8. Patki, P. S., J. Singh, S. V. Gokhale, P. M. Bulakh, D. S. Shrotri, B. Patwardhan. Efficacy of potassium and magnesium in essential hypertension: A double blind, placebo controlled, crossover study. *Br. Med. J.* 301:521–3 (1990).

9. Tobian, L., T. M. Jahner, and M. A. Johnson. High K diets markedly reduce athero-sclerotic cholesterol ester deposition in aortas of rats with hypercholesterolemia and hypertension. *Am. J. Hypertension* 3:133–5 (1990).

10. Tobian, L. Potassium protection against lesions of the renal tubules, arteries, and glomeruli and nephron loss in salt-loaded hypertensive Dahl S rats. *Hypertension* 6(suppl I):I-170–I-176 (1984).

11. Messerli, F. H., U. R. Kaesser, and C. J. Losem. Effects of antihypertensive therapy on hypertensive heart disease. *Circulation* (suppl IV) 80(6): IV-145–IV-150 (1989).

12. Tobian, L. High potassium diets reduce stroke mortality and arterial and renal tubular lesions and sometimes even the blood pressure in hypertension. In *The Regulation of Potassium Balance,* ed. D. W. Seldin and G. Giebisch. New York: Raven Press (1989).

13. Priddle, W. W. Hypertension—sodium and potassium studies. *J. Assoc. Med. Can.* 86:1–9 (1962).

14. Gordon, D. B., and D. R. Drury. The effect of potassium on the occurrence of petechial hemorrhages in renal hypertensive rabbits. *Circ. Res.* 4:167–72 (1956).
15. Meneely, G. R., and C. O. T. Ball. Experimental epidemiology of chronic sodium chloride toxicity and the protective effect of potassium chloride. *Am. J. Med.* 25:713–25 (1958).
16. Dahl, L. K., G. Leitl, and M. Heine. Influence of dietary potassium and sodium/ potassium molar ratios on the development of salt hypertension. *J. Exp. Med.* 136:318–30 (1972).
17. See 12.
18. Vieth, I. *The Yellow Emperor's Classic in Internal Medicine* (Translated from Huang ti Nei thing Su Wen, 2600 BC) Berkeley, Calif.: Berkeley University Press (1966).
19. Kramer, S. N., and M. Levry. The oldest medical text in man's recorded history: A Sumerian physician's prescription book of 4000 years ago. In *Illustrated London News* 226:370. Strand: Ingram House (1955).
20. Ambard, L., and Beaujard. Causes de l'hypertension arterielle. *Arch. Gen. Med.* (Paris) 81:520–33 (1904).
21. Addison, W. L. T. The use of sodium chloride, potassium chloride, sodium bromide and potassium bromide in cases of arterial hypertension which are amenable to potassium choloride *Can. Med. Assoc. J.* 18:281–5 (1928).
22. Addison, W. L. T. The use of calcium chloride in arterial hypertension. *Can. Med. Assoc. J.* 14:1059–61 (1924).
23. Resnick, L. Calcium effective for low-renin hypertension. *Cardiology Observer* 1(3):4 (1984); and Resnick, L. M., J. P. Nicholson, and J. H. Laragh. Calcium metabolism and the renin-aldosterone system in essential hypertension. *J. Cardiovasc. Pharmacol.* 7 (Suppl.6):5187–93 (1985).
24. McCarron, D. A., and C. D. Morris. Blood pressure response to oral calcium in persons with mild to moderate hypertension. *Ann. Intern. Med.* 103:825–31 (1985).
25. See 21.
26. Addison, W. L. T., and H. G. Clark, Calcium and potassium chlorides in the treatment of arterial hypertension. *Can. Med. Assoc. J.* 15:913–15 (1925).
27. Priddle, W. W. Observations on the management of hypertension. *Can. Med. Assoc. J.* 25:5–8 (1931).
28. McQuarrie, I., W. H. Thompson, and J. A. Anderson. Effects of excessive ingestion of sodium and potassium salts on carbohydrate metabolism and blood pressure in diabetic children. *J. Nutr.* 11:77–01 (1936).
29. Kempner, W. Treatment of hypertensive vascular disease with rice diet. *Am. J. Med.* 4:545–77 (1948).
30. Dahl, L. K. Salt and hypertension. *Am. J. Clin. Nutr.* 25:231–44 (1972).
31. See 11; and Dole, V. P., L. K. Dahl, G. C. Cotzias, H. A. Eder, and M. E. Krebs. Dietary treatment of hypertension: Clinical and metabolic studies of patients on rice-fruit diet. *J. Clin. Invest.* 29:1189–1206 (1950).
32. Pritikin, N. Optimal dietary recommendations: A public health responsiblity. *Preventive Med.* 11:733–9 (1982).
33. Beard, T. C., W. R. Gray, H. M. Cooke, and R. Barge. Randomized controlled trial of a no added sodium diet for mild hypertension. *Lancet* 2:455–8 (1982).

34. Siani, A., P. Strazzullo, A. Giacco, D. Pacioni, E. Celentano, and M. Mancini. Increasing the dietary potassium intake reduces the need for antihypertensive medication. *Ann. Intern. Med.* 115(10):753–59 (1991).

35. MacGregor, G. A., N. D. Markandu, F. E. Best, D. M. Elder, J. M. Cam, G. A. Sagnella, and M. Squires. Double-blind randomized crossover trial of moderate sodium restriction in essential hypertension. *Lancet* 1:351–55 (1982); and MacGregor, G. A., S. J. Smith, N. D. Markandu, R. A. Banks, and G. A. Sagnella. Moderate potassium supplementation in essential hypertension. *Lancet* 2:567–70 (1982).

36. See 35, first reference.

37. See 35, second reference.

38. Iimura, O., T. Kijima, K. Kikuchi, A. Miyama, T. Ando, T. Nakao, and Y. Takigami. Studies on the hypotensive effect of high potassium intake in patients with essential hypertension. *Clin. Sci.* 61:77s–80s (1981).

39. Morgan, T., and C. Nowson. Comparative studies of reduced sodium and high potassium diet in hypertension. *Nephron* 47(suppl 1):21–26 (1987).

40. Intersalt Cooperative Research Group. Intersalt: An international study of electrolyte excretion and blood pressure. Results for 24 hour urinary sodium and potassium excretion. *Br. Med. J.* 297:319–28 (1988).

41. Krishna, G. G., and S. C. Kapoor. Potassium depletion exacerbates essential hypertension. *Ann. Intern. Med.* 115:77–83 (1991).

42. Krishna, G. G., E. Miller, and S. C. Kapoor. Increased blood pressure during potassium depletion in normotensive men. *N. Engl. J. Med.* 320:1177–82 (1989).

43. McCarron, D. A., C. D. Morris, H. J. Henry, and J. L. Stanton. Blood pressure and nutrient intake in the United States. *Science* 224:1392–8 (1984).

44. Gruchow, H. W., K. A. Sobocinski, and J. J. Barboriak. Alcohol, nutrient intake, and hypertension in U.S. adults. *J. Am. Med. Assoc.* 253:1567–70 (1985).

45. Overlack, A., K. O. Stumpe, B. Mocha, A. Olig, R. Kleinmann, H-M. Müller, R. Kolloch, and F. Krück. Hemodynamic, renal, and hormonal responses to changes in dietary potassium in normotensive and hypertensive man: Long-term antihypertensive effect of potassium supplementation in essential hypertension. *Klin. Wochenschr.* 63:352–60 (1985).

46. Ibid.

47. Cappuccio, F. P., and G. A. MacGregor. Does potassium supplementation lower blood pressure? A meta-analysis of published trials. *J. Hypertension* 9(5):465–73 (1991).

48. Working Group Report on Primary Prevention of Hypertension. National High Blood Pressure Education Program: National Heart, Lung, and Blood Institute. *Arch. Intern. Med.* 153:186–208 (1993).

49. Stamler, R. Implications of the Intersalt study. *Hypertension* 17(suppl I):I-16–I-20 (1991).

50. Parfrey, A. S., M. S. Vandenbury, P. Wright, et. al. Blood pressure and hormonal changes following alteration in dietary sodium and potassium in mild essential hypertension. *Lancet* 1(8211):59–63 (1981).

51. Siani, A., P. Strazzullo, L. Russo, S., Guglielmi, L., Iacoviello, L. A., Ferrara, and M. Mancini. Controlled trial of long term oral potassium supplements in patients with mild hypertension. *Br. Med. J.* 294:1453–6 (1987).

52. Richards, A. M., M. G. Nicholls, E. A. Espiner, H. Ikram, A. H. Maslowski, E. J. Hamilton, and J. E. Wells. Blood-pressure response to moderate sodium restriction and to potassium supplementation in mild essential hypertension. *Lancet* 1:757 (1984).

53. Smith, S. J., N. D. Markandu, G. A. Sagnella. Moderate potassium chloride supplementation in essential hypertension: Is it additive to moderate sodium restriction? *Br. Med. J.* 290:110–13 (1985).

54. Grimm, R. H., J. D. Neaton, P. J. Elmer, et al. The influence of oral potassium chloride on blood pressure in hypertensive men on a low-sodium diet. *N. Engl. J. Med.* 322(9):569–74 (1991).

55. Meneely, G. R., and H. D. Battarbee. High sodium-low potassium environment and hypertension. *Am. J. Cardiol.* 38:768–85 (1976).

CHAPTER 7

1. Reaven, G. M. Role of insulin resistance in human disease. *Diabetes* 37:1595–1607 (1988).

2. Ibid.

3. Krotkiewski, M., K. Mandroudas, L. Sjostrom, L. Sullivan, H. Wetterqvist, and P. Bjorntorp. Effects of long-term physical training on body fat, metabolism, and blood pressure in obesity. *Metabolism* 28:650–58 (1979); and Bjorntorp, P., K. de Jounge, L. Sjostrom, and L. Sullivan. The effect of physical training on insulin production in obesity. *Metabolism* 19:631–38 (1970).

4. Welborn, T. A., A. Breckenridge, A. H. Rubinstein, C. T. Dollery, and T. Russell Frazer. Serum-insulin in essential hypertension and in peripheral vascular disease. *Lancet* 1:1336–37 (1966).

5. Moore, R. D. Effects of insulin upon ion transport. *Biochim. Biophys. Acta* 737:1–49 (1983).

6. Haffner, S. M., D. Fong, H. P. Hazuda, J. A. Pugh, and J. K. Patterson. Hyperinsulinemia, upper body adiposity, and cardiovascular risk factors in non-diabetics. *Metabolism* 37(4):338–45 (1988); and Flack, J. M. Epidemiologic and clinical aspects of insulin resistance and hyperinsulinemia. *Am. J. Med.* 91(suppl. 1A):11S–21S (1991).

7. King, D. S., G. P. Dalsky, W. E. Clutter, D. A. Young, M. A. Staten, P. E. Cryer, and J. O. Holloszy. Effects of exercise and lack of exercise on insulin sensitivity and responsiveness. *J. Appl. Physiol.* 64(5):1942–46 (1988).

8. Devlin, J. T., and Horton, E. S. Effects of prior high intensity exercise on glucose metabolism in normal and insulin-resistant men. *Diabetes* 34:973–79 (1985).

9. King, D. S., G. P. Dalsky, M. A. Staten, W. E. Clutter, D. R. Van Houten, and J. O. Holloszy. Insulin action and secretion in endurance-trained and untained humans. *J. Appl. Physiol.* 63(6):2247–2252 (1987).

10. Landsberg, L., and J. B. Young. Diet and the sympathetic nervous system: Relationship to hypertension. *Int. J. Obesity* 5 (supp 1):79–90 (1981).

11. Rowe, J. W., J. B. Young, K. L. Minaker, A. L. Stevens, J. Pallotta, and L. Landsberg. Effect of insulin and glucose infusions on sympathetic nervous system activety in normal man. *Diabetes* 30:219–25 (1981).

12. Mineur, P., and J. Kolanowski. Changes in blood pressure and cardiovascular indices of adrenergic activity in obese subjects undergoing total starvation. *J. Obesity Weight Regul.* 2:69–79 (1983).

13. Kolanowski, J. Pathophysiology of hypertension in overweight subjects. *Medicographia* 7:29–31 (1985).

14. Reisin, E., R. Abel, M. Modan, D. S. Silverberg, H. E. Eliahou, and B. Modan. Effect of weight loss without salt restriction on the reduction of blood pressure in overweight patients. *N. Engl. J. Med.* 298:1–6 (1978); and Eliahou, H. E., A. Iaina, T. Gaon, J. Shochat, and M. Modan. Body weight reduction necessary to attain normotension in the overweight hypertensive patient. *Int. J. Obesity* 5(suppl 1):157–63 (1981).

15. MacMahon, S. W., G. J. Macdonald, L. Bernstein, G. Andrews, and R. B. Blacket. Comparison of weight reduction with metroprolol in treatment of hypertension in young overweight patients. *Lancet* 1:1233–6 (1985).

16. J. M. Hagberg. Exercise, fitness, and hypertension. In *Exercise, Fitness, and Health: A Consensus of Current Knowledge*, ed. C. Bouchard, R. J. Shephard, T. Stephens, J. R. Sutton, and B. D. McPherson, 455–466. Champaign, Ill.: Human Kinetics Books (1989).

17. Ibid.

18. Ibid.

19. Cononie, C. C., J. E. Graves, M. L. Pollock, M. I. Phillips, C. Sumners, and J. M. Hagberg. Effect of exercise training on blood pressure in 70- to 79-year old men and women. *Med. Sci. Sports Exercise* 23(4):505–11 (1991).

20. Krotkiewski, M., K. Mandroukas, L. Sjostrom, L. Sullivan, H. Wetterqvist, and P. Bjorntorp. Effects of long-term physical training on body fat, metabolism, and blood pressure in obesity. *Metabolism* 28:650–58 (1979); and Cade, R., D. Mars, H. Wagemaker, C. Zauner, D. Packer, M. Privette, M. Cade, J. Peterson, and D. Hood-Lewis. Effect of aerobic exercise training on patients with systemic arterial hypertension. *Am. J. Med.* 77:785–90 (1984).

21. See 20, first reference.

22. Martin, J. E., and P. M. Dubbert. Controlled trial of aerobic exercise in hypertension. *Circulation* 72(suppl III):III–13(abstr.) (1985).

23. See 20, second reference.

24. See 22.

25. Bogardus, C. E., E. Ravussin, D. C. Robbins, R. R. Wolfe, E. S. Horten, and E. A. H. Sims. Effects of physical training and diet therapy on carbohydrate metabolism in patients with glucose intolerance and non-insulin dependent diabetes mellitus. *Diabetes* 33:311–18 (1984).

26. See 9.

27. See 20, first reference.

28. Stamler, J., E. Farinaro, L. M. Mojonnier, Y. Hall, D. Moss, and R. Stamler. Prevention and control of hypertension by nutritional-hygienic means. *J. Am. Med. Assoc.* 243:1819–23 (1980).

CHAPTER 8

1. Cooke, K. M., G. W. Frost, I. R. Thornell, and G. S. Stokes. Alcohol consumption and blood pressure: Survey of the relationship at a health-screening clinic. *Med. J. Aust.* 1:65–69 (1982); and Kromhout, D., E. D. Bosschieter, and C. de L. Coulander. Potassium, calcium, alcohol intake and blood pressure: The Zutphen study. *Am. J. Clin. Nutr.* 41:1299–1304 (1985).

2. Klatsky, A. L., G. D. Friedman, A. B. Siegelaub, and M. J. Gerard. Alcohol consumption and blood pressure. *N Engl. J. Med.* 296:1194–1200 (1977).

3. MacMahon, S. Alcohol consumption and hypertension. *Hypertension* 9 (2):111–121 (1987).

4. Knutsson, E., and S. Katz. The effect of ethanol on the membrane permeability to sodium and potassium ions in frog muscle fibres. *Acta Pharmacol. Toxicol.* 25:54–64 (1967).

5. Seelig, M. S. *Magnesium Deficiency in the Pathogenesis of Disease.* New York: Plenum (1980).

6. Potter, J. F., and Beevers, D. G. Pressor effect of alcohol in hypertension. *Lancet* 1:119–122 (1984).

7. Puddey, I. B., L. J. Beilin, R. Vandongen, I. L. Rouse, and P. Rogers. Evidence for a direct effect of alcohol consumption on blood pressure in normotensive men: A randomized controlled trial. *Hypertension* 7:707–713 (1985).

8. Puddey, I. B., L. J. Beilin, and R. Vandongen. Regular alcohol use raises blood pressure in treated hypertensive subjects. *Lancet* 1:647–651 (1987).

9. Ibid.

10. Working Group Report on Primary Prevention of Hypertension. National High Blood Pressure Education Program: National Heart, Lung, and Blood Institute. *Arch. Intern. Med.* 153:186–208 (1993).

11. Dawson, E. B., M. J. Frey, T. D. Moore, and W. J. McGanity. Relationship of metal metabolism to vascular disease mortality rates in Texas. *Am. J. Clin. Nutr.* 31:1188–97 (1978).

12. Altura, B. M., B. T. Altura, A. Gebrewold, H. Ising, and T. Gunther. Magnesium deficiency and hypertension: Correlation between magnesium-deficient diets and microcirculatory changes in situ. *Science* 223:1315–17 (1984).

13. Haddy, F. J. Local effects of sodium, calcium, and magnesium upon small and large blood vessels of the dog forelimb. *Circ. Res.* VIII:57–70 (1960).

14. Altura, B. M., B. T. Altura, and A. Carella. Magnesium deficiency-induced spasms of umbilical vessels: Relation to preeclampsia, hypertension, growth retardation. *Science* 221:376–78 (1983).

15. Albert, D. G., M. Yoshikazu, and L. T. Iseri. Serum magnesium and plasma sodium levels in essential hypertension. *Circulation* XVII:761–64 (1958).

16. Resnick, L. M., J. H. Laragh, J. E. Sealey, M. H. Alderman. Divalent cations in essential hypertension. *N. Engl. J. Med.* 309:888–91 (1983).

17. Resnick, L. M., R. K. Gupta, and J. H. Laragh. Intracellular free magnesium in red blood cells of essential hypertension: Relation to blood pressure and serum divalent cations. *Proc. Natl. Acad. Sci. U.S.A.* 81:6511–15 (1984).

18. Whang, R., and J. K. Aikawa. Magnesium deficiency and refractoriness to potassium repletion. *J. Chron. Dis.* 30:65–68 (1977); and Dyckner, T., and P. O. Wester. Intracellular potassium after magnesium infusion. *Br. Med. J.* April 1:822–23 (1978).

19. Hollenberg, N. K. Management of hypertension and cardiovascular risk. *Am. J. Med.* 90(suppl 2A):2S–6S (1991).

20. Berthelot, A., and J. Esposito. Effects of dietary magnesium on the development of hypertension in the spontaneously hypertensive rat. *J. Am. Coll. Nutr.* 4:343–53 (1983).

21. Lim, P., and E. Jacob. Magnesium deficiency in patients on long-term diuretic therapy for heart failure. *Br. Med. J.* Sept. 9:620–22 (1972).

22. Blackfan, K. D., and B. Hamilton. Uremia in acute glomerular nephritis. *Boston Med. Surg. J.* 193:617–28 (1925).

23. Conradt, A., H. Weidinger, and H. Algayer. Evidence that magnesium deficiency could be a causal factor of (essential) gestosis. In *Recent Advances in Pathophysiological Conditions in Pregnancy,* ed. J. G. Schenker, E. T. Rippmann, and D. Weinstein, 36–39. Amsterdam: Elsevier Science (1984).

24. Dyckner, T., and P. O. Wester. Effect of magnesium on blood pressure. *Br. Med. J.* 286:1847–49 (1983).

25. Addison, W. L. T. The use of calcium chloride in arterial hypertension. *Can. Med. Assoc. J.* 14:1059–61 (1924).

26. Johnson, N. E., E. L. Smith, and J. L. Freudenheim. Effects on blood pressure of calcium supplementation of women. *Am. J. Clin. Nutr.* 42:12–17 (1985).

27. Resnick, L., as reported in: Calcium effective for low-renin hypertension. *Cardiol. Observer* 1(3):4 (1984).

28. Belizan, J. M., J. Villar, A. Zalazar, L. Rohas, D. Chan, and G. F. Bryce. Preliminary evidence of the effect of calcium supplementation on blood pressure in normal pregnant women. *Am. J. Obstet. Gynecol.* 146:175–80 (1983).

29. Strazzullo, P., V. Nunziata, M. Cirillo, R. Giannattasio, L. A. Ferrara, P. L. Mattioli, and M. Mancini. Abnormalities of calcium metabolism in essential hypertension. *Clin. Sci.* 65:137–41 (1983).

30. Kesteloot, H., J. Geboers, and R. Van Hoof. Epidemiological study of the relationship between calcium and blood pressure. *Hypertension* 5(suppl II):II52–56 (1983).

31. Ibid.

32. McCarron, D. A. Calcium, magnesium, and phosphorus balance in human and experimental hypertension. *Hypertension* 4(suppl III):III27–33 (1982).

33. Kotchen, T. A., R. G. Luke, C. E. Ott, J. H. Galla, and B. G. S. Whitescarver. Effect of chloride on renin and blood pressure response to sodium chloride. *Ann. Intern. Med.* 98(Part 2):817–22 (1983); and Kurtz, T. W., and R. C. Morris. Dietary chloride as a determinant of "sodium-dependent" hypertension. *Science* 222:1139–41 (1983).

34. Addison, W. L. T. The use of sodium chloride, potassium chloride, sodium bromide and potassium bromide in cases of arterial hypertension which are amenable to potassium chloride. *Can. Med. Assoc. J.* 18:281–85 (1928).

35. Banks, T., N. Ali, and K. Dais. Dietary management of the patient with atherosclerosis: Are the new national cholesterol education panel recommendations enough? *J. Natl. Med. Assoc.* 81(5):493–495 (1989).

36. Iacono, J. M., R. M. Dougherty, and P. Puska. Reduction of blood pressure associated with dietary polyunsaturated fat. *Hypertension* 4(suppl III):III34–42 (1982); and Puska, P., J. M. Iacono, A. Nissinen, H. J. Korhonen, E. Vartiainen, P. Pientinen, R. Dougherty, U. Leino, M. Mutanen, S. Moisio, and J. Huttunen. Controlled, randomized trial of the effect of dietary fat on blood pressure. *Lancet* 1:1–5 (1983).

37. Fleischman, A. I., M. L. Bierenbaum, A. Stier, S. H. Somol, P. Watson, and A. M. Naso. Hypotensive effect of increased dietary linoleic acid in mildly hypertensive humans. *J. Med. Soc. New Jersey* 76:181–83 (1979).

38. Tobian, L., M. Ganguli, M. A. Johnson, and J. Iwai. Influence of renal prostaglandins and dietary linoleate on hypertension in Dahl S rats. *Hypertension* 4(suppl II):II-149–II-53 (1982).
39. Iacono, J. M., P. Puska, R. M. Dougherty, P. Pietinen, E. Vartiainen, U. Leino, M. Mutanen, and S. Moisio. Effect of dietary fat on blood pressure in a rural Finnish population. *Amer. J. Clin. Nutr.* 38:860–69 (1983).
40. Summarized in Sacks, F. M., and E. H. Kass. Low blood pressure in vegetarians: Effects of specific foods and nutrients. *Am. J. Clin. Nutr.* 48:795–800 (1988).
41. Berry, E. M., and J. Hirsch. Does dietary linoleic acid influence blood pressure. *Am. J. Clin. Nutr.* 44:336–340 (1986).
42. Banks, T., N. Ali, and K. Dais. Dietary management of the patient with atherosclerosis: Are the new national cholesterol education panel recommendations enough? *J. Am. Med. Assoc.* 81(5):493–495 (1989).
43. Medical Research Council Working Party. MRC trial of treatment of mild hypertension: Principal results. *Br. Med. J.* 291:97–104 (1985).
44. Editorial accompanying British MRC report, by A. Breckenridge. Treating mild hypertension. *Br. Med. J.* 291:89–97 (1985).
45. Stanton, J. L., L. E. Braitman, A. M. Riley Jr., C.-S. Khoo, and J. L. Smith. Demographic, dietary, lifestyle, and anthropometric correlates of blood pressure. *Hypertension* 4 (suppl. III):III-136–I-142 (1982).
46. Skrabal, F., J. Aubock, H. Hortnagl, H. Braunsteiner. Effect of moderate salt restriction and high potassium intake on pressor hormones, response to noradrenaline and baroreceptor function in man. *Clin. Sci.* 59:157–60s (1980).
47. Seer, P. Psychological control of essential hypertension: review of the literature and methodical critique. *Psychological Bull.* 86:1015–43 (1979).
48. Aoki, K., K. Sato, S. Kondo, C. B. Pyon, and M. Yamamoto. Increased response of blood pressure to rest and handgrip in subjects with essential hypertension. *Jap. Circ. J.* 47:802–9 (1983).
49. See 47.
50. Brennan, P. J., G. Greenberg, W. E. Miall, and S. G. Thompson. Seasonal variation in arterial blood pressure. *Br. Med. J.* 285:919–23 (1982).
51. Working Group Report on Primary Prevention of Hypertension. National High Blood Pressure Education Program: National Heart, Lung, and Blood Institute. *Arch. Intern. Med.* 153:186–208 (1993).

INTRODUCTION TO PART THREE

1. Working Group Report on Primary Prevention of Hypertension. National High Blood Pressure Education Program: National Heart, Lung, and Blood Institute. *Arch. Intern. Med.* 153:186–208 (1993).

CHAPTER 9

1. World Health Organization (WHO) and the International Society of Hypertension (ISH). 1986 Guidelines for the Treatment of Mild Hypertension: Memorandum from the WHO/ISH. *Hypertension* 8(10):957–961 (1986).

CHAPTER 10

1. Eaton, S. B., and M. Konner. Paleolithic nutrition. *N. Engl. J. Med.* 312:283–89 (1985).
2. Phillipson, B. E., D. W. Rothrock, W. E. Conner, W. S. Harris, and D. R. Illingworth. Reduction of plasma lipids, lipoproteins, and apoproteins by dietary fish oils in patients with hypertriglyceridemia. *N. Engl. J. Med.* 312:1210–16 (1985); and Kromhout, D., E. B. Bosschieter, and C. de L. Coulander. The inverse relation between fish consumption and 20-year mortality from coronary heart disease. *N. Engl. J. Med.* 312:1205–09 (1985).
3. Johnson, N. E., E. L. Smith, and J. L. Freudenheim. Effects on blood pressure of calcium supplementation of women. *Am. J. Clin. Nutr.* 42:12–17 (1985).
4. Conradt, A., H. Weidinger, and H. Algayer. On the role of magnesium in fetal hypotrophy, pregnancy induced hypertension, and pre-eclampsia. *Magn. Bull.* 2:68–76d (1984).
5. Lipid Research Clinics Program. The lipid research clinics coronary primary prevention trial results. *J. Am. Med. Assoc.* 251:351–74 (1984).
6. Ornish, D. *Dr. Dean Ornish's Program for Reversing Heart Disease.* New York: Random House (1990).
7. Singer, P., W. Jaeger, M. Wirth, S. Voigt, E. Naumann, S. Zimontkowski, I. Hajdu, and W. Goedicke. Lipid and blood-pressure-lowering effect of mackerel diet in man. *Atherosclerosis* 49:99–108 (1983).
8. See 2, first reference.
9. See 2, second reference.
10. Jacobson, M., B. F. Liebman, and G. Moyer. *Salt: The Brand Name Guide to Sodium Content.* New York: Workman (1983).
11. Ledger, H. P. Body composition as a basis for a comparative study of some east African mammals. *Symp. Zool. Soc. Lond.* 21:289–310 (1968).
12. The Editors of Rodale Press. *How to Fight 10 Common Diseases,* 6. Emmaus, Pa.: Rodale Press (1986).
13. Henningsen, N. C., L. Larson, and D. Nelson. Hypertension, potassium, and the kitchen. *Lancet* 1:133 (1983).
14. Silva, P., J. F. Hayslett, and F. H. Eptstein. The role of Na-K-activated adenosine triphosphate in potassium adaptation. *J. Clin. Invest.* 52:2665–71 (1973).
15. See 12.

CHAPTER 11

1. Cade, R., D. Mars, H. Wagemaker, C. Zauner, D. Packer, M. Privette, M. Cade, J. Peterson, D. Hood-Lewis. Effect of aerobic exercise training on patients with systemic arterial hypertension. *Am. J. Med.* 77:785–90 (1984).
2. Parillo, M., A. Coulston, C. Hollenbeck, and G. Reaven. Effect of a low fat diet on carbohydrate metabolism in patients with hypertension. *Hypertension* 11(3):244–48 (1988); and Krotkiewski, M., K. Mandroukas, L. Sjöström, L. Sullivan, H. Wetterqvist, and P. Björntorp. Effects of long-term physical training on body fat, metabolism, and blood pressure in obesity. *Metabolism* 28:650–58 (1979).

3. Yeater, R. A., and I. H. Ullrich. The role of physical activity in disease prevention and treatment. *West Virginia Med. J.* 81:35–39 (1985).

4. Blair, S. N., N. N. Goodyear, L. W. Gibbons, and K. H. Cooper. Physical fitness and incidence of hypertension in healthy normotensive men and women. *J. Am. Med. Assoc.* 252:487–90 (1984).

5. Hanson, P., and R. Kochan. Exercise and diabetes. *Primary Care* 10:653–62 (1982).

6. See 5.

7. Billman, G. E., P. J. Schwartz, and H. L. Stone. The effects of daily exercise on susceptibility to sudden cardiac death. *Circulation* 69:1182–89 (1984).

8. Medical Research Council Working Party. MRC trial of treatment of mild hyperension: Principal results. *Br. Med. J.* 291:97–104 (1985).

9. Cooper, K. H. *Running With Fear: How to Reduce the Risk of Heart Attack and Sudden Death During Aerobic Exercise.* New York: M. Evans (1985).

10. See 9.

11. Thompson, P. D., E. J. Funk, R. A. Carleton, and W. Q. Sturner. Incidence of death during jogging in Rhode Island from 1975 through 1980. *J. Am. Med. Assoc.* 247:2535–38 (1980).

12. Siscovick, D. S., N. S. Weiss, R. H. Fletcher, and T. Lasky. The incidence of primary cardiac arrest during vigorous exercise. *N. Engl. J. Med.* 311:874–77 (1984).

13. Ragosta, M. Death during recreational exercise in the state of Rhode Island. *Med. Sci. Sports Exercise* 16:339–42 (1984).

14. Vuori, I., M. Makarainen, and A. Jaaskelainen. Sudden death and physical activity. *Cardiology* 63:287–304 (1978).

15. See 9.

16. Sheenan, G. Live to win. The Keynote Address at the Wellness Strategies Conference, Trenton, New Jersey, June 1985.

17. Pritikin, N. *The Pritikin Promise: 28 Days to a Longer Healthier Life,* 9. New York: Simon and Schuster (1983).

18. Lamb, L. E. *The Health Letter* 13:1–4 (1979).

19. Paffenbarger, R. S., Jr., A. L. Wing, and R. T. Hyde. Physical activity as an index of heart attack risk in college alumni. *Am. J. Epidemiol.* 108:161–75 (1978).

20. Paffenbarger, R. S., Jr., R. T. Hyde, A. L. Wing, and C. H. Steinmetz. A natural history of athleticism and cardiovascular health. *J. Am. Med. Assoc.* 252:491–95 (1984).

21. See 12.

22. Blair, S. N., H. W. Kohl III, R. S. Paffenbarger, D. G. Clark, K. H. Cooper, and L. W. Gibbons. Physical fitness and all-cause mortality: A prospective study of healthy men and women. *J. Am. Med. Assoc.* 262(17):2395–1401 (1989).

23. Frisch, R. E., G. Wyshak, N. L. Albright, T. E. Albright, I. Schiff, K. P. Jones, J. Witschi, E. Shiang, E. Koff, and M. Marguglio. Lower prevalence of breast cancer and cancers of the reproductive system among former college athletes compared to nonathletes. *Br. J. Cancer* 52:885–91 (1985).

24. See 12.

25. Blair, S. N., et al. Running and the incidence of osteoarthritis. *Med. Sci. Sports Exercise* 22:116 (1990); and Smith, E. L., et al. Exercise, fitness, osteoarthritis and osteoporosis. In *Exercise, Fitness and Health,* ed. C. Bouchard, R. J. Shepard, T. Stephens, J. R. Sutton, and B. D. McPherson. Champaign, Ill.: Human Kinetics Books (1990).

26. Nabokov, P. *Indian Running.* Santa Barbara, Calif.: Capra Press (1981).
27. Yeater, R. A., and R. B. Martin. Senile osteoporosis. The effects of exercise. Postgrad. Med. 75:147–59 (1984).
28. Hagberg, J. M. Exercise, fitness, and hypertension. In *Exercise, Fitness and Health;* and Smith, E. L. et al. Exercise, fitness, osteoarthritis and osteoporosis. In *Exercise, Fitness and Health,* ed. C. Bouchard, R. J. Shepard, T. Stephens, J. R. Sutton, and B. D. McPherson. Champaign, Ill.: Human Kinetics Books (1990).
29. Cononie, C. C., J. E. Graves, M. L. Pollock, M. I. Phillips, C. Sumners, and J. M. Hagberg. Effect of exercise training on blood pressure in 70- to 79-year old men and women. *Med. Sci. Sports Exercise* 23(4):505–11 (1991).
30. MacDougall, J. D., Tuxen, D. G. Sale, J. R. Moroz, and J. R. Sutton. Arterial blood pressure responses to heavy resistance exercise. *J. Appl. Physiol.* 58:785–90 (1985).
31. Freedson, P. More on hypertension and lifting. *Physician Sports Med.* 12(10):21 (1984).
32. Dr. Rachel A. Yeater, University of West Virginia, personal communication.
33. Shephard, R. J. *Endurance Fitness.* Toronto: University of Toronto Press (1977).
34. White, M. K., R. A. Yeater, R. B. Martin, et al. The effects of aerobic dancing and walking on the cardiovascular and muscular systems of post-menopausal females. *J. Sports Med. Phys. Fitness* 24:159–66 (1984); and Milburn, S., and N. K. Butts. A comparison of the training responses to aerobic dance and jogging in college females. *Med. Sci. Sports Exercise* 15:510–13 (1984).
35. Blair, S. N., H. W. Kohl III, R. S. Paffenbarger, D. G. Clark, K. H. Cooper, and L. W. Gibbons. Physical fitness and all-cause mortality: A prospective study of healthy men and women. *J. Am. Med. Assoc.* 262(17):2395–1401 (1989).
36. See 14.
37. Allen, C. J., M. A. Craven, D. Rosenbloom, and J. R. Sutton. Beta-blockade and exercise in normal subjects and patients with coronary artery disease. *Physician Sportsmed.* 12:51–63 (1984).
38. American College of Sports Medicine. Position statement on the recommended quantity and quality of exercise for developing and maintaining fitness in healthy adults. *Am. Coll. Sports Med.* 10:1–4 (1978).
39. Ibid.
40. Seals, D. R., and J. M. Hagberg. The effect of exercise training on human hypertension: A review. *Med. Sci. Sports Exercise* 16:207–215 (1984).
41. See 9.
42. See 38.
43. Ibid.
44. Krotkiewski, M., K. Mandroukas, L. Sjostrom, L. Sullivan, H. Wetterqvist, and P. Bjorntorp. Effects of long-term physical training on body fat, metabolism, and blood pressure in obesity. *Metabolism* 28:650–58 (1979).
45. See 1.
46. Holloszy, J. O., J. Schultz, J. Kusnierkiewicz, J. M. Hagberg, and A. A. Ehsani. Effects of exercise on glucose tolerance and insulin resistance: Brief review and some preliminary results. *Acta Med. Scand. Suppl.* 711:55–65 (1986).
47. See 16.
48. Sheehan G. A. *Running and Being. The Total Experience.* New York: Simon and Schuster (1978).
49. See 9.

CHAPTER 12

1. The Fifth (1993) Report of the Joint National Committee on the Detection, Evaluation, and Treatment of High Blood Pressure. *Arch. Intern. Med.* 153:154–183 (1993).
2. Sims, E. A. H. Diabesity and obitension: Common mechanisms and common management. In *Controversies in Obesity*, ed. B. C. Hansen. New York: Praeger (1983); and Kolanowski, J. Pathophysiology of hypertension in overweight subjects. *Medicographia* 7:29–31, 51 (1985).
3. Reisin, E., R. Abel, M. Modan, D. S. Silverberg, H. E. Eliahou, and B. Modan. Effect of weight loss without salt restriction on the reduction of blood pressure in overweight patients. *N. Engl. J. Med.* 298:1–6 (1978); and Eliahou, H. E., A. Iaina, T. Gaon, J. Shochat, and M. Modan. Body weight reduction necessary to attain normotension in the overweight hypertensive patient. *Int. J. Obesity* 5(suppl 1):157–63 (1981).
4. Presta, E., J. Wang, G. G. Harrison, P. Bjorntorp, W. H. Harker, and T. B. van Itallie. Measurement of total body electrical conductivity: A new method for estimation of body composition. *Am. J. Clin. Nutr.* 37:735–39 (1983).
5. Ismail-Beigi, F., and I. S. Edelman. Mechanism of thyroid calorigenesis: Role of active sodium transport. *Proc. Natl. Acad. Sci. U.S. A.* 67:1071–78 (1970).
6. Remington, D. W., A. G. Fisher, and E. A. Parent. *How to Lower Your Fat Thermostat.* Provo, Utah: Vitality House International (1983).
7. Clausen, T., O. Hansen, K. Kjeldsen, and A. Norgaard. Effect of age, potassium depletion and denervation on specific displaceble [^{3}H]ouabain binding in rat skeletal muscle *in vivo. J. Physiol.* 333:367–81 (1982); and Kjeldsen, K., A. Norgaard, and T. Clausen. Effect of K-depletion on ^{3}H-ouabain binding and Na-K contents in mammalian skeletal muscle. *Acta Physiol. Scand.* 122:103–17 (1984).
8. Kolata, G. Why do people get fat? *Science* 227:1327–28 (1985).
9. Oscai, L. B., M. M. Brown, and W. C. Miller. Effect of dietary fat of food intake, growth and body composition. *Growth* 48:415–24 (1984).
10. Flatt, J. P. The biochemistry of energy expenditure. *Recent Adv. Obes. Res.* II:211–18. (1978); and Flatt, J. P. Energetics of intermediary metabolism in substrate and energy metabolism in man. *Int. J. Obes.* 9(suppl 2):58–69 (1985).
11. Danforth, E., Jr. Diet and obesity. *Am. J. Clin. Nutr.* 41:1132–45 (1985).
12. Hanson, P., and R. Kochan. Exercise and diabetes. *Primary Care* 10:653–62 (1983).
13. Rowe, J. W., J. B. Young, K. L. Minaker, A. L. Stevens, J. Palotta, and L. Landsberg. Effect of insulin and glucose infusions on sympathetic nervous system activity in normal man. *Diabetes* 30:219–25 (1981).
14. Fagerberg, B., O. Andersson, U. Nilsson, T. Hedner, B. Isaksson, and P. Bjorntorp. Weight-reducing diets: Role of carbohydrates on sympathetic nervous activity and hypotensive response. *Int. J. Obesity* 8:237–43 (1984).
15. See 6.

CHAPTER 14

1. Toffler, A. Science and change. Foreword to *Order out of Chaos* by I. Prigogine and I. Stengers. Toronto: Bantam Books (1984).

2. Guttmacher, S., M. Teitelman, G. Chapin, G. Garbowski, and P. Schnall. Ethics and preventive medicine: The case of borderline hypertension. *Hastings Center Report* 12–20 (Feb. 1981).
3. Dahl, L. K. Salt and hypertension. *Am. J. Clin. Nutr.* 25:231–44 (1972).
4. See 3.
5. Messerli, F. H., U. R. Kaesser, and C. J. Losem. Effects of antihypertensive therapy on hypertensive heart disease. *Circulation* (suppl IV) 80(6): IV-145–IV-150 (1989)
6. Moore, R. D. The case for intracellular pH in insulin action. In *Molecular Basis of Insulin Action,* ed. M. P. Czech, 145–70. New York: Plenum (1985).

CHAPTER 15

1. Sigurdsson, J. A., and C. Bengtsson. Urinary findings and renal function in hypertensive and normotensive women. From the Korpilampi Hypertension Meeting, 1980. *Acta Med. Scand.* (suppl 646):51–3 (1981).
2. Lever, A. F., C. Beretta-Piccoli, J. J. Brown, D. L. Davies, R. Fraser, and J. I. S. Robertson. Sodium and potassium in essential hypertension. *Br. Med. J.* 283:463–68 (1981); and Beretta-Piccoli, C., D. L. Davies, K. Boddy, J. J. Brown, A. M. M. Cumming, B. W. East, R. Fraser, A. F. Lever, P. L. Padfield, P. F. Semple, J. I. S. Robertson, P. Weidmann, and E. D. Williams. Relation of arterial pressure with body sodium, body potassium and plasma potassium in essential hypertension. *Clin. Sci.* 63:257–70 (1982).
3. Bulpitt, C. J., M. J. Shipley, and A. Semmence. Blood pressure and plasma sodium and potassium. *Clin. Sci.* 61:85s–87s (1981).
4. Usehima, H., M. Tanigaki, M. Ida, T. Shimamoto, M. Konishi, and Y. Komachi. Hypertension, salt, and potassium. *Lancet* 1:504 (1981).
5. Maxwell, M. H., E. Fitzsimmons, R. Harrist, J. Hotchkiss, H. G. Langford, G. H. Payne, K. A. Schneider, and P. Varaday. Baseline laboratory examination characteristics of the hypertensive participants. *Hypertension* 5(Part II):IV-133–59 (1983).
6. Ericsson, F. Intracellular potassium in man. *Scand. J. Clin. Lab. Invest.* 42(suppl 163):1–58 (1982); and Ericsson, F., B. Carlmark, and K. Eliasson. Whole body and skeletal muscle potassium in untreated primary hypertension. In *Potassium, Blood Pressure and Cardiovascular Disease.* Amsterdam: Excerpta Medica (1983).
7. Veniero, J. C., and R. K. Gupta. NMR measurement of intracellular free potassium in the perfused normotensive and spontaneously hypertensive rat aorta by a multinuclear subtraction procedure. *Am. J. Hypertension* 5:733–739 (1992).
8. See 2, first reference.
9. See 2, second reference.
10. Sasaki, N. High blood pressure and the salt intake of the Japanese. *Jap. Heart J.* 3:313–24 (1962).
11. Walker, W. G., P. K. Whelton, H. Saito, R. P. Russell, and J. Hermann. Relation between blood pressure and renin, renin substrate, angiotensin II, aldosterone and urinary sodium and potassium in 574 ambulatory subjects. *Hypertension* 1:287–91 (1979).

12. Watson, R. L., H. G. Langford, J. Abernethy, T. Y. Barnes, and M. J. Watson. Urinary electrolytes, body weight, and blood pressure: Pooled cross-sectional results among four groups of adolescent females. *Hypertension* 2(Part 2):93–98 (1980).

13. Grim, C. E., F. C. Luft, J. Z. Miller, G. R. Meneely, H. D. Battarbee, C. G. Hames and L. K. Dahl. Racial differences in blood pressure in Evans County, Georgia: Relationship to sodium and potassium intake and plasma renin activity. *J. Chron. Dis.* 33:87–94 (1980).

14. See 12.

15. Langford, H. G. Dietary potassium and hypertension: Epidemiologic data. *Ann. Intern. Med.* 98(part 2):770–72 (1983).

16. Sever, P. S., D. Gordon, W. S. Peart, and P. Beighton. Blood pressure and its correlates in urban and tribal Africa. *Lancet* 2:60–64 (1980).

17. Stressen, J., K. Jagard, P. Lynsn, A. Amery, C. Bulpitt, and J. V. Joossens. Salt and blood pressure in Belgium. *J. Epidemiol. Commun. Health* 35:256–61 (1981).

18. Meneely, G. R., and C. O. T. Ball. Experimental epidemiology of chronic sodium chloride toxicity and the protective effect of potassium chloride. *Am. J. Med.* 25: 713–25 (1958).

19. Dahl, L. K, G. Leitl, and M. Heine. Influence of dietary potassium and sodium/potassium molar ratios on the development of salt hypertension. *J. Exp. Med.* 136:318–30 (1972).

20. Battarbee, H. D., D. P. Funch, and J. W. Dailey. The effect of dietary sodium and potassium upon blood pressure and catecholamine excretion in the rat. *Proc. Soc. Exp. Biol. Med.* 161:32–37 (1979).

21. Treasure, J., and D. Ploth. Role of dietary potassium in the treatment of hypertension. *Hypertension* 5:864–72 (1983).

22. Haddy, F. J. Minireview. Potassium and blood vessels. *Life Sci.* 16:1489–98 (1975).

23. Webb, R. C., and D. F. Bohr. Potassium relaxation of vascular smooth muscle from spontaneously hypertensive rats. *Blood Vessels* 16:71–79 (1979).

24. Tannen, R. L. Effects of potassium on blood pressure control. *Ann. Intern. Med.* 98(part 2):773–80 (1983).

25. Keith, M. N., and M. W. Binger. Diuretic action of potassium salts. *J. Am. Med. Assoc.* 105:1584–91 (1935); and Smith, S. J., N. D. Markandu, G. A. Sagnella, L. Poston, P. J. Hilton, and G. A. MacGregor. Does potassium lower blood pressure by increasing sodium excretion? A metabolic study in patients with mild to moderate essential hypertension. *J. Hypertension* 1(suppl 2):27–30.

26. Fujita, T., Y. Sato, and K. Ando. Role of sympathetic nerve activity and natriuresis in the antihypertensive actions of potassium in NaCl hypertension. *Jap. Circ. J.* 47:1227–31 (1983); and see 20.

27. Tannen, R. L. Effects of potassium on blood pressure control. *Ann. Intern. Med.* 98(part 2):773–80 (1983).

28. Dustin, H. P. Mechanisms of hypertension associated with obesity. *Ann. Intern. Med.* 98(Part 2):860–64 (1983); and Havlik, R. J., H. B. Hubert, R. R. Fabsitz, and M. Feinleib. Weight and hypertension. *Ann. Intern. Med.* 98(Part 2):855–59 (1983).

29. Eliahou, H. E., A. Iaina, T. Gaon, J. Shochat, and M. Modan. Body weight reduction necessary to attain normotension in the overweight hypertensive patient. *Int. J. Obesity* 5 (Suppl. 1):157–163 (1981).

30. Mineur, P., and J. Kolanowski. Changes in blood pressure and cardiovascular indices of adrenergic activity in obese subjects undergoing total starvation. *J. Obesity Weight Regul.* 2:69–79 (1983).

31. Nizet, A., P. Lefebvre, and J. Crabbe, Control by insulin of sodium-potassium and water excretion by isolated dog kidneys. *Pflug. Arch.* 323:11–20 (1971).

32. DeFronzo, R. A., R. Sherwin, M. Dillingham, R. Hendeler, W. Tamborlane, and P. Felig. Influence of basil insulin and glucagon-secretion on potassium and on sodium metabolism—studies with somatostatin in normal dogs and in normal and diabetic human beings. *J. Clin. Invest.* 61:472–479 (1978).

33. Sims, E. A. H. Diabesity and obitension: Common mechanisms and common management. In *Controversies in Obesity,* ed. B. C. Hansen, New York: Praeger (1983) 193–212.

34. Moore, R. D. Effect of insulin on ion transport. *Biochem. Biophys. Acta* 737:1–49 (1983).

35. Berchtold, P., and E. A. H. Sims. Obesity and hypertension: Conclusions and recommendations. *Int. J. Obesity* 5(suppl 1):183–184 (1981).

36. Dr. Wayne Gavryck, personal communication.

37. See 29 and 30.

38. Rowe, J. W., J. B. Young, K. L. Minaker, A. L. Stevens, J. Palotta, and L. Landsberg. Effect of insulin and glucose infusions on sympathetic nervous system activity in normal man. *Diabetes* 30:219–225 (1981).

39. Besarab, A., P. Silva, and L. Landsberg. Effect of catecholamines on tubular function in the isolated perfused rat kidney. *Am. J. Physiol.* 233:F39–F45 (1977); and Gullner, H.-G. The role of the adrenergic nervous system in sodium and water excretion. *Klin. Wochenschr.* 61:1063–66 (1983).

40. Marks, P., B. Wilson, and A. Delassalle. Aldosterone studies in obese patients with hypertension. *Am. J. Med. Sci.* 289:224–28 (1985).

41. Krotkiewski, M., P. Bjorntorp, G. Holm, V. Marks, L. Morgan, U. Smith, and G. E. Feurle. Effects of physical training on insulin, connecting peptide (C-peptide) gastric inhibitory polypeptide (GIP) and pancreatic polypeptide (PP) levels in obese subjects. *Int. J. Obesity* 8:193–99 (1984); and Bjorntorp, P., K. De Jounge, L. Sjostrom, and L. Sullivan. The effect of physical training on insulin production in obesity. *Metabolism* 19:631–38 (1970).

42. Haddy, F. J. Mechanism, prevention and therapy of sodium-dependent hypertension. *Am. J. Med.* 69:746–58 (1980).

43. Ibid.

CHAPTER 16

1. Conn, J. W. The mechanism of acclimatization to heat. *Adv. Intern. Med.* 3:373–93 (1949).

2. Thomas, W. A. Health of a carnivorous race. A study of the Eskimo. *J. Am. Med. Assoc.* 88:1559–60 (1927).

3. Dahl, L. K. Salt and hypertension. *Amer. J. Clin. Nutr.* 25:231–44 (1972).

4. Ibid.

5. Dole, V. P., L. K. Dahl, G. C. Cotzias, H. A. Eder, and M. E. Krebs. Dietary treatment

of hypertension: Clinical and metabolic studies of patients on rice-fruit diet. *J. Clin. Investig.* 29:1189–1206 (1950).

6. Smith, S. E., and P. D. Aines. Salt requirements of dairy cows. *New York Agric. Exp. Sta. Ithaca Bull.* 938:1–26 (1959).

7. Babcock, S. M. The addition of salt to the ration of dairy cows. *Wisc. Agric. Exp. Sta. Annu. Rep.* (1905), p. 129; and Cox, R. F., and E. F. Smith. *Salt for beef cattle and sheep.* Chicago: Salt Institute (1957).

8. Tobe, J. H. *Salt and Your Health,* 37. New York: Hearthside Press (1965).

9. Patton, A. R. Letter. *Nutr. Rev.* 11:159 (1953).

10. Watt, B. K., and A. L. Merrill, *Composition of Foods.* Agriculture Handbook No. 8, U.S. Dept. of Agriculture, Washington D.C.: U.S. Government Printing Office (1975); and Altman, P. L., and D. S. Dittmer, eds. *Biological Handbooks. Blood and Other Body Fluids,* 455–58. Washington, D.C.: FASEB (1961).

11. Beauchamp, G. K., M. Bertino, and K. Engelman. Modification of salt taste. *Ann. Intern. Med.* 98(Part 2):763–69 (1983).

CHAPTER 17

1. Dahl, L. K., M. Heine, and K. Thompson. Genetic influence of the kidneys on blood pressure. Evidence from chronic renal homografts in rats with opposite predispositions to hypertension. *Circ. Res.* 34:94–100 (1974).

2. See 1; and Bianchi, G., U. Fox, G. F. Di Francesco, A. M. Giovanetti, and D. Pagetti. Blood pressure changes produced by kidney cross-transplantation between spontaneously hypertensive rats and normotensive rats. *Clin. Sci. Mol. Med.* 47:435–48 (1974).

3. Ibid.

4. Tobian, L. Salt and hypertension. In *Hypertension, Physiopathology and Treatment,* ed. J. Genest, O. Kuchel, P. Hamet, and M. Cantin, 73–83. New York: McGraw-Hill (1983).

5. Guyton, A. C., T. G. Coleman, and H. J. Granger. Circulation: Overall regulation. *Annu. Rev. Physiol.* 34:13–46 (1972); and Guyton, A. C., T. G. Coleman, W. W. Cowley, R. D. Manning, R. A. Norman, and J. D. Ferguson. A systems analysis approach to understanding long-range arterial blood pressure control and hypertension. *Circ. Res.* 35(2):159–176 (1974).

6. Hamlyn, J. M., P. D. Levinson, R. Ringel, P. A. Levin, B. P. Hamilton, M. P. Blaustein, and A. A. Kowarski. Relationships among endogenous digitalis-like factors in essential hypertension. *Fed. Proc.* 44:2782-88 (1985); and de Wardener, H. E., and G. A. MacGregor. The relation of a circulating sodium transport inhibitor (the natriuretic hormone?) to hypertension. *Medicine* 62:310–26 (1983).

7. Moore, R. D. Effect of insulin upon sodium pump in frog skeletal muscle. *J. Physiol.* 232:23–45 (1973).

8. Nizet, A., P. Lefebvre, and J. Crabbe. Control by insulin of sodium potassium and water excretion by the isolated dog kidney. *Pflugers Arch.* 323:11–20 (1971).

9. Laragh, J. H. The role of aldosterone in man: Evidence for regulation of electrolyte balance and arterial pressure by renal-adrenal system which may be involved in malignant hypertension. *J. Am. Med. Assoc.* 174:293–95 (1960).

10. Laragh, J. H. Biochemical and physiological aspects of the renin-angiotensin system: A journey through darkest hypertension. In *Hypertension: Physiological Basis and Treatment,* ed. H. H. Ong and J. C. Lewis, 49–93. New York: Academic Press (1984).

11. Garvaras, H., H. R. Brunner, and J. H. Laragh. Renin and aldosterone and the pathogenesis of hypertensive vascular damage. *Prog. Cardiovasc. Dis.* 17:39–49 (1974).

12. See 10.

13. Landsberg, L., D. R. Krieger. Obesity, metabolism, and the sympathetic nervous system. *Am. J. Hypertension* 2:125S–132S (1989).

14. Young, D. B. Analysis of long-term potassium regulation. *Endocr. Rev.* 6(1):24–44 (1985).

15. Lin, H., and D. B. Young. Impaired control of renal hemodynamics and renin release during hyperkalemia in rabbits. *Am. J. Physiol.* 254:F704–F710 (1988); and Lin, H., D. B. Young, and M. J. Smith. Stimulation of renin release by hyperkalemia in the nonfiltering kidney. *Am. J. Physiol.* 260:F170–F176 (1991).

16. Vander, A. J. Control of renin release. *Physiol. Rev.* 47:359–382 (1967).

17. See 5, first reference.

18. See 10.

19. See 14.

20. See 5, first reference.

CHAPTER 18

1. The Joint National Committee of Detection, Evaluation, and Treatment of High Blood Pressure. The 1984 report of the Joint National Committee of Detection, Evaluation, and Treatment of High Blood Pressure. *Arch. Intern. Med.* 144:1045–57 (1984); and Baker, C. E., Jr. *Physicians' Desk Reference* (PDR), 34th ed. Oradell, N.J.: Medical Economics (1980).

2. Bennett, W. M., W. J. McDonald, E. Kuehnel, M. N. Hartnett, and G. A. Porter. Do diuretics have antihypertensive properties independent of natriuresis? *Clin. Pharmacol. Ther.* 22:499–504 (1977).

3. Edmonds, C. J., and B. Jasani. Total-body potassium in hypertensive patients during prolonged diuretic therapy. *Lancet* 2:8–12 (1972).

4. See 3; and Wilkinson, P. R., H. Issler, R. Hesp, and E. B. Raftery. Total body and serum potassium during prolonged thiazide therapy for essential hypertension. *Lancet* 1:759–62 (1975).

5. Schwartz, W. B. Potassium and the kidney. *N. Engl. J. Med.* 253:601–08 (1955).

6. Morgan, T. O., W. R. Adam, M. Hodgson, and R. W. Gibberd. Failure of therapy to improve prognosis in elderly males with hypertension. *Med. J. Aust.* 2:27–31 (1980).

7. Lim, P., and E. Jacob. Magnesium deficiency in patients on long-term diuretic therapy for heart failure. *Br. Med. J.* 3:620–22 (1972).

8. Gilman, A. G., L. S. Goodman, and A. Gilman, ed. *Goodman and Gilman's The Pharmacological Basis of Therapeutics,* 6th ed. New York: Macmillan (1980).

9. See 1.

10. See 8.

11. See 8.
12. See 8.
13. See 8.
14. Brantigan, C. O., N. Joseph, and T. A. Brantigan. Effect of beta blockade and beta stimulation on stage fright. *Am. J. Med.* 72:88–94 (1982).
15. Weinberger, M. H. Cardiovascular risk factors and antihypertensive therapy. *Am. J. Med.* 84(suppl 4A):24–29 (1988).
16. Laragh, J. H. Biochemical and physiological aspects of the renin-angiotensin system: A journey through darkest hypertension. In *Hypertension: Physiological Basis and Treatment*, ed. H. H. Ong and J. C. Lewis, 49–93. New York: Academic Press (1984).
17. Lewis, G. R. J. Lisinopril versus placebo in older congestive heart failure patients. *Am. J. Med.* 85(suppl 3B):48–54 (1988).
18. Ferris, T. F., and E. K. Weir. Effect of captopril on uterine blood flow and prostaglandin E synthesis in the pregnant rabbit. *J. Clin. Invest.* 71:809–815 (1983).
19. Anonymous. Are ACE-inhibitors safe in pregnancy? *Lancet* 2:482–483 (1989).
20. Messerli, F. H., S. Oren, and E. Grossman. Effects of calcium channel blockers on systemic hemodynamics in hypertension. *Am. J. Med.* 84(suppl 3B):8–12 (1988).
21. Weinberger, M. H. Cardiovascular risk factors and antihypertensive therapy. *Am. J. Med.* 84(suppl 4A):24–29 (1988); and Zawada, E. T. Metabolic considerations in the approach to diabetic hypertensive patients. *Am. J. Med.* 87(suppl 6A):34S–38S (1989).
22. See 21, second reference.

CHAPTER 19

1. The Fifth Report of the Joint National Committee on Detection, Evaluation, and Treatment of High Blood Pressure. *Arch. Intern. Med.* 153:154–183 (1993).
2. Kaplan, N. M. Hypertension: Prevelance, risks, and effect of therapy. *Ann. Intern. Med.* 98:705–09 (1983).
3. The Joint National Committee of Detection, Evaluation, and Treatment of High Blood Pressure. The 1984 Report of the Joint National Committee of Detection, Evaluation, and Treatment of High Blood Pressure. *Arch. Intern. Med.* 144:1045–57 (1984).
4. The Joint National Committee of Detection, Evaluation, and Treatment of High Blood Pressure. The 1988 report of the Joint National Committee of Detection, Evaluation, and Treatment of High Blood Pressure. *Arch. Intern. Med.* 148:1023–38 (1988).
5. See 1.
6. Multiple Risk Factor Intervention Trial Research Group. Multiple risk factor intervention trial. Risk factor changes and mortality results. *J. Am. Med. Assoc.* 248:1465–77 (1982).
7. See 2.
8. Medical Research Council Working Party. MRC trial of treatment of mild hypertension: Principal results. *Br. Med. J.* 291:97–104 (1985).
9. Sims, E. A. H., and P. Berchtold. Obesity and hypertension. Mechanisms and implications for management. *J Am. Med. Assoc.* 247:49–52 (1982).
10. See 1.
11. Working Group Report on Primary Prevention of Hypertension National High Blood Pressure Education Program. National Heart, Lung, and Blood Institute. *Arch. Intern. Med.* 153:186–208 (1993).

12. Schwartz, S. M., G. R. Campbell, and J. H. Campbell. Replication of smooth muscle cells in vascular disease. *Circ. Res.* 58(4):427–444 (1986); and Lever, A. F. Editorial review: Slow pressor mechanisms in hypertension: A role for hypertrophy of resistance vessels? *J. Hypertension* 4(5):515–524 (1986).

13. Khaw, K.-T., and E. Barrett-Connor. Dietary potassium and stroke-associated mortality: A 12-year prospective population study. *N. Engl. J. Med.* 316(5):235–240 (1987).

14. Silva, P., J. F. Hayslett, and F. H. Eptstein. The role of Na-K-activated adenosine triphosphate in potassium adaptation. *J. Clin. Invest.* 52:2665–71 (1973); and DeFronzo, R. Extrarenal K^+ regulation. A talk at the Eleventh Yale Symposium on Membrane Transport Processes, New Haven, Conn., April 1985.

15. McMahon, F. G. The role of diet in the management of essential hypertension. *Management of Essential Hypertension.* Kisco, N.Y.: Futura (1978).

16. See 14, second reference.

17. Moore, R. D. Effects of insulin upon ion transport. *Biochim. Biophys. Acta* 737:1–49 (1983).

18. See 14, second reference.

19. Clausen, T., O. Hansen, K. Kjeldsen, and A. Norgaard. Effect of age, potassium depletion and denervation of specific displaceable [^{3}H]ouabain binding in rat skeletal muscle *in vivo. J. Physiol.* 333:367–81 (1982).

20. See 1.

21. Kaplan, N. M. Misdiagnosis of systemic hypertension and recommendations for improvement. Editorial. *Am. J. Cardiol.* 60:1383–1386 (1987).

22. The Joint National Committee of Detection, Evaluation, and Treatment of High Blood Pressure. The 1988 report of the Joint National Committee of Detection, Evaluation, and Treatment of High Blood Pressure. *Arch. Intern. Med.* 148:1023–38 (1988).

23. See 1.

24. Breckenridge, A. Editorial accompanying British MRC report. Treating mild hypertension. *Br. Med. J.* 291:89–97 (1985).

25. Iimura, O., T. Kijima, K. Kikuchi, A. Miyama, T. Ando, T. Nakao, and Y. Takigami. Studies on the hypotensive effects of high potassium intake in patients with essential hypertension. *Clin. Sci.* 61:77–80 (1981).

26. Hunt, J. C. Sodium intake and hypertension: A cause for concern. *Ann. Intern. Med.* 98:724–28 (1983).

27. Siani, A., P. Strazzullo, A. Giacco, D. Pacioni, E. Celentano, and M. Mancini. Increasing the dietary potassium intake reduces the need for antihypertensive medication. *Ann. Intern. Med.* 115(10):753–759 (1991).

28. The Joint National Committee of Detection, Evaluation, and Treatment of High Blood Pressure. The 1988 report of the Joint National Committee of Detection, Evaluation, and Treatment of High Blood Pressure. *Arch. Intern. Med.* 148:1023–38 (1988).

29. Kuller, L. H., P. H. Stephen, B. Hulley, J. D. Cohen, and J. Neaton. Unexpected effects of treating hypertension in men with electrocardiographic abnormalities: A critical analysis. *Circulation* 73:114–23 (1986).

30. The Joint National Committee of Detection, Evaluation, and Treatment of High Blood Pressure. The 1988 report of the Joint National Committee of Detection, Evaluation, and Treatment of High Blood Pressure. *Arch. Intern. Med.* 148:1023–38 (1988).

31. Sterns, R. H., M. Cox, P. U. Feig, and I. Singer. Internal potassium balance and the control of the plasma potassium concentration. *Medicine* 60:339–54 (1981).

32. Hollenberg, N. K. Management of hypertension and cardiovascular risk. *Am. J. Med.* 90(suppl 2A):2S–6S (1991).
33. Weber, M. A. Antihypertensive treatment: Considerations beyond blood pressure control. *Circulation* (suppl) 80:120–127 (1989).
34. See 32.
35. Struthers A. D., R. Whitesmith, J. L. Reid. Prior thiazide diuretic treatment increases adrenaline-induced hypokalaemia. *Lancet* 1:1358–60 (1983); and Kaplan, N. M. Our appropriate concern about hypokalemia. *Am. J. Med.* 77:1–4 (1984).
36. Holland, O. B., J. V. Nixon, and L. Kuhnert. Diuretic-induced ventricular ectopic activity. *Am. J. Med.* 70:762–768 (1981).
37. Nordrehaug, J. E., and G. von der Lippe. Hypokalaemia and ventricular fibrillation in acute myocardial infarction. *Br. Heart J.* 50:525–529 (1983).
38. Hollenberg, N. K. Cardiovascular therapeutics in the 1980s: "An ounce of prevention." *Am. J. Med.* 82(suppl 3A):1–3 (1987).
39. See 32.
40. See 36.
41. See 35, second reference.
42. See 1.
43. Schoenberger, J. A. Epidemiology and evaluation: Steps toward hypertension treatment in the 1990's. *Am. J. Med.* 90(suppl 4B):3–7 (1991).
44. See 43.
45. Andren, L. General considerations in selecting antihypertensive agents in patients with type II diabetes mellitus and hypertension. *Am. J. Med.* 87(suppl 6A):39–41 (1989).
46. Weinberger, M. H., Cardiovascular risk factors and antihypertensive therapy. *Am. J. Med.* 84(suppl 4A):24–29 (1988).
47. See 1.
48. Ibid.
49. Ibid.
50. Ibid.

Index

Aboriginals, 88, 89, 90, 91–95, 137
ACE (Angiotensin Converting Enzyme), 54
ACE-inhibitors, 28, 54, 294, 308, 309, 310, 313
  contraindicated in pregnancy, 309
  diabetes and, 327
  elevate plasma potassium levels, 310, 321, 323, 328
  severe cough and, 301
Acid, cellular extrusion of by the Na$^+$/H$^+$ exchange pump, 66–68
  function in hypertension, 68–73
  insulin and, 72–73
Acidosis, 324
Addison, W. L. T., 10, 83, 107–9, 130, 132, 256, 257
Addison's disease, 291
ADH (antidiuretic hormone), 289
Adrenal-gland tumor, 22, 148, 291
Adrenal gland
  EDLS, 290
  adrenaline, 307
  aldosterone, 290, 293
  aldosterone and angiotensin II, 307
  aldosterone and potassium, 296
Adrenaline, 68, 135, 215, 221, 222, 268, 271
Adrenaline-like, 139
Adrenergic inhibitors, 54
  caution about discontinuing, 299
  centrally acting, 304–5
  peripherally acting, 305
  propranolol, 301
Adrenergic blockers, 306
Adrenergic nervous system, function of, 295
Adult-type diabetes, (NIDDM), 6, 51, 52, 55, 77, 78, 85, 119, 120, 211, 258, 271, 327
Adventists, Seventh-Day, 92, 93
Aerobic exercise, 184–88
  arguments against, 188

  arguments for, 192–93, 195
  beta blockers and, 198
  blood lipids reduced by, 193, 203, 186
  blood pressure reduced by, 185, 195
  blood triglyceride reduced by, 193
  calories burned in, 192
  dangers of, 194
  definition of, 196
  and fatigue, 187
  guidelines for, 196
  heart, electrical activity of, stabilized through, 186, 193, 202, 204
  high-density lipoprotein cholesterol (HDL-C) increased by, 186, 193
  hormone balance restored through, 185, 203
  medical evaluation of patient before, 197
  prevention of high blood pressure through, 203
  program for, 196
  progressive resistance exercise compared with, 196
Africa, studies in
  diet of primitive groups correlated with hypertension, 88
  urinary K Factor correlated with hypertension, 266
American Heart Association (AHA), 158, 174
Aita people, Solomon Islands, 90
Alcohol consumption
  need to reduce, 1–6, 9, 29, 31, 39, 145, 223, 315, 320, 329, 330
  role in hypertension, 128, 137, 142, 227
Aldosterone
  magnesium deficiency and, 129
  sodium retention caused by, 290–91
Aldosteronism, primary (Conn's syndrome), 148, 291, 325
Algorithm, treatment for hypertension, 29, 30, 31
Almonds, 233

Alpha-blockers, 54, 135, 300, 306, 307, 309, 313, 327
Ambard-Beaujard report, 107, 256,
Ambrosioni, 79
Amino acids, 67, 156, 169, 174, 287
Anaerobic, 187
Anchovies, 161
Anemia, severe, 149
ANF (atrial natriuretic factor), 294
Angina, and beta blockers, 32, 150, 328
Angiography, 191
Angiotensin, 54, 73, 77, 138, 140, 271, 272, 291, 292, 293, 294, 296, 297, 301, 307, 308
Animal studies relating K Factor to hypertension, 102–5
Anthropological evidence of cultures without hypertension, 88, 95–97
Aorta, 148, 285
Appetite, 148, 161, 218, 221, 280, 301
Apples, effect upon blood pressure, 98, 264
Apricots, 156, 165, 168, 180, 183, 230, 231
Arrhythmias, 302, 310, 316, 324, 326
Arterioles
  beta blocker effect on, 307
  calcium maintains muscle tone around, 66
  peripheral, resistance at the, 74–76
  potassium's effect on muscle surrounding the, 268–69
  sympathetic innervation of muscle surrounding the, 305–6
Arteriosclerosis, 149
Atherosclerosis, 158, 190, 245, 280
ATP, 59, 64, 67
Australian studies, 33, 35, 84, 90, 93, 110, 116
Australian aborigines, 90
Autonomic nervous system, 295
Avocado, 130, 181, 231

Bacon, Francis, 258
Bacon (pork), 160, 161, 166, 177, 232
Baconian (Roger) philosophy, 252, 253
Baking soda (sodium bicarbonate), 132, 164
Balance, 47, 122, 171
Banana
  magnesium and, 130, 158
  potassium and, 10, 156, 165, 231, 317
  and stroke prevention, 6, 42, 101
Barley, 157, 228
Barrett-Connor, 101, 102, 352, 375

Beans 157, 158
  canned, 160
  dried, 156, 165
  fat content, 219
  frozen, 160
Bean sprouts, 168
Beard, Trevor, 110
Beef, 160, 162, 217, 232, 233, 234, 280, 281
Beer, 128, 178, 227, 228, 238
Beet salad, 183
Benedictine monks, 93, 94
Beta blockers
  blacks and, 308, 309
  danger of sudden withdrawal of, 150, 198, 328
  diabetes and, 53, 327
  exercise capability and, 31, 198, 201, 308
  heart rate and, 198, 201
  potassium regulation affected by, 321, 323, 328
  triglyceride increase and, 32, 53, 54, 309, 327
Beta-endorphins, stimulated with exercise, 187
Binge eating, 222
Biofeedback, 136
Biophysics, cell, detailed explanation at the level of, 56–87, 268–70
Bitters, 164
Blacks and hypertension, 16, 32, 89, 96, 97, 115, 265, 266
Black-eyed peas, 130
Blaustein, Mordecai, 69, 70
Blind faith, 252, 253
Blindness, 4, 5, 8, 16
Blind study
  double blind, 103, 131
  single blind, 37
Blood pressure
  alcohol and, 128
  biofeedback and, 136
  calcium and, 130, 131
  collagen and, 68
  cuff, description of the, 20, 241, 242
  death rate correlated with, 23–25
  diastolic, 4, 20–25
  equipment for measuring, 20, 241–43
  exercise and, 121, 123–26
  fasting and, 121, 122
  fish oils and, 159

health improved even without reduction of, 101–4
high. *See* Hypertension
insulin and, 77, 78, 290
insulin-resistance and, 52, 54, 68–70, 76, 78, 80, 82, 119, 121, 122, 203, 271, 327
K Factor causal chain, 79
kidneys and. *See* Blood pressure regulation
magnesium reducing, 129, 130
mechanical model, 76
measurement of, 20, 240–44
monitoring your, 329
sodium-hydrogen exchange pump and, 66–68
nerves and. *See* Blood pressure regulation
normal, 3, 14, 22–25, 139
regulation of. *See* Blood pressure regulation
as symptom, 26, 49, 50, 68, 136, 148, 153, 226, 309
sugar and increase of, 121, 221, 290
systolic, 20–22, 25, 220–24
triglycerides and, 52–55
weight loss and, 122, 125, 210, 211
why potassium doesn't always lower, 113–18
Blood pressure regulation
aldosterone, 290
angiotensin and renin, 292–94
calcium and, 82
chain of events, 82–84
EDLS, 83, 289
K Factor, 297
kidneys and, 283–86
nervous system, 295
obesity and diabetes, 78, 119–26
strokes and, 82
Blood triglycerides
abdominal obesity and, 120
ACE-inhibitors and, 54
beta blockers and, 32, 53, 54
exercise and, 123, 151, 186
insulin and, 52, 70, 77, 86, 125
prazosin decreases, 55
"Syndrome X" and, 49–53, 76, 119, 120, 125, 127
thiazide diuretics and, 32, 299, 30
Blood vessel dilators. *See* Vasodilators
Blueberries, 168, 183, 229, 231

Body fat. *See* Obesity
Boiling food and potassium removal, 7, 159, 171, 172, 278
Bologna, 79, 160, 166, 232
Bones, 89, 131, 194, 195, 199
Borderline hypertension, 18, 39, 50, 53, 79, 124, 140, 253, 254, 303, 312
Botswana natives, studies of, 90, 96
Bouillon, 180
Brain
blood pressure regulation, 295, 304
damage to, 293
EDLS and, 80, 269, 290
hypertension and, 8, 66, 271, 308
influence of, 136, 187
strokes and, 82
Bran, 157, 175, 229
Brazilian Indians, studies of, 90, 92, 96, 279
Bread
commercially baked, 160
sodium-free, 160
Breakfast
guidelines for preparing, 167, 168, 176–83
importance of, 167
recommended foods for, 155, 162, 167–68
in restaurants, 170
Broccoli, 168, 176, 180, 219, 234, 310
Broiling, 168, 172
Broth, 162, 182
Brown fat cells, 214
Brussels sprouts, 182, 234
Buckwheat, 130, 157, 175
Burrito, 233
Butter, 14, 155, 158, 159, 160, 165, 166, 168–71, 177, 179–82, 217, 218, 230, 233

Cade, Robert, 123, 184, 185, 203, 204
Calcium (Ca)
foods containing, 156–58
hypertension and, 68, 70, 130, 131
muscle contractions and, 66
oxalic acid and, 169
positive role of, 66
recommended dietary allowance (RDA) of, 156
sodium battery regulation of, 64, 65
sodium exchange with, 64
See also Calcium pump

Calcium-channel blockers, 54, 309, 310
Calcium pump, 64–67
Calisthetics, 199
Calories
    burning off in exercise, 212
    calculating fat percentage in diet, 219, 245
    content of various foods, 217, 218
    in menu plan, 180–83
    restricting intake of, 219
    where they go, 59, 212, 215
Cancer
    dietary fat and, 132, 134, 166
    exercise and, 192, 193
    fruits and vegetables, 145
Cantaloupe, 231
Carbohydrates
    complex, 156, 170, 219
    simple, 170, 217, 221
Carbonic anhydrase inhibitors, 325
Cardiac arrhythmia and potassium, 316,
    324, 326
Cardiovascular disease, 3, 5, 24, 97, 139, 151
Carotid sinus, 295
Carrots, 168, 172, 180–183, 219, 235
Catsup, 163, 176
Cauliflower, 168, 180, 235
Celery, 219, 235
Cell membrane, 56–87, 268
    acid (hydrogen ion) exchange at the, 66–68
    calcium-sodium exchange at the, 64–66
    leakiness of the, 62, 66, 82, 83, 128
    potassium-sodium exchange at the,
        58–60
    voltage regulation at the, 61–64
Cellulose and digestion, 217
Centrally acting adrenergic inhibitors, 304
Cereals, recommended, 162, 165, 175, 219
Chain, causal, 80, 81, 82
Charles, 208
Chart progress, 146, 152, 175, 226, 240,
    245, 246
Cheesecake, 161
Cheeses, 157, 161–63, 165, 166, 168–70,
    175–77, 229, 232, 234, 236–38
Chemical potential of sodium at cell
    membrane, 62, 63, 64
Cherries, 177, 182, 230, 231
Chick-peas, 235
Chicken, 157, 160, 162, 165, 166, 168, 170,
    171, 175, 177, 217, 232,
Chicken soup, 238

Chili, 91, 109, 164, 165, 169
China
    groups with hypertension and stroke, 97
    groups without hypertension, 90
Chinese cabbage, 164
Chips (potato), 161, 163, 166, 170, 233
Chloride (Cl⁻),
    affect upon blood pressure, 132, 133
    role in kidney, 288, 289
Cholesterol
    ACE-inhibitors and, 54
    beta blockers and, 54
    chance of death correlated with specific
        amounts of, 186
    channel-blockers, 54
    dietary saturated fat and, 34
    exercise and, 122, 125
    fish oils and, 159
    unsaturated fats and, 133
    insulin and, 77
    metabolic disturbance part of hyperten-
        sion, 2, 6, 47, 51–53, 93, 120
    medical recommendations concerning,
        158
    monitoring, 150
    potassium effect upon, 3, 103, 104
    prazosin and, 55
    thiazide diuretics and, 32, 53
Cholesterol-filled, 188
Cholesterol-promoting, 104
Cider, 171
Cigarettes, 42, 128, 151, 192, 202
Clams, 157, 165, 230
Clausen, Torben, 317, 318
Climate and hypertension, 8, 10, 11, 136,
    279, 280
Climbing, 305
Club soda, 228
Coarctation, 148
Coconut oil, 104, 159, 162
Cod, 157, 231
Coffee, 128, 172, 218, 228, 230
Cold, 10, 160, 162, 176
Collaboration, 150
Collagen, 68, 76, 273
Commercially processed food, 5, 13, 89, 91,
    93, 155, 159, 160, 163, 219, 319, 322
Complex carbohydrates, 156, 170, 217, 219,
    221, 245
Conductivity test for fat, 211
Congestive heart disease, 31, 303, 309

Conservation of Energy Law, 212
Contraceptive therapy, 148
Controlled studies. *See* Statistical evidence
Cookbooks recommended, 172, 174
Cooking
  planning recommendations for, 167–70
  tips for, 172
  See also Commercially processed food;
    Food preparation
Cool-down, 198, 205, 206
Cooper, Kenneth, 152, 189, 191, 201, 205,
  328
Cooperation, a key to success, 13, 112, 144,
  149–50, 253
Corn, 91, 109, 132, 159, 160, 165, 166, 168,
  169, 170, 176, 180, 229, 235
Cornbread, 172, 180
Cornstarch, 163, 219
Coronary artery heart disease, 19, 151–52,
  190–91, 199
Cottage cheese, 157, 161, 162, 163, 166,
  171, 179, 232
Cow, sodium needs of, 281
Crabbe, Jean, 270, 290
Cracked wheat, 229
Crackers, 161, 163, 165, 170, 182, 183, 229
Cranberry, 181, 228
Cream equals fat, 158
Creamers, nondairy, 245
Creatinine serum, indicator of kidney
  function, 150, 318, 319
Cucumber, 235
Cultural evidence of groups without
  hypertension, 88–99
Cuna Indians, 90, 91
Curry, 164, 165
Cushing's syndrome, 148, 325

Dahl, Lewis, 10, 17, 102, 106, 109, 250,
  256, 267, 280, 284
Dairy cattle, sodium needs of, 281
Dance, aerobic, 196, 197, 203, 208
Death, chance of
  blood pressure and, 23–25
  cholesterol level and, 186
  exercise and, 188–94
Decongestants, 148
Deepfrying, 159
DeFronzo, Ralph, 270, 317, 318
Desserts, 160, 161, 219, 229
Diabetes mellitus

hypertension and, 51, 60, 119–20
recommendations to physicians
  concerning, 327
Diagnosis
  criteria, 319
  early, 140
  importance, 149
  mistaken, 319
Dialogue, 330
Diastolic blood pressure, 20
Diet
  break-in period necessary for, 173
  compensating for mistakes in,
    236–38
  exercise and, 110, 189–92, 202
  hypertension, key factor in, 86–87, 89,
    92–99
  monitoring your, 227
  See also Dietary fat
Dietary approach. *See* Nutritional therapy
Dietary fat
  blood pressure and, 132, 158
  foods high in, 218
  Greenland Eskimos and, 280
  health and, 132
  monitoring your, 245
  obesity and, 134
  polyunsaturated, 133, 219
  saturated, 132
  See also Nonfat and low-fat foods
Digitalis, 61, 80, 105, 302, 324, 326
Digitalis-like substance. *See* EDLS
Dilators of blood vessels. *See* Vasodilators
Dill pickles, 161, 166, 235–37
Dining out, recommendations for, 170
Dinner (evening meal)
  guidelines for preparing, 168–70
  in restaurants, 170–71
  See also Lunch
Dip, preparing a, 170
Discharged "sodium battery," 66, 82, 87, 290
Diuresis, 107
Diuretics, 10, 17, 27, 33, 302–4,
  furosemide, 300
  hypokalemia and, 325
  introduction of, 17
  mechanics of, 299
  potassium-sparing, 303
  sodium and, 10
  See also Thiazide diuretics
DNA, 72

Doctor
  collaboration with your, 13, 147–52
  information for the, 312–30
Double blind study, 131
Dried fruit, 156, 157, 165, 168, 179–82
Drinking, 3, 39, 128, 145, 162, 239, 316
Drugs for hypertension
  ACE-inhibitors, 54, 294, 301, 308, 309
  adrenergic inhibitors, 300, 304
  atrial natriuretic factor (ANF), 294
  beta blockers, 54, 307–8
  calcium entry blockers, 54, 309
  demanded by patients, 255
  diuretics, 27–28, 31, 300, 302–3
  failure of, to restore body's balance, 315
  generic names of, 299
  mechanics of, 26
  medical recommendations about
    withdrawal of, 150, 328, 329
  money spent each year on, 41
  side effects of, 27, 31, 299, 309, 310
  table of, 299–301
  trade names of, 299–301
  types of, 302–9
  vasodilators, 301, 308
  See also Drug therapy
Drug therapy
  abnormal electrocardiograms and, 34
  borderline hypertension and, 34, 39
  early dissent from, 35
  first evidence effectiveness of, 28, 34
  for mild cases, recommendations against,
    28, 39
  ignorance (doctors') of programs other
    than, 252
  justification for, 33, 34
  medical embrace of, 27
  mild hypertension and, 28, 35, 37, 39,
    313
  origin of, 253
  regarded as high tech, 253
  stepped-care procedure, 28
  sudden discontinuance, danger of, 150,
    328, 329
  summary of arguments against, 35, 41
  See also Drugs for hypertension;
    Nutritional therapy; Pharmaceutical
    industry
Dry milk, 163, 180, 217

Eating, time of, 167, 222

Eating out, 170–71
Ectopic heart beat, 32, 326
Edema, 301
EDLS (Endogenous Digitalis Like
  Substance), 61, 69, 80, 83, 289, 290, 294
Eggplant, 235
Eggs, 94, 169
Ehrlich's "magic bullet," 253
Ejaculation, 300, 301, 307
EKG. See Electrocardiogram
Elderly people and exercise, 199
Electrical energy as part of medical theory,
  resistance to, 253
Electrical signaling between heart
  chambers, block of, 149
Electrical voltage regulation at the cell
  membrane, 60
Electrical eel research, 64
Electrocardiogram
  before beginning exercise program, 151,
    327
  drug therapy and abnormal, 35, 324
  fallibility of, 152, 190
  with stress test, 151, 191, 194, 202
Electrochemical potential, 64
Endocrine, 283, 298
Energy, 6, 41, 57–59, 62–67, 121, 132, 138,
    187, 196, 198, 203–4, 211–18, 221,
    223, 253, 274, 287–88
Entropy, 57, 274
Epidemiological evidence of groups without
  hypertension, 88–99
Epinephrine, 68
Equilibrium, 78, 261, 274
Erections, inhibition by drugs, 310
Eskimos, 90, 136, 280
Essential hypertension, 22, 149, 313. See
  also Primary hypertension
Estrogen, 148
Euphoria and exercise, 187
Examination, physical, need for a complete,
  147–49, 191–92
Exercise
  aerobic, definition of, 196
  arguments against, 188–91
  arguments for, 184–88, 193, 195
  dangers of, 194
  guidelines for, 196
  insulin and the lack of, 185–86
  medical evaluation of patient before, 151–52
  monitoring, 197–208

smoking and, 187
time of meals and, 222
weight reduction and, 185–86, 219–22
See also Aerobic exercise
Extrarenal regulation of potassium, 316–19

Falafel, 233
Family involvement in a high-K Factor diet, 171
Fast foods, 155, 159, 171
Fasting, 122, 270–71
Fat. *See* Dietary fat; Nonfat foods; Obesity; Weight reduction
Fat-burning, 221
Fat-free, 219
Fatigue
exercise and, 187
resistance to, 187
Fattening foods, 169, 217
FDA, labeling requirements of, 13, 163
Feedback, 82, 223, 240
Females
and exercise, 199, 201
and hypertension, 266
Fiber-containing foods, 91, 145, 156, 166, 170, 217, 218, 223
Fibrillation
exercise and, 187
hypokalemia and, 326
Fibroblasts, 73
Fidelman, Mark, 50, 51
Fifth Joint National Committee on Detection, Evaluation, and Treatment of High Blood Pressure, 4, 7, 210, 280, 312, 313, 326, 330
Financial costs of present approach, 12, 13, 41, 320
First Law of Thermodynamics, applied to weight reduction, 212, 223
Fish oil. *See* Omega-3 polyunsaturated fatty acids
Fitness. *See* Exercise; Weight reduction
Fixx, Jim, reasons for death, 152–91
Flawed studies, 7, 38
Flour, 130, 157, 165, 170, 180, 229
Food
caloric output of, 212–16
detailed recommendations, 153–62
fiber-containing, 91, 145, 156, 166, 170, 217, 218, 223
key factor in hypertension, 47–48, 94–95

selecting the best, 153–59
table with the K Factor value in various, 228–35
See also Food preparation
Food and Drug Administration, US labeling requirements of, 13, 163
Food preparation
detailed plans for, 167–70
K Factor reduction in typical, tips for, 172
See also Commercially processed food
Four-step program, 142
Fourteen-day menu plan, 176–83, 227
Fragmented view of reality, 8, 9, 11
Framingham study, 53, 186
Frankfurters, 160, 166
Fresh vegetables and fruits, 155, 156, 167–70, 217
Fried food, limiting, 155, 159
Frozen fruits, 157–60
Frozen juice concentrates, 165
Frozen vegetables, 160
Fructose, 217
Fruit
canned, 159, 160, 166
dried, 156
fresh, 156
frozen, 157, 160
ices, 161
juice concentrates, 157, 161

Galactose, 217
Garbanzo beans, 156, 233, 235
Garlic, 163, 164, 165, 169
Gavryck, Wayne, 271
Gelatin, 161, 163
Generator, of electricity in cell, 57, 58, 59, 63
Genetic weakness for hypertension, 91, 96, 138
Georgia, low K Factor and high rate of strokes, 97, 265
Germany, 114
GFR (Glomerular Filtration Rate), 296, 318
Gibbs' Free Energy, 274
Glomerulonephritis, 324
Glomerulus, 287
Glucagon, 345, 370
Glucose, testing for serum levels of, 150
Glutamate, 82
Glycosuria, 302
Goal of hypertension treatment, 12, 18, 49, 142, 146, 163, 312, 314, 315

Goulash, 183
Gout, 302
Grains whole, 155, 158, 169, 217
Granolas, 162
Grapefruit, 156, 170, 180, 181, 182, 183, 228, 231
Grapes, 156, 179, 231
Gravy, 155, 217, 218
Green beans, 160, 172, 219, 234
Greenland Eskimos, health and diet of, 90, 136, 280
Green peppers, 163, 165, 238
Grocery lists
    healthy, 165
    unhealthy, 166
Gupta, Raj, 70, 264
Guyton, Arthur, 284–86, 296, 297
Gymnastics, 203

H$^+$, cellular expulsion of, 66, 67
Haddock, 231
Halibut, 157, 231
Ham, 160, 166, 232
Hamburger, 169, 176, 180, 181, 234, 304
HANES studies, 134, 270
"Hardening of the arteries," 19, 190
Harmony, 9, 253
Hawaii, 98
HDL-cholesterol, 32, 52–55, 76, 82, 120, 122, 150, 185–86, 189, 193
Health-care, cost due to lack of, 11, 12, 16, 17
Heartbeat, 32, 53, 307
Heart disease
    block of electrical signaling between chambers, 149
    dietary fat and, 158
    exercise and, 191
    fish oils and, 159
    hypertension and, 3–5, 8, 13, 16, 19
    Kempner rice-fruit diet and, 109
    silent, 190
Heart-healthy meals, 170
Heart output
    body's regulation of, 283
    thiazide diuretics' effect on, 272
Heart rate
    during exercise, 196, 198, 200, 201–4
    predicted maximum (PMHR), 201
    at rest, 208, 209
Hematocrit, testing for, 150
Hemoglobin, testing for, 150

Hemorrhagic strokes, 42, 101, 103
Hereditary tendency for hypertension, 127
Hg (hydragyrum), meaning of, 20
High-density lipoprotein cholesterol (HDL-C) increased by exercise, 186
High-energy-density foods, 216–18
High-fat, 189, 190, 202
High-K, 109, 156, 268, 303
High-stress lifestyle, 189, 190, 202
High-tech not the automatic answer, 5, 9, 252
Hippocratic oath, 8
Hodgkin, Alan, 64
Holistic (wholistic), 6, 46, 137, 252, 273, 329
Honey, 179, 217, 233
Hopi Indians, 195
Hormones
    aldosterone, sodium retention and potassium loss caused by, 290, 296
    angiotensin, part of kidney-hypertension causal chain, 291, 296
    antidiuretic (ADH), urine production regulated by, 289
    balance restored through exercise, 121, 125
    kidney regulation through, 294, 298
    natriuretic (sodium-excreting), 294
    prostaglandins, 295
    renin, part of kidney-hypertension causal chain, 291, 293
    thyroid, calories turned into heat by, 214
    See also Insulin
Horseradish, 164, 165, 170
Hot cereals, 162, 165
Hot dogs, 160
Hot fudge banana split, 161
Human milk, 98, 233
Human studies relating K Factor to hypertension, 88–99, 100–102, 107–18
Hummus, 233
Hunter-gatherers, 88, 97, 348
Hydrogen ions, (H$^+$), cellular expulsion of 66, 67
Hydrogenated, 159
Hyperinsulinemia, 270
Hyperkalemia
    "dangers" of, 316
    extrarenal mechanisms and, 316–19
    side effect of some drugs, 300–301, 323–24, 328
    See also Hypokalemia; Potassium
Hyperplasia, congenital adrenal, 148

Hypertension is a "Syndrome," 49, 71, 76, 134, 271, 314, 327

Hypertension
adrenergic nervous system and, 135
alcohol consumption and, 128
apparent inevitability of, 99
biofeedback and, 136
biophysical evidence concerning, 56–79
blacks and, 96–97, 113, 265–66
calcium and, 68–70, 107, 128–31
children developing, 91, 171
chloride and, 131–32
civilization and, 89, 92
climate and, 136
collagen and, 68
complications of, 31, 104
curing with high-K Factor diet, 48, 100–102, 107–18
diabetes and, 51, 119, 271, 327
diagnosis of, 21, 22, 147, 148
diet and, 91–99, 106, 107, 155–83
essential, 22, 111, 112, 116, 123, 149, 184, 286, 302
exercise and, 99, 120, 121, 184, 209, 271, 327
fatty foods and, 121–25, 132–34
genetic weakness for, 76, 91, 96–97, 99
goal of treatment, 26, 142
"hardening of the arteries" and, 75–77, 272
heart disease and, 32
holistic approach to, 27, 30, 31, 109
hyperrenin, hypokalemia and, 129, 279, 293, 294, 316, 325, 326
hypertrophy and, 76, 100, 104, 272, 273
incidence of, in US, 16
Kempner rice-fruit diet and, 109, 256, 280
K Factor connected to, 95, 98, 266
kidney function and, 283–86
magnesium deficiency and, 69, 84, 128–30
medical recommendations for physicians in treating, 28–31, 320, 321, 326–28
meditation and, 135
microscopic evidence concerning, 56
the nervous system's relationship to, 135, 295, 296
noninevitability of, 91, 99
number of sufferers, 24
obesity and, 120–26, 210–23, 270, 271
overwork and, 136

plasma potassium level correlated with, 80–81, 98, 239, 263, 324
populations with low incidence of, 88, 279, 280
potassium level in patients with, 79, 96–97, 263, 264
potassium-sodium exchange, problems associated with, 60, 61
preventing with high K-Factor diet, 48, 100–102, 107–18
primary, 22, 75
primitive people with high incidence of, 89, 91, 280
program for treating, 143–45, 147
relaxation and, 76
secondary, 22
sodium concentration in white blood cells associated with, 79
studies demonstrating connection of K Factor to, 58, 69, 79, 88–99, 100–113,
the sympathetic nervous system and, 121
as symptom, 26, 49, 50, 68, 136, 148, 153, 226, 309
"Syndrome X" and, 119, 120, 271
systolic, 20, 21, 24, 95, 115
types of, 22
urinary K Factor correlated with, 264–66
See also Drugs for hypertension

Hypertriglyceridemia, 76, 120
Hypoinsulinemia, 318, 326
Hypokalemia, 322, 325, 326
Hypomagnesemia, 325
Hypotension, 301
Hypothalamus, 271, 290

Ice, fruit, 161
IDDM (Insulin Dependent Diabetes Mellitus), 51
Imbalances within the body in hypertension, 2, 45, 49, 50, 55, 76, 80, 86, 88, 314
Indians, American
diet and blood pressure, 91
exercise and, 194–95
Infarction, myocardial, 34, 37, 188, 326
Inherited tendency toward hypertension, 91, 96, 138
Inhibitors of sympathetic nerve function.
See Adrenergic inhibitors
Injuries and exercise, 196–97, 199, 203, 206

Insipidus, diabetes, 289
Insulin
  abdominal obesity and, 120, 327
  blood pressure and, 123, 271
  drugs that can affect insulin function,
    53–55
  effect upon blood cholesterol and
    triglycerides, 122, 125, 186,
  high-energy-density foods and, 217–18
  hypertension involves abnormal function
    of, 2, 47, 50–52, 70, 77–78, 119–20
  hypothalamus affected by, 271
  insulin function improved by exercise,
    121, 123–24, 185, 203
  kidney reabsorption of sodium affected
    by, 271, 289–90
  link between adult type (NIDDM)
    diabetes and hypertension, 55, 60, 119,
    270, 327
  obesity and, 119–20, 214–15, 221, 270
  potassium and, 80, 317–18, 327
  regulation of cellular acid by, 73, 77
  the sodium-potassium pump stimulated
    by, 60, 120, 270
  the sympathetic nerves stimulated by, 221
  "Syndrome X" and, 119, 271, 314
Intersalt study, 113, 115
Interventionist versus natural philosophy, 9,
    34, 252–54
Intravenous pyelogram, 150
Iodized, 157
Iron
  foods and supplements containing, 156,
    157
  women's need for supplemental, 174
Irregularities, cardiac, 32, 300, 303, 326
Irreversible, 76, 140
Isometric exercise, 272
Isotonic exercise, 272

"J" shape curve and heart attacks, 38
Jam, 177
Joint National Committee on Detection,
    Evaluation, and Treatment of High
    Blood Pressure
  Third Report (1984), 27, 39, 210, 312
    stepped-care reccommendations of, 28
  Fourth Report (1988), 18, 312, 320
    adds nondrug approach as first step,
      28, 40

Fifth Report (1993), 4, 7, 18, 22, 148,
    280, 312, 313–14, 326
  definition of high blood pressure,
    22, 148
  redefinition of healthy blood pressure, 24
  further emphasizes nondrug
    approaches, 29–30
  and legal implications, 255
Jogging. See Aerobic exercise
Joints and exercise, 194–95, 197, 199–200
Juice, 157, 161, 162, 164, 165, 166, 167,
    168, 170, 171, 176, 177, 178, 179,
    180, 181, 182, 228, 256, 279
Junk foods, 144, 155, 159, 161, 169, 175

K (kalium), 95. See also Potassium
Kaplan, Norman, 100, 312, 319
Kempner, Walter, 10, 17, 27, 109, 256, 257,
    280, 329
Kenya natives, 90
Kepler, 251
Ketchup, 165
Khaw, Kay-Tee, potassium protects against
    strokes, 101, 102
Kickball, 91, 194
K Factor
  adequate time to take effect, 114, 115
  animal studies verifying effectiveness of
    diet high in 102–6
  arteries strengthened by diets high in, 84
  biophysical evidence supporting
    importance of, 79–83
  blood potassium analysis to estimate
    your, 239–40
  blood pressure connected to, 80–83
  blood pressure and increase of, 272–73
  calculating the, 236–40
  cautions concerning, 236–38
  cellular natural level of, 78–79
  desirable value of dietary, 96, 98, 114,
    116, 117, 118, 126, 321, 329
  "gray" area, 114, 116, 297, 298
  determining from a label, 163
  diet high in, detailed description of a,
    165–70, 176–93, 227–40
  discovery of, 105–6
  exercise and, 144–45
  failure to refute influence of, 113, 117
  family involvement with diet high in, 171
  fat set point and, 214–18

human studies verifying effectiveness of diet high in, 100–102, 107–12

hypertension frequency correlated with, in various populations, 95–97

Kempner rice-fruit diet high in, 10, 109

least value to prevent hypertension, 96, 100–102

low-energy density foods high in, 218

measurement of, 176–83

microscopic evidence supporting importance of the, 69, 78–80

monitoring your, 227, 239–40

muscle tone influenced by, 317

natural value in body, 58–60

populations with diets high in, 88–95

Priddle and McQuarrie studies of diets high in, 105, 109

primitive groups with diets low in, 92

protects against strokes, 100–102

reduction in food preparation, 172

selecting foods with a high, 154–57

sodium-potassium pump's role in maintaining natural, 58–60, 138

statistical studies verifying effectiveness of diet high in, 110–13

table of values, 228–35

threshold for, 114, 321

of urine, correlated with hypertension, 239

weight loss, connection with, 125–26

values of foods, 228–35

See also Nutritional therapy; Potassium, diet high in; Sodium, diet low in

Kidney
blood pressure influenced by the, 283–86

excretion of excess sodium from, 268–69

explanation of the workings of, 286–89

hormone regulation of, 289–95

narrowing of artery to, 283

sodium reabsorption by, 287, 289

See also Kidney disease

Kidney disease, 318–19
blacks and, 97

potassium and, 318–19

prevention and potassium, 104

Knee, 194, 195, 199, 207

Kochan Robert, 201

Korean study, 131

!Kung, 96

Label, determining K Factor from, 159, 162–64, 172

Laboratory animals, studies with, 102–6

Labrador Eskimos, health and diet of, 280

Lactose, 157, 217

Lactovegarians, 92

Lappé, Frances Moore, 169

Laragh, John, 293, 294, 297

Lard, 159

LDL-cholesterol, 52, 53, 54, 55, 70, 77, 82, 186, 193

Leakiness of cell membrane
alcohol and, 128

calcium and, 83, 129

magnesium and, 129

role in strokes, 82

Legumes, 111, 133, 156, 169, 182

Lemon, 161, 164, 165, 168–70, 178–79, 230

Lentils, 156, 165, 169, 182, 235, 238

Lettuce, 168, 170, 177–78, 181, 183, 219, 235–37

Licorice, 325

Lifestyle, summary of arguments supporting changes in, 137–39

Lifespan and exercise, 188

Ligaments, 194, 195, 197, 199

Lima beans, 130, 234

Lime, 170, 177, 178

Linguine, 156

Linoleic acid, 132, 133, 219, 295

Linolenic acid, 132, 133, 134

Lipid reduction caused by exercise, 186

Lipoproteins, 52, 185, 186

Listening to your body, 200, 204

List, grocery
healthy, 165

unhealthy, 166

Lobster, 231

London experiments, 111, 115, 262

Loop diuretics and hypokalemia, 325

Low-calorie, 157, 221

Low-density, 186

Low-energy-density food, 216, 217, 218

Low-fat food, 145, 155, 156–58, 161. 163, 167, 170, 192, 217, 218
so-called, 155

"Low-sodium" on label, 161

Lunch
  guidelines for preparing, 168
  in restaurants, 170–71
Lung disease, 151
Lysosomes, 82

Macaroni, 156
Machine, nature and the body viewed as, 8,
    11, 26, 44–46, 194, 195
Macrobiotic diet, 92
Magic bullet concept, 27, 253–54, 259
Magnesium (Mg), 129–30
  alcoholism associated with decreased
      levels of, 128
  foods containing, 95, 130
  hypokalemia and deficiency of, 32, 129
  irregular heart beat and, 32
  potassium replenishment helped by,
      129–30
  preeclampsia of pregnancy treated with, 130
  recommended dietary allowance (RDS)
      of, 130
  sodium control helped by, 84, 129
  thiazide diuretics deplete, 32, 129
MAKING THE TRANSITION, 173
Malignant hypertension, 325
Mangoes, 156
Maple syrup, 168, 180, 233
Marathon, 188, 190, 205
Margarine, 217, 218, 230
Mayonnaise, 178, 181, 230, 236, 237
Meal preparation, detailed
    recommendations for, 167–70
Meatless, 108, 179
Meats, processed, 160
Meat eating, relationship to hypertension,
    93–95
Medical examination, need for a complete,
    147–52
Medical paradigm ("medical model"), the,
    26, 44, 72, 194, 223
Medical studies relating K Factor to
    hypertension
  contradicting reports, flaws in, 113–17
  historical, 107–10
  protects against strokes, 101
  with control groups, 110–12
Medicines, nonprescription, sodium in, 162
Medicines, prescription. See Drugs for
    hypertension; specific drugs by name
Meditation and hypertension, 135, 222

Mellitus, diabetes, 51, 78, 85, 151, 289–90,
    324, 327
Menu plan, 173–83
Meringues, 161
Meta-analysis, 113, 115, 116, 117
Metabolic disease, 151
Mexican food, 178
Microwave, 168, 169, 172
Mild hypertension (now Stage 1), 22, 23,
    28, 33, 35, 36, 40, 103, 111, 112, 114,
    116, 129, 133, 134, 187, 189, 222,
    302, 312, 320
Milk
  human, 98, 233
  nonfat dry, 155, 163
  potatoes compared with, 155–56
  skim, 156, 165, 170, 179–83
Mineral-poor soil and water, 129
Minnesota studies, 10, 97, 102, 167, 314
Misdiagnosis, 319
Mitochondria, 187
Moderate hypertension (now Stage 2), 3,
    22, 23, 38, 40, 110, 111, 112, 116,
    123, 161, 164, 168, 193, 195, 203,
    221, 268, 322, 329
Molecular, 72, 252, 284
Monasteries, hypertension in, 93
Monitoring your progress, 144, 204, 227,
    239, 329
Monks and hypertension, 92, 93
Moore, 77, 169, 270, 330
Morbidity, 5, 37, 38, 39, 312, 314, 329
Mortality, 3, 23, 33, 35, 36, 37, 38, 39, 42,
    102, 140, 193, 257, 301, 312, 313,
    314, 329
Mothers milk, 98, 233
Motivation for exercise, 208
MRC (British Medical Research Council
    study), 37, 313
MRFIT (Multiple Risk Factor Intervention
    Trial), 34, 35, 37, 313, 326
Muffins
  corn, 176–77, 180
  mixes for, 180
Muffins, 160, 166, 172, 180, 181, 183
Mullins, Dr. Lorin, 10
Munford, Dr. John, 50, 60
Muscle
  calcium concentration and, 82
  diabetes associated with sodium
      concentration in, 61

potassium's effect on arteriolar smooth, 268–69
strain, preventing, 194–95, 206–8
sympathetic innervation of smooth, 304–6
Mushrooms, 163, 165, 177, 182, 235, 238
Music and aerobic exercise, 197, 208, 222
Mustard, 163, 164, 165, 168, 177, 180

Na-K-Cl and kidney function, 288
National Heart, Lung and Blood Institute recommendations, 1–2, 18, 39, 128, 142, 158, 314,
National High Blood Pressure Education Program (NHBPEP), 2–4, 7, 8, 13, 24, 25, 115, 142, 314
National Institutes of Health (NIH) MRFIT study. See MRFIT.
"Natural" steps to good health, 1
Nature's diuretic, 79
Navy beans, 156, 234
Neg-entropy, 57
Neonatal danger of drugs, 309
Nephrons, 286–88, 303
Nerves
blood pressure regulation by, 295
insulin's stimulation of, 296
sodium and the transmission along, 64
Neurotransmitter, 82
New Zealand studies, 42, 188
Newton, Isaac, 251
NHANES study, 16
Niacin, 156
NMR (Nuclear Magnetic Resonance), 70, 264
No-fat, 157
Nonathletic, 203
Nonchloride, 132
Nondairy, 233, 245
Nondiabetics, 356
Nondrug, 40, 255
Nonfat dairy products, 144, 163
Nonfat and low-fat foods, 144, 158–59, 163, 217
books about, 174.
See also Dietary fat
Non-insulin-dependent diabetes mellitus (NIDDM), 51, 78, 119
Nonprescription drugs, sodium in, 162
Nonpharmacological approaches
for borderline cases, 312

before drugs, 18, 29, 320
in obese patients, 210, 326
for Stages 1 and 2, 329
during "step down" therapy, 30
Non-vegetarians, 92, 96, 98
Non-westernized, 135
Noodles, 156, 165, 179, 183, 229
Noradrenalin
beta blockers and, 307–8
guanethidine and, 305
obesity and, 271
potassium and, 269
reserpine and rauwolfia alkaloids and, 305
Norepinephrine. See Noradrenalin
Normal blood pressure, definition of, 22, 24
Normotensive (have "normal" blood pressure), 3, 5, 24, 39
No-salt, 161, 170, 349
No-sodium, 161
No-sugar, 161
Nutritional therapy
Kempner, 10, 17, 27, 109
medical resistance to, 33–39, 113–18
Pritikin, 91, 109
studies indicating effectiveness of, 107–13
summary of arguments supporting, 118
Nuts, 133, 144, 158, 161, 168, 170, 175, 217, 218, 227

Oatmeal, 162, 170, 177, 178, 179, 229
Obesity
alcohol and, 217
controlling, recommendations for, 1, 4, 210
exercise and, 121, 123, 220, 221
hypertension and, 3, 39, 48, 60, 119, 120–25, 136, 137, 210, 211, 215, 270, 327
insulin and, 120, 122, 215, 270, 271
noradrenalin and, 271
program for curing, 210, 216–22
recommendations to physician for treating, 223, 326
stress and, 222
testing for, 211, 212
time of eating and, 222
See also Weight reduction
Olives, 161, 166, 226, 231
Omega-3 polyunsaturated fatty acids, 157, 159

Onions, 163–65, 168–69, 177, 183, 235, 238
Orange, 157, 165, 167, 170, 171, 176, 177,
    178, 179, 180, 181, 182, 228, 230,
    231, 279
Ornish, Dean, 158
Orthopedic, 195, 197, 200
Osmotic diuretics and hypokalemia, 325
Osteoarthritis, 194
Osteoporosis, preventing, 195
Ouabain, potassiums artery dilation
    capabilities inhibited by, 61, 268
Overbeck, Henry, 60, 61
Overdrinking, 135
Overeating, 126, 135, 145, 212, 218,
    222, 223
Overexertion during exercise, 197, 198, 200
Overindulgence, 19, 158
Overweight. See Obesity
Oxalic acid in spinach, 169, 170
Oysters, 157, 165, 231

Paffenbarger study, 192
Palm oil, 159, 162, 244
Panamanian Indians, 90, 91
Pancakes, 165, 168, 170, 180
Pancreas, 290
Paradigm (conceptual framework), 194,
    216, 223, 252, 253, 257
Participating with your doctor, 13, 147–52
Pasta, 156, 165, 168, 217, 245
Pastrami, 177
Pathophysiological, 323, 325
Peaches, 156, 168, 178
Peanut, 161, 165, 168, 171, 233
Pears, 156, 232
Peas, 94, 130, 156, 157, 160, 165, 166, 169,
    172, 180, 235
Pecans, 230, 233
Penis, 310
Peripheral resistance
    body's regulation of, 283
    magnesium deficiency associated with,
    129
    muscle tone and, 74–75, 82
Perspiration, sodium in, 279
pH, 71–73, 85, 138, 315,
Pharmaceutical industry, 251, 252, 254, 258
Pheochromocytoma, 148
Physical examination, need for a complete,
    147–49, 191–92

Physician
    diagnosis of hypertension, 147, 148
    information for, 312–30
    physical exam by, 147
    physician-nutritionist, 216
    ruling out secondary hypertension, 148
    working with your, 147–52
Physics, 11, 57, 212, 253, 274
Pickles, 161, 166, 226, 235
Piggyback pumps, 288, 289
Pillsworth, Tom (Good Time Charley's
    friend), 60
Pima Indians, 52, 120
Pineapple, 156, 170, 232
Pita, 170
Pituitary gland, 289
Pizza, 160, 166, 171, 234, 238
Placebos, experiments using, 33, 35, 37,
    103, 111, 113, 115, 130, 131
Plant-eaters, 278
Platelets, blood, 71, 73, 85
Plasma potassium. See Serum potassium
Plums, 156, 232
PMHR (predicted maximum heart rate), 201
Polyunsaturated fats. See Dietary fat
Popcorn, 157, 159, 170
Pork, 160, 166, 178, 232
Postexercise, 124
Postmenopausal, 157
Postsynaptic, 306
Potash, 109, 267
Potassium (K)
    Addison's study of diet high in, 107–9
    aldosterone and loss of, 129
    arteriolar smooth muscle affected by,
    129, 135, 268
    blood pressure reduction by diet high in,
    100, 113–17
    cardiac arrhythmia and, 32, 316
    at the cell membrane, 59, 62
    content of various foods, 228–35
    Dahl's studies of diet high in, 102, 109
    dangers of, 316
    diet high in, detailed recommendations
    for, 95, 98, 102
    doctors' fear of, reasons for, 316
    extrarenal regulation of, 317
    Gordon and Drury's studies of diet high
    in, 105
    insulin blood levels stimulated by, 103, 314

intolerance for, 173, 317–18
Kempner rice-fruit diet high in, 17, 27, 109
kidney disease and, 102, 104, 130, 318–19
on label, 13, 112, 163
low-fat high-P/S ratio diet's success partly due to, 133
magnesium deficiency and, 84, 128–30
nature's diuretic, 79
noradrenalin decrease associated with, 77, 271
plasma level of, correlated with hypertension, 80, 98, 261–64
Priddle and McQuarrie's studies of diet high in, 105, 109
relaxation of arteries by, 74, 268–70
restoration of deficiency of, 173, 317–18
sodium and. See K Factor
sodium exchange with, 58–60
    See also Sodium-potassium pump
sodium excretion stimulated by, 107
sodium-potassium pump and blood level of, 83, 269
statistical studies of diets high in, 102–18
stomach ulcer and, 316
stress and, 135
supplements, medical recommendations concerning, 317, 318, 322
sympathetic nerves relaxed by, 135
testing for serum levels of, 32, 324, 325
thiazide diuretics and loss of, 129, 323
Tobian's studies of diet high in, 102, 104, 105, 314, 315
tolerance for, 173, 317–18
total body level of, 264, 265
in urine, 32, 264
    See also K Factor; Sodium-potassium pump
Potassium chloride, dangers of, 318–19, 322–24
Potassium-containing salt substitutes, 163–64
Potassium-sparing diuretics, 32, 37, 151, 164, 303, 321, 323
Potato
    at breakfast, 168
    a magnesium source, 130
    milk compared with, 156
    yogurt with, 169, 171
Potential (chemical) of sodium at cell membrane, 62, 63, 64

Powdered milk, 161, 233
Power weight lifting, 196
Prazosin, 54, 55, 301, 306, 307, 309, 327
Pre-eclampsia, magnesium used to treat, 130
Predictions that are confirmed, 7, 85, 86, 264, 298
Preformed urine, 287, 288, 290, 294, 296, 303
Pregnancies, 131
Pregnancy
    ACE-inhibitors dangerous in, 309
    calcium and, 131, 157
    magnesium and, 157
Prehistoric diet, estimate of K Factor in, 95
Presynaptic, 305
Pretzels, 170, 176
Preventive medicine, 13, 149
Primary hypertension, 22, 149, 313
Primitive societies and hypertension, 47, 89, 91–93, 95, 97, 99
Pritikin, Nathan, 91, 109, 191
Program for treating hypertension, 141–45
Progress, 226–48,
Progress chart, 247–48
Proof, burden of, 140
Prostaglandins, 133, 295, 324
Protein
    combining foods to make complete, 169
    manufacture of, in body, 68, 72, 84, 87
    sodium battery's maintenance of, 67, 87
Prove, 37, 78, 285
    nothing ever totally proven, 139
Prunes, 178
Psychological stress, 99, 135, 209, 296
Puffed rice or wheat, 162, 165, 182, 229
Pump. See Calcium pump; Sodium-potassium pump
Pumping iron, 196
Pumpkin, 230
Push-pull, potassium-sodium balance, 275
Pyelogram, intravenous, 150

Qash'qai in Iran and hypertension, 92
Quantum, 344

Rabbits with hypertension, 105
Racquetball, 196
Radishes, 168
Raisins, 156, 165, 168, 179, 181, 183, 229, 230, 232

Rats
  calcium diets for, 70, 107
  hormone for sodium excretion discovered
    in, 69
  potassium-poor diets for, 268
  potassium-rich diets for, 102, 104–5
  sodium-rich diets for, 102, 105–6
RDA, recommended dietary allowances,
  130, 155, 156, 157, 174
Reading this book, ix, x, 6, 14,
Readings
  blood pressure, 105, 135, 242, 243, 244,
    245, 319, 321
  serum potassium, 325
Reality,
  behind facts, 257
  fragmented view of, 9, 11
Reaven, Gerald, 78, 119
Rebalancing, 40, 136, 186
Rebound hypertension, 150, 198, 300, 328
Receptors, 270, 271, 295, 305, 306, 307, 327
Recharge "sodium-battery," 83, 87
Recipes
  comments on, 109, 159, 163, 169, 172,
    174
Reciprocal relation between sodium and
    potassium, 6, 78, 79, 81, 273
Records of progress, keeping, 226–45, 247–48
Red blood cells, concentration of sodium in,
    79
Relaxation therapy, 39, 135, 222
Renin
  beta blockers and, 307
  magnesium deficiency associated with, 129
  part of kidney-hypertension causal chain,
    291–94,
  potassium and, 296–97
Renin-secreting tumor, 148
Resnick, Lawrence, 68, 76, 107, 130
Restaurant, selecting meals in, 170–71, 178
Rethinking hypertension, 18, 39, 45, 327
Revolution in hypertension, 1, 2, 3, 10, 13
Rhubarb, 183
Rice-fruit diet, 17, 27, 109, 252, 256, 280
Ricotta chese, 157, 163, 165
Rigidity of the arteries, 149
Rogaine, 308
Runner's high, 187
Running, 123, 188–97, 202, 203, 206–8,
    215. See also Aerobic exercise

Safflower oil, 132, 133, 159, 165, 168, 295
Salads, 14, 164, 168
Salami, 160
Salmon, 157, 177, 231
Salt. See Sodium chloride
Salt substitutes, 111–12, 144, 151, 163–64,
    167–68, 170, 172, 289, 316, 318–19, 322
Salt-free products, 162, 164, 172
Sardines, 161, 231
Sasaki, Naosuke, 264
Saturated fats. See Dietary fat
Sauerkraut, 235
Sausage, 160, 166, 177, 232, 234, 238
Scallops, 231
Science
  as means to dominate nature, 251, 253–54
  technology confused with, 252
Scotland, potassium and heart disease, 97
Seafood, 157, 170, 230
Seasoning, 162, 164, 170, 281
Secondary hypertension, 22, 148–49
Seeholzer, Steven, 50
Self-regulating, 44, 45
Self-renewing, 194, 195
Semmelweiss, 257
Senior citizens and exercise, 199
Serum potassium
  hypertension incidence correlated with,
    80, 98, 261–64
  monitoring, 32, 324, 325
  "normal" value of, set too low, 263
  sodium-potassium pump depends upon
    level of, 59–60, 80–83, 269
Set point, applied to weight reduction
  changing the, 214–15, 222–23
  exercise according to, 203
Severe (Stage 3) hypertension, 22
Servomechanism, 285
Seventh-Day Adventists, 92, 93
Sexual dysfunction
  drugs and, 300, 301, 307, 310
Sheehan, George, 191, 197, 201, 205, 207
Sherbet, 161, 165, 230
Sherry, 228
Shopping list
  healthy, 165
  unhealthy, 166
Shrimp, 158, 231, 234
Side-effects, 101, 313
Silent heart disease, 190

Sims, Ethan, 270, 313
Simple carbohydrates, 170, 217, 221
Single-blind, 35
Skin fold test for fat, 212
Smoking, 31, 34, 36, 39, 40, 42, 134, 137,
     145, 159, 185, 187, 190, 192, 202,
     320, 327
Snacks, guidelines for prepairing, 170
Socrates, 12
Sodium (Na)
     Addison's studies of relationship of
          hypertension to, 107–9
     appetite for, origin of our, 109, 282
     athlete's supposed need for extra, 279
     "battery," 61–69
     blood presssure reduced by diet low in,
          113–17, 272–73
     body's need for, amount of, 289
     calcium exchange with, 64, 65, 69
     at the cell membrane, 56–87, 268–70
     conserving mechanism for, 278, 279, 289
     content in various foods, 228–35
     Dahl's studies of diet low in, 106, 109, 280
     dairy cattle's need for, 281
     diabetes and, 51, 64, 67
     diet low in, detailed recommendations
          for, 95, 98, 102
     diuretic prescriptions and, 256
     excretion of, 61, 79, 107, 283–96, 302
     function of, 59, 61–64
     human milk, amount in, 233
     Kempner's rice-fruit diet and, 17, 27, 109
     kidneys and, 104, 286–89, 294, 302
     on label, 112
     magnesium deficiency and, 68, 129, 130
     in muscle cells, 60, 62
     peripheral resistance and, 83,
     perspiration and, 279
     potassium and. See K Factor
     potassium exchange with, 58, 60. See
          also Sodium-potassium pump
     Priddle and McQuarrie's studies of diet
          low in, 105–9
     reabsorption of, 61, 77, 286–89
     red blood cell concentration of, 71, 79
     statistical studies of diets low in, 102–18
     in urine, correlated with hypertension,
          264–66
     white blood cell levels of, associated
          with hypertension, 79

     See also K Factor; Sodium battery;
          Sodium chloride; Sodium-potassium
          pump
Sodium battery
     calcium regulation in cells by the, 64–65
     nerve transmission function of the, 64
     protein maintenance by, 68
     sodium necessary for the, 58, 82
     sodium-potassium pump charges the, 64,
          67
Sodium chloride (NaC1)
     appetite for, origin of our, 280–82
     experimental diet (for rats) high in, 105
     poisoning, 316
     sodium bicarbonate, comparison with,
          131–32
     substitutes for, 163–64
     See also Sodium
Sodium-potassium pump, 58–60
     calcium pump's connection to, 64–66
     calories turned into heat by, 214
     insulin's stimulation of, experiments
          confirming, 60
     muscle tone influenced by the, 68–69
     natriuretic hormone's depression of the, 61
     nerve transmission function of the, 64
     potassium level in blood influences, 80,
          268–69
     retardation of, 80
     sodium battery charged by the, 61–64
Sodium-retaining hormones, 290
Softeners, water, 129, 162, 239
Sole, 157, 171, 231
Solomon Island natives, 90
Sour cream, 14, 155, 158, 166, 169, 218
South American natives, 88, 279
South African natives, 90
Southeastern U.S. blacks and dietary
     K Factor, 97
Soy sauce, 14, 161, 166
Spaghetti, 156, 164, 165, 179, 229
Spices, 164, 169, 238
Spinach, 165, 169, 170, 177, 181, 182, 235
     conteracting oxalic acid in, 169
Spiritual aspect of science, 251
Split peas, 156
Sprains, 195
Sprouts, 168, 179, 182, 234
Squash, 91, 109, 179, 235, 238
Starch, 217

Statistical evidence
  on diet's relationship to hypertension,
    110–12
  on exercise, 192–93
Steaming, 113, 171, 172, 175, 179, 180, 181
Step-care, 29, 33, 34, 313
Step-down from drugs, 28, 40, 312, 328, 329
Steroid hormones, 61, 290
Stethoscope, buying and using, 241–44
Stir-frying, 171, 172
Stone age diet, 89, 94, 95, 97, 99
Strawberries, 168, 177, 180–82, 232
Stress, 8, 27, 39, 92, 135, 145, 151–152,
    190, 191–95, 198–202, 209, 222–23,
    272, 296, 307–8, 328
Stress test, 151, 152, 179, 190, 191, 192,
    194, 198, 199, 200, 202, 328
Stretching, benefits of, 197, 206–8, 294
Stroke
  mechanism, 82
  "normal" blood pressure and, 139
  prevention of, 100–103
Substitutes for salt. See Salt substitutes
Sucrose, 121, 168, 217
Sudden death and exercise, 189–95, 198,
    202, 293
Sugar
  blood pressure and, 121
  nutrition and, 160, 161, 165, 168, 170,
    177, 178, 179, 180
  weight loss and, 213, 217, 218, 219, 221,
    223
Sun, cellular order connected to, 57
Sunflower seeds, 157, 165, 168
Supper
  guidelines for preparing, 168, 169
  in restaurants, 170
Supplement (potassium) medical recom-
    mendations regarding, 318, 322, 323
Supermarket, making the right selections,
    144, 154–62
Surgery, secondary hypertension may
    require, 149, 291
Sweat glands, sodium conservation by, 278,
    279, 282, 291
Sweet potatoes, 168, 169, 179, 181
Swimming, 190, 196, 197, 202, 204, 208, 220
Swiss cheese, unsalted, 157, 163, 165, 168,
    178, 232, 236, 237
Symmetry, 12

Sympathectomy, 27
Sympathetic nerves
  inhibitors of. See Adrenergic inhibitors
  innervation of artriolar smooth muscle
    diagrammed, 306
  insulin's stimulation of, 121–22
  potassium's effect on, 269–70
Synaptic transmission, 305
Systems approach, 214, 216, 252, 261, 273,
    284, 285, 296, 298, 315
Systolic hypertension, 149

Tabasco, 164
Table of K Factor values of foods, 228–35
Tacos, 169, 233
Tahini, 233
Tangerine, 179
Tapioca, 161, 163, 230
Tarahumara Indians, 90, 91, 109, 194
Technologies, 254
Technology, blind faith in, 252–54
Teflon cooking ware, 159
Tendonitis, 194, 206
Tennessee, 105, 266
Tennis, 195, 196, 206
Tenoretic, 299
Texas, 100, 319
Theory, importance of, 145, 214, 253
Therapeutic, 33, 36, 49, 118, 134, 255, 320
Thermodynamics, 57, 212, 223, 274
Thiazide diuretics
  cardiac output and, 301
  caution note about, 323
  cholesterol level and, 303
  digitalis users and, 302,
  hypokalemia and, 322
  list of, 299
  magnesium and, 303
  mechanics and side effects of, 302–303, 310
  potassium loss and, 302, 310
  potassium supplements and, 322
  uric acid level and, 299, 302
Threshold for K Factor, 114, 321
Thyroid hormone, calories turned into heat
    by, 214, 215
Thyrotoxicosis, 149
Timing of eating and exercise, 222
Tobacco smoking and strokes, 42
Tobian, Louis, 10, 97, 100, 102, 104, 105,
    106, 256, 302, 314, 315

Tofu, 233
Tomatoes, 159, 166, 182
  juice, 161, 166, 167
  paste, 163, 166, 180, 238
Toronto, 107
Tortillas, 170
Tranquilizers, 135
Transition to higher K Factor diet, 173, 176, 246, 322, 323
Trappist monks, 92–94, 349, 350
Treadmill stress test, 151, 190–92, 196, 200, 201, 309
Triglycerides
  beta blockers and, 53
  blood pressure and, 122
  exercise program and, 150–51
Tuna, 160, 168, 171, 172, 178, 181, 231
Turkey, 157, 160, 164, 165, 168, 170, 171, 177, 181, 234
Turnips, 182
Tumor and secondary hypertension, 22, 148, 291

Ugandan natives, 90
Ulcer (stomach), potassium and, 316
Ultrafiltrate
  chloride necessary for, 289
  in obese people, 121
  sodium reabsorbed from, 287–89
Unboiled, 92
Underwater immersion test for fat, 211
Uric acid levels, 299, 302
Urinalysis, 150, 318
Urinary tract obstruction, 150
Urine
  hormone regulation of, 289–92, 294
  measurement of, 239
  sodium reabsorbed from, 121, 132, 287–89
U.S. Food and Drug Administration
  labeling requirements of. See FDA

Variables implicit in new paradigm, 45, 46, 106
Vasodilation, 205
Vasodilators, 108, 301
Vegetarians, rarity of hypertension, 47, 92–97, 99
Ventricular fibrillation
  decreased chance of, 186–87
  hypokalemia and, 326

Vicious cycle, 216
Vinegar, 165, 168, 178, 179, 182
Vitamin A, 156
Vitamin B_1 and B_2, 156
Vitamin C, 134, 156, 280
Vitamin D, 134
Vitamin E, 134
VLDL cholesterol, exercise and, 186
Voltage regulation at cell membrane, 60
Vuori study on exercise and sudden death, 198, 364

Walking, 123, 152, 195–200, 202–5, 214, 221–22
Walnuts, 133, 158, 161, 182, 233
Warm-down, 205
Warm-up, 198, 205
Warnings before exercise, 200
Watermelon, 232
Webb, Dr. George, 1, 10
Weight reduction
  comprehensive program for, 216–22
  control systems theory applied to, 213–16
  diastolic blood pressure and, 122, 185
  exercise and, 123–25, 184–209, 220, 222
  group and professional support for, 223
  insulin level and, 210
  K Factor and, 211
  monitoring your, 240
  time of eating and, 222
  See also Obesity
Weight training
  dangers of, 196
  recommendations about, 227
Well-being, 142, 146, 210
Wheat
  bran, 157
  bulgar, 157
  puffed or shredded, 162, 229
White blood cells
  elevated sodium in, 79
  elevated Na^+/H^+ exchange in, 71
  hypertension associated with, 71, 79
White fat cells, calories into fat by, 214
Whitefish, 231
Wild rice, 157
Wine, 163, 165, 178, 227, 228
Wisdom, 11, 12, 41, 45, 100
WITHDRAWAL, dangers of sudden drug withdrawal, 150, 305, 328

Women, 16, 23, 32–33, 35–37, 92, 97,
    101–3, 113, 123–24, 130–31, 155–57,
    167, 173–74, 185–86, 193–95, 201,
    211, 220–21, 257, 262, 265–66
Worcestershire, 164
Workaholism and hypertension, 136

X-ray, chest, 150, 191

Yanomamo Indians, 90, 92, 96, 280
Yeast, 160, 170, 172

Yeater, Rachael, 199
Yin-yang, 87, 136, 275
Yoga, 207, 208, 222
Yogurt, low-fat or no-fat, 155–57, 165, 167,
    169–71, 217, 233
Young's computer simulation, 297

Zierler, Ken, 60, 70
Zucchini, 168, 177, 235